药理学实验

双语版

赵春贞　李成檀　王雅娟　主编

清华大学出版社

北京

内 容 简 介

本书为全国普通高等医学、药学院校医药学专业的《药理学》课程配套实验教材。全书分为六个模块：药理学总论、传出神经系统药理、中枢神经系统药理、心血管系统药理、激素内脏药理、化疗药物药理。围绕国内高校广泛开设的药理学经典教学实验，深入探讨和解释实验理论、技术、现象等方面的问题，并将相关领域的前沿知识融入其中。同时每个实验配套练习题、思考题和与实验相关的课程思政素材，本书兼具实验指导和实践育人双重功能。本书的特色之一是通过数字技术将实验操作中的难点演示视频、知识拓展素材与纸质媒体融合，有效提升了本书的知识容量，又与现代学生的学习方式契合。

本书适用于全国高等医学、药学院校的医学、药学专业以及相关专业学生使用。

本书供医学院校护理学专业教学使用，也可供医护相关行业人员参考使用。

图书在版编目（CIP）数据

药理学实验：双语版 / 赵春贞, 李成檀, 王雅娟主编. —— 北京：清华大学出版社，2024. 11.

ISBN 978-7-302-67622-5

Ⅰ . R965.2

中国国家版本馆CIP数据核字第2024YG1002号

责任编辑：孙　宇
封面设计：钟　达
责任校对：李建庄
责任印制：刘海龙

出版发行：清华大学出版社
　　　　网　　　址：https://www.tup.com.cn, https://www.wqxuetang.com
　　　　地　　　址：北京清华大学学研大厦 A 座　　邮　　编：100084
　　　　社 总 机：010-83470000　　邮　　购：010-62786544
　　　　投稿与读者服务：010-62776969, c-service@tup.tsinghua.edu.cn
　　　　质量反馈：010-62772015, zhiliang@tup.tsinghua.edu.cn
印 装 者：三河市君旺印务有限公司
经　　销：全国新华书店
开　　本：185mm×260mm　　　　印　张：27.75　　字　　数：366 千字
版　　次：2024 年 12 月第 1 版　　　　印　　次：2024 年 12 月第 1 次印刷
定　　价：89.00 元

产品编号：106373-01

编 委 会

主　编　赵春贞　李成檀　王雅娟

副主编　成　敏　叶夷露　王姿颖　房春燕　崔晓栋

编　委（按姓氏笔画排序）

　　　　王　琳（山东第二医科大学）

　　　　王　蕾（安徽大学）

　　　　王姿颖（山东大学）

　　　　王琳琳（山东第二医科大学）

　　　　王雅娟（安徽中医药大学）

　　　　王舒舒（安徽中医药大学）

　　　　方　辉（山东第二医科大学）

　　　　叶夷露（杭州医学院）

　　　　史立宏（山东第二医科大学）

　　　　成　敏（山东第二医科大学）

　　　　孙志朋（山东第二医科大学）

　　　　李　鑫（山东第二医科大学）

　　　　李文涛（山东第二医科大学）

　　　　李成檀（杭州师范大学）

　　　　邹莹莹（安徽中医药大学）

　　　　张朋飞（山东第二医科大学）

　　　　周　倩（杭州医学院）

　　　　房春燕（山东第二医科大学）

赵　超（山东第二医科大学）

赵春贞（山东第二医科大学）

钟　恺（杭州医学院）

高　伟（山东第二医科大学）

崔晓栋（山东第二医科大学）

韩　雪（杭州医学院）

童骏森（杭州师范大学）

潘瑞艳（山东第二医科大学）

序　言

在当今信息技术与教育深度融合的背景下，新形态教材建设不但顺应时代发展趋势，而且是高等教育推进数字化转型工作的改革要求。该书的编写，注重理论知识与实践相结合、医学药学知识相结合，重在强化培养学生的实践能力和创新能力。

该书的主要特点如下：

1. 契合教学实际、突显内容针对性和适应性

该书的编写从国内各高校教学实践的实际需求出发，坚持围绕教学和人才培养的需求，保证教材内容具有较强的针对性和适应性。

2. 双语教学、实践导向

该书为英汉双语版，供学生理解和学习，方便有双语教学需求的课程使用。完善案例分析和实验设计内容，培养学生的综合素质和创新思维能力。

3. 互动学习、模块化教学

该书内容按模块划分，围绕素质和能力为核心，通过提供丰富的练习题、思考题等教学资源，供学生课后自学，提高学习兴趣。

4. 科学前沿、思政同行

该书内容紧跟学科发展，联系科学前沿开展思政设计，满足医药学教育教学适应医药卫生事业发展要求。

5. 丰富教学资源，促进信息化教学

该书在出版纸质教材的同时，还配套教学课件、图片、视频、练习题等，使教学资源更加丰富、多样化和立体化，为提高教育教学水平和质量提供支撑。

该书编写注重实用性和可读性，力求使复杂的药理学知识变得易于理解和记忆，是药理学实验学习指导和教学参考的宝贵资源。感谢该书的编写团队所付出的辛勤和努力，期待该书成为引导学习者深入探索药理学奥秘的重要向导。

陈哲生

2024 年 11 月 1 日

目　录

第一章 药理学总论

第一节 实验动物的基础知识

【实验动物的定义】

实验动物指经人工饲育，遗传背景明确或者来源清楚的，用于科学研究、教学、生产、鉴定以及其他科学实验的动物。实验中通常对其携带的微生物实施监控。

实验用动物泛指用于实验的动物，其只表明该类动物被用于实验这一用途属性，不表明该类动物的质量属性或其使用的规范性。实验动物具有如下特征：①遗传背景明确；②对携带微生物和寄生虫实施监控；③在特定的环境条件下进行人工繁殖；④应用范围明确；⑤具有政府制定法律法规进行监管的许可证制度和质量监督制度等。

【实验动物的种类】

实验动物是现代生命科学研究的重要组成部分，是生命科学特别是生物医学研究的基础和重要支撑条件，功能验证和安全评价离不开实验动物，其发挥着其他研究技术和手段无法替代的作用。根据国家标准，实验动物分为普通级、清洁级、无特定病原体级和无菌级四个等级。

普通级动物指不携带所规定的人兽共患病病原和动物烈性传染病病原的实验动物。

清洁级动物指除了普通级动物应排除的病原体外，不携带对动物危害大和对科学研究干扰强的病原的实验动物。

无特定病原体动物（specific pathogen free animal，SPF）指除了清洁级应排除的病原外，不携带主要潜在感染或条件性致病，以及对科学实验干扰强的病原的实验动物。

无菌动物是不携带任何以现有手段可检出的微生物和寄生虫的实验动物。

【实验动物的特点】

动物实验方法是药理学研究中不可缺少的重要手段，常用的实验动物有蟾蜍、小鼠、大鼠、豚鼠、家兔、猫和犬等。

1. **蟾蜍**　属两栖纲、无尾目、蟾蜍科。蟾蜍离体心脏能持久有节律地收缩，常用来观察心脏的生理功能及药物对心脏的影响。蟾蜍腓肠肌和坐骨神经样本用来观察药物对周围神经、骨骼肌及神经肌肉接头的作用。蟾蜍腹直肌标本还能用来观察胆碱能药物的作用。

2. **小鼠**　属脊椎动物门、哺乳动物纲、啮齿目、鼠科、小家鼠种。在各种药理学实验中，以小鼠应用最为普遍。目前有 500 多个远交群和近交系，是当今世界上研究最详尽的哺乳类实验动物，常用的小鼠品系有昆明小鼠、C57BL/6 小鼠、BALB/c 小鼠、129 小鼠等。小鼠与人类的基因相似度为 90% ~ 99%，且易于大量繁殖、价格低廉，适用于药物筛选、各种毒性实验（急性实验、亚急性和慢性毒性实验，半数致死量的测定等）等。小鼠为夜行性动物，其饮食与活动在夜间会增加，雄性好斗，群居优势明显，对外界环境反应敏感。

3. **大鼠**　属脊椎动物门、哺乳动物纲、啮齿目、鼠科、家鼠属、褐家鼠种。外观与小鼠相似，但个体较大。常用的大鼠品系有 Wsitar 大鼠、Sprague Dawley（SD）大鼠等，广泛应用于医药学、生物学、毒理学和营养学研究。Wistar 大鼠是我国引进最早的大鼠品种，性情温顺、繁殖力强，对传染病的抵抗力较强，自发肿瘤发生率较低；SD 大鼠生长发育较 Wistar 大鼠快，抗病能力尤其是对呼吸系统疾病的抵抗力强，自发肿瘤发生率低，对性激素感受好。

4. **豚鼠**　又名荷兰猪、天竺鼠、葵鼠、几内亚猪。属哺乳纲、啮齿目、豚鼠科、豚鼠属。豚鼠来源于南美洲的安第斯山脉。实验动物豚鼠是由野生豚鼠驯化而来，毛色多样，有白色、黑花、沙白等。豚鼠性情温顺，性早熟，抗缺氧能力强，过敏反应灵敏，体温调节能力较差，对环境温度的变化较为敏感。因豚鼠对组胺特别敏感而易被抗原性物质所致敏，常被用来观察平喘药、抗组胺药物以及抗过敏药物的反应和过敏性休克实验研究，为过敏反应实验首选动物。

5. **家兔**　属哺乳纲、啮齿目、兔科、真兔属。繁殖力高，适应性好，抗病力强。家兔性情温顺，便于灌胃、静脉注射、取血等实验操作，可用于直接记录呼吸、血压、心电图、体温等实验研究，常用于观察药物对心脏、肺部的影响以及有机磷农药中毒和解救实验，也可用于药物对中枢神经系统的作用、体温、热原检查以及避孕药实验等。家兔为药品质控中热原检查的指定动物。

6. **猫** 属哺乳纲、食肉目、猫科。猫天生胆怯和谨慎，对陌生人、陌生环境多疑不安。猫对外科手术的耐受性强，血压相对比较稳定，但价格较高，且极具攻击性，常用于去大脑僵直、下丘脑以及血压等方面的实验研究。猫为药品质控中降压物质检查的指定动物。

7. **犬** 属哺乳纲、食肉目、犬科。犬嗅觉、视觉、听觉灵敏，对外界环境适应力强。其血液循环、神经和消化系统均与人类接近。常用于观察药物对心脏泵血功能和血流动力学的影响，降压药和抗休克药的研究。犬还可以通过训练，用于慢性实验研究，如条件反射、胃肠蠕动、分泌实验和中枢神经系统实验等。

【实验动物的选择】

在药理学实验中，实验动物的选择是否恰当直接关系到课题质量的高低与实验结果的正确性，是动物实验中首先要考虑的问题。为了获得理想的实验结果，必须根据实验目的选择适宜的观察对象。实验动物的选择应符合下列基本原则：

（1）选择对刺激因素较为敏感且与人类相似的实验动物，包括结构、代谢、健康状况与疾病特点等方面的相似性。

（2）根据实验目的、内容等选择相适应的标准化动物。

（3）选择解剖、生理特点等符合实验要求的动物，即充分利用不同品种、品系动物具有的某些解剖、生理特点及存在的特殊反应。

（4）在符合实验目的与不影响实验结果的前提下，选择易获得、易饲养与管理的实验动物。

实验动物对人类疾病的表达程度和施加因素的反应情况，除了与动物自身的生理特征有关外，还受动物的状态，如是否饥饿、是否睡眠充足、是否患有其他疾病等因素的影响。另外，环境因素对实验动物也有明显的影响，在实验时应选择与受试动物自然生活尽量一致的实验环境或人为地将实验环境控制到符合条件的程度。

实验动物的选择和应用还需遵循国际上对待动物的"3R"原则：减少（reduction）、优化（refinement）、替代（replacement），并应注意符合相应的国际实验室操作规范（good laboratory practice，GLP）和标准操作规程（standard operating procedure，SOP）。

【练习题】

1. 过敏反应试验首选动物是 _____。

A. 豚鼠   B. 小鼠   C. 大鼠   D. 家兔

2.根据国家标准，将实验动物分为 ＿＿＿＿ 个等级。

A. 一　　　　　　　B. 二　　　　　　　C. 三　　　　　　　D. 四

3.关于小鼠描述不正确的是 ＿＿＿＿ 。

A. 易于繁殖、价格低廉

B. 对外科手术耐受性强，血压稳定，常用于血压实验

C. 与人类基因同源性高

D. 用于药物筛选、毒性实验等

【思考题】

（1）实验动物与实验用动物有何区别？

（2）对于动物实验，我们应该如何做才能保证既达到实验目的又最大限度减轻动物的痛苦呢？

【知识拓展】

实验的"小白鼠"

提到实验动物，你第一时间想到的是什么呢？大家常说："不要做实验用的小白鼠哦。"但你真的了解"小白鼠"吗？可供选择的实验动物那么多，科学家为什么偏偏盯上了"小白鼠"呢？小白鼠学名"小鼠"，数量庞大，全世界有1700多种鼠类，分布在世界各地，比人类数量还要多。早在16世纪，已有部分科学家利用小鼠进行科学研究。20世纪初，因孟德尔遗传定律的研究需不同物种进行验证，小鼠成为重要研究对象，1912年美国的哈希·巴格经多代近交培育，获得品系为BALB/c的白化小鼠品系，自此小鼠正式登上实验研究的历史舞台。

（赵春贞）

第二节　实验动物的常用技术

【实验动物的编号】

在动物实验中，常用多只动物同时进行实验，并对实验动物进行适当的分组，为了便于观察、辨别并记录动物的变化情况，需要在实验前对动物进行编号标记。标记

的方法有很多，良好的标记方法应满足标号清晰、易辨、简便、耐久的要求。常用的标记方法有染色法、烙印法和耳缘剪孔法等。

1. **染色法** 使用有色染料在动物明显体位被毛上进行涂染，并用不同染色来区分各组动物。这种标记方法在实验室最常用也最方便。常用的染料有 3% ~ 5% 苦味酸溶液（黄色）、0.5% 中性品红（红色）、2% 硝酸银溶液（咖啡色）。标记时用棉签或毛笔蘸取上述溶液，在动物体表的不同部位涂上斑点，以表示不同号码。编号的原则：先左后右，从上到下。如图 1-2-1 所示，一般把涂在左前腿上的记为 1 号，左侧腰部记为 2 号，左后腿记为 3 号，头顶部记为 4 号，背部正中记为 5 号，尾根部记为 6 号，右前腿记为 7 号，右侧腰部记为 8 号，右后腿记为 9 号。若动物编号超过 10 或者更大数字时，可使用两种颜色不同的溶液，即把一种颜色作为个位数，另一种颜色作为十位数，这种交互使用可编到 99 号。例如品红染色作为十位数，苦味酸染色作为个位数，如图 1-2-1 所示"31 号"。这种标记方法对于实验周期短的动物实验较为合适，时间长了染料易褪色，应及时再次涂染标记。

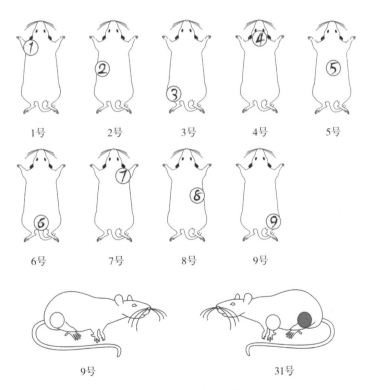

图 1-2-1　小鼠的编号方法

2. **烙印法** 用刺数钳（又称耳号钳）在动物耳朵上刺上号码，然后用棉签蘸取溶在食醋里的黑墨水涂抹。烙印打号前需用酒精对烙印部位进行消毒，烙印操作宜轻巧、敏捷。该法适用于耳朵比较大的兔、狗等动物。也可将号码烙印在方形或圆形金属牌上，或将号码按实验分组编号烙在动物的皮带上，将皮带固定在动物颈部。此法也叫号牌法，适用于兔、猫、狗等较大的动物。

3. 耳缘剪孔法 用打孔器在动物耳的一定位置打扎编号，根据打孔的位置和孔的数量来区别实验动物的方法（也称打孔法）。也可用剪刀剪缺口，注意应在剪后用滑石粉捻一下，以免剪口闭合（也称剪缺口法）。

4. 针刺法 去除动物被毛，用针头蘸取少量碳素墨水，在动物的耳部、前后肢或尾部等刺入皮下组织，在受刺部位留下黑色标记。

5. 被毛法 用剪毛刀在动物身体一侧或背部剪除所标记号码形状的被毛，适用于大、中型的实验动物，如兔、狗等。此法标记清楚可靠，仅限于短期观察使用。

【实验动物的捉拿与固定】

1. 蟾蜍 通常以左手握持，用食指和中指夹住前肢，将下肢拉直，用无名指及小指夹住下肢，同时用拇指按压背部。

2. 小鼠 右手提起尾部，放在鼠笼盖或者其他粗糙面上，向后上方轻拉，此时小鼠前肢紧紧抓住粗糙面，迅速用左手拇指和食指捏住小鼠颈背部皮肤并用小指和手掌尺侧夹持其尾根部固定手中。也可仅用单手操作，先用拇指和食指抓住小鼠尾部，再用手掌尺侧及小指夹住尾根部，然后用拇指及食指捏住其颈部皮肤。

3. 大鼠 大鼠易被激怒伤人，捉持时左手应戴防护手套或用厚布盖住大鼠。左手的拇指和中指从大鼠背部绕到腋下抓住大鼠。此时若用右手，可把食指放在右前肢的前方，与中指夹住右前肢则易于捉持。对于 1 ~ 2 周龄或体积较小的大鼠可轻轻捏住背部皮肤抓起，抓住其整个身体并固定其头部以防咬伤。

4. 家兔 捉拿时一手抓住其颈背部皮肤，轻轻将家兔提起，另一手托住其臀部，使家兔呈坐位姿势。

5. 豚鼠 豚鼠性情温顺，可用左手直接从背侧握持前部躯干，体重小者用单手捉持，体重大者宜用双手，右手托住臀部。也可用固定器固定豚鼠或将豚鼠四肢固定在木板上。

6. 猫 若猫较为温顺，可用一只手抓住猫的颈部皮肤，另一只手托起四肢抱起。对于较凶的猫，将手慢慢伸入笼内，轻抚猫的背、头、颈部，一只手抓住猫的颈部，出笼后，另一只手抓住从背到腰部的皮肤。若猫对手接触其皮肤出现明显抵触时，可戴皮手套捉拿。

7. 犬 对于未经驯服的犬，用捕犬叉夹住犬颈将其按倒，以绳索捆扎犬嘴。绑嘴时，绳带先从嘴角绕到鼻上方打一结，再将绳带绕到嘴下方打一结，然后将绳带拉到耳后颈部打结固定，方可给药。对于驯养的犬，可先对其轻抚，逐渐接近动物，给狗戴好嘴罩固定，分别把狗的四肢用带子捆绑好。

【实验动物的麻醉】

在一些动物实验中，特别是动物手术等试验，为便于操作，常需对动物采取必要的措施。动物麻醉可选择全身麻醉和局部麻醉，不同的麻醉方式，选择的药物也不同。

1. 常用的麻醉药

1）局部麻醉药 普鲁卡因、利多卡因等，起效快，常用于局部浸润麻醉。

2）全身麻醉药

（1）乙醚：乙醚吸入麻醉适用于各种动物，其优点为麻醉作用剂量和致死量差距大，所以安全性也大，动物麻醉深度容易掌握，麻醉后容易苏醒。缺点是局部刺激大，可使得上呼吸道黏液分泌增加，通过神经反射可影响呼吸、血压和心跳活动，且易引起窒息。

（2）戊巴比妥钠：常用 1% ~ 3% 戊巴比妥钠生理盐水溶液，一次给药麻醉有效时间可延续 3 ~ 5 h。麻醉使用方便，麻醉过程较平稳，动物无明显挣扎现象，缺点是苏醒较慢。

（3）硫喷妥钠：常用浓度为 1% ~ 5%。此药注射后，可迅速进入脑组织，故麻醉诱导快，但苏醒也很快，一次给药的麻醉时效仅维持 0.5 ~ 1 h。

2. 麻醉方法

1）全身麻醉

（1）吸入麻醉法：麻醉药以蒸气或者气体状态经呼吸道吸入而产生麻醉，常用乙醚，可用于大鼠、小鼠、家兔的麻醉。具体方法：将动物放入玻璃麻醉箱内，把装有浸润乙醚棉球的小烧杯放入麻醉箱。

（2）腹腔注射和静脉给药麻醉法：常用的麻醉药有戊巴比妥钠、硫喷妥钠等。采用腹腔注射和静脉注射进行麻醉，操作简单，是实验室最常用的方法之一。腹腔给药麻醉多用于大鼠、小鼠和豚鼠，较大的动物如兔、狗等则多用静脉给药麻醉。

2）局部麻醉

用局部麻醉药阻滞周围神经末梢或神经干、神经节、神经丛的冲动传导，产生局部麻醉作用，其特点是动物保持清醒，对重要器官功能干扰轻微，麻醉并发症少。猫的局部麻醉一般注射 0.5% ~ 1.0% 盐酸普鲁卡因溶液；家兔进行眼球手术时，可于结膜囊滴入 0.02% 盐酸可卡因溶液，数秒钟即可出现麻醉。

【实验动物的给药】

1. 腹腔注射 用大小鼠进行实验时，左手固定动物，使腹部向上，头呈低位使内脏移向上腹，右手将注射针于右（左）下腹刺入皮肤，并以45°角穿过腹肌，在此处保持针尖不动的状态下，回抽针栓，如无回血或尿液，缓慢注入药液。若实验动物为家兔，进针部位为下腹部腹白线旁开1 cm为宜。

2. 灌胃给药 适用于小鼠、大鼠、豚鼠、家兔等动物。以小鼠为例，左手抓住颈背部皮肤将动物固定，右手持灌胃针插入动物口中，沿咽后壁徐徐插入食管。动物应固定成垂直体位，针插入时应无阻力，若感到阻力或动物挣扎时，应立即停止进针或将针拔出，以免损伤或穿破食管甚至误入气管。小鼠常用的灌胃量为0.2 ~ 1 mL，大鼠为1 ~ 4 mL，豚鼠为1 ~ 5 mL。

3. 静脉注射

（1）尾静脉注射：小鼠和大鼠一般采用尾静脉注射。注射时将动物固定在尾静脉注射装置内或者固定在鼠筒内，使尾巴露出，尾部用45 ~ 50℃的温水浸润半分钟或者用75%的乙醇溶液擦拭，使血管扩张、表皮角质软化。以左手拇指和食指捏住鼠尾两侧，使静脉充盈，用中指从下面托起尾巴，以无名指和小指夹住尾巴的末梢，右手持针使针头与尾静脉平行（小于30°），从尾下1/4处（距尾尖2 ~ 3 cm）进针。先缓慢注入少量药液，如无阻力，可继续注入至完毕。

（2）耳缘静脉注射：家兔一般采用耳缘静脉注射。将家兔放入固定盒内，首先拔去耳缘静脉注射部位的被毛，用手指弹动或轻揉耳，使静脉充盈。左手食指和中指夹住静脉近端，拇指绷紧静脉远端，无名指及小指垫在下面，右手持注射器从远端刺入血管，并沿血管平行方向深入，移动手指于针头上以固定针头，放开食指和中指，将药液注入，然后拔出针头，用棉球压迫针孔片刻即可。

4. 肌内注射 多选择肌肉发达、无大血管神经通过的部位，一般多选臀部。注射时垂直刺入肌肉，回抽针栓如无回血，即可进行注射。给大鼠、小鼠等小动物进行肌内注射，可将药液注入后腿上部外侧肌肉。

5. 皮下注射 注射时以左手拇指和食指提起皮肤，将注射器针头刺入皮下，缓慢注入药液，拔出针头后，用手指轻压注射部位，以防药液漏出。不同实验动物注射部位有所不同，小鼠通常在背部，犬、猫多在大腿外侧。

6. 颅内注射 用于观察作用于大脑病变部位的药物作用。针对小动物如需精确进针位置和深度，可采用脑立体定位仪进行辅助注射。小鼠、大鼠、豚鼠、兔等进行颅内注射时，须先用穿颅钢针穿透颅骨，再用注射器针头刺入脑部。

【实验标本的采集】

1. 尾静脉取血 主要用于需血量很少的大鼠或小鼠实验。固定动物并露出鼠尾，用 45 ~ 50℃温水浸泡或用二甲苯擦拭鼠尾使血管扩张充血，用手术刀片切开尾静脉，血液即自行流出。也可采用剪除尾尖法（剪去尾尖 3 ~ 5 mm）取血。

2. 球后静脉丛取血 取血时左手捏住鼠两耳间的颈背部，头皮轻轻向下压迫背部两侧，以阻断头部静脉回流而使眼球外凸。右手持毛细采血管（0.5 ~ 1 mm），从眼睑与眼球插入，使毛细管与眶壁平行地向喉头方向推进 4 ~ 5 mm，即达到球后静脉丛，血液会自行流入管内。小鼠每次可采血 0.2 ~ 0.3 mL，大鼠每次可采血 0.4 ~ 0.6 mL，此法可连续取血多次。

3. 眼眶静脉取血 将鼠倒持压迫眼球，使其充血后突出，用止血钳迅速摘除眼球后，眼眶内很快有血液流出，将血液滴入有抗凝剂的试管里即可。

4. 心脏取血 主要用于家兔、犬等较大动物。将动物仰卧固定在手术台上，剪去心前区的毛，用 75% 的乙醇溶液消毒皮肤，用左手触摸胸骨左缘第 3、4 肋间隙，选心脏跳动最明显处作穿刺点。右手持注射器，将针头刺入心脏，随心脏的搏动血液自动进入注射器。

5. 耳缘静脉取血 多用于家兔取血。取血部位局部用手轻弹耳廓或涂二甲苯，使血管扩张，后用乙醇擦净，再用粗针头刺入耳缘静脉取血。

6. 断头取血 主要用于大鼠、小鼠的大量采血。左手固定动物，并使头略向下倾，右手用剪刀迅速剪掉动物头部，让血液快速滴入试管内（含抗凝剂）。

【实验动物的处死】

根据动物伦理学规定，当实验中途停止或结束时，应对实验动物实施安乐死。实验动物安乐死方法的选择取决于动物的种类与研究的课题，为尽可能减少实验动物的痛苦和恐惧，推荐对实验动物麻醉后再处死。

1. 蟾蜍 用刺蛙针插入枕骨大孔，破坏脑、脊髓等方法处死，或者用粗剪刀剪断头处死。

2. 大鼠和小鼠 ①颈椎脱臼法：右手抓住鼠尾用力向后上拉，同时左手拇指与食指用力向下按住鼠头，将脑与脊髓断离，鼠立刻死亡，这是小鼠最常用的处死方法。②断头法：持剪刀于鼠颈部将鼠头剪掉。③击打法：右手抓住鼠尾，提起，用力摔击其头部，鼠痉挛后立即死亡；或用小木槌用力击打鼠头部也可致死。④急性失血法：可采用鼠眼眶动脉和静脉急性大量失血方法使鼠立刻死亡。

3. 犬、猫、兔、豚鼠 ①空气栓塞法：向动物静脉内注入一定量的空气，使之发生栓塞而死。②急性失血法：先使动物麻醉，暴露股三角区或腹腔，再切断股动脉或腹主动脉，立刻喷出血液，用自来水不断冲洗流血，3～5 min即可死亡。③击打法：对家兔用木槌用力击打其后脑部，损伤延脑，造成死亡。④开放气胸法：将动物开胸，造成开放性气胸，使动物窒息而死。

【练习题】

1. 实验动物编号最常用的方法是 _____。

A. 染色法　　　　　B. 号牌法　　　　　C. 烙印法　　　　　D. 被毛法

2. 大鼠处死常用的方法不包括 _____。

A. 急性失血法　　　B. 击打法　　　　　C. 断头法　　　　　D. 破坏脊髓

3. 小鼠少量取血可选择 _____。

A. 断头取血　　　　B. 尾静脉取血　　　C. 心脏取血　　　　D. 股动脉取血

【思考题】

动物实验前需进行哪些准备？

【知识拓展】

克隆小鼠"小小"

2009年中国科学家首次利用iPS细胞成功克隆出活体小鼠"小小"，这只小鼠的诞生，向世界宣告中国人的智慧，并延续克隆羊"多利"的传奇，该成果发表在 Nature 杂志上。iPS细胞全称为诱导性多功能干细胞，是由体细胞诱导而成的干细胞，具有和胚胎干细胞类似的发育多潜能性。iPS细胞具有和胚胎干细胞类似的功能，绕开了胚胎干细胞研究面临的伦理和法律等诸多屏障，医疗领域应用前景非常广阔，但因此前未能培育出完全由iPS细胞发育而来的活体哺乳动物，其全能性一直受到怀疑。中国科学家克隆小鼠"小小"，在世界上首次证明了iPS细胞与胚胎干细胞一样具有全能性，该研究成果是从干细胞研究迈向实际医疗过程的一大步，对于细胞全能性机理研究、器官移植、药物筛选、基因治疗等临床应用研究有重要价值。这一成果受到国际干细胞研究界的高度重视，Nature 杂志网站称赞中国科学家"为克隆成年哺乳动物开辟了一条全新道路"。

（赵春贞）

第三节 实验动物伦理

【实验动物福利与保障】

实验动物伦理是从道德层面审视实验动物是否以及如何获得道德对待和道德关怀，并约束和规范人类对实验动物的使用行为。实验动物也是动物的一分子，因而从广义上讲，实验动物福利也属于动物保护主义的一部分。动物保护主义于 20 世纪 60 年代在西方首先兴起，动物伦理的研究也日益兴盛。近年来关于动物保护主义的多种观点逐渐浮现，但有些理论过于偏激或极端。因此，我们需结合中国实际国情，正确认识实验动物伦理，这关系到我国生命科学和医学的发展。

动物福利指人类采取各种措施避免对动物造成不必要的损害，防止虐待动物，使动物在健康舒适的状态下生存。按照国际上通认的说法，动物福利的主要内容包括五大理念（"5F"）：享有不受饥渴的自由，享有生活舒适的自由，享有不受痛苦，伤害和疾病的自由，享有生活无恐惧和无悲伤的自由，享有表达天性的自由。

实验动物福利并不意味着就是绝对地保护实验动物不受任何伤害，而是在兼顾科学问题探索和在可能的基础上最大限度地满足实验动物维持生命、维持健康和提高舒适程度的需要。研究实验动物生活环境条件、实验动物"内心感受"、人道的实验技术等是科学的实验动物福利的主要内容。我们在进行与实验动物相关的活动时，要本着为科学服务的目的尽可能地减少给实验动物带来的伤害。

目前，实验动物福利问题已引起世界各国和国际组织的广泛重视。现在凡涉及动物实验的科研论文发表或者申报科学研究课题，必须出示由"动物伦理委员会"提供的证明，确保该动物实验研究符合动物福利准则。

【实验动物伦理的基本要求】

为了解决生命伦理学与动物实验的冲突，我们需遵守动物福利的"3R"原则和五大理念（"5F"）。

"3R"原则指：①"减少"（reduction）：尽可能地减少实验中所用动物的数量，提高实验动物的利用率和实验的精确度；②"优化"（refinement）：改善实验条件，减少动物的精神紧张和痛苦；③"替代"（replacement）：不使用活体动物进行实验，而以单细胞生物、微生物或细胞或其他非动物模型进行替代。

动物福利的五大理念为：①享有不受饥渴的自由（freedom from hunger and thirst，

生理福利）；②享有生活舒适的自由（freedom from discomfort，环境福利）；③享有不受痛苦、伤害和疾病的自由（freedom from pain, injury and disease，卫生福利）；④ 享有生活无恐惧和无悲伤的自由（freedom from fear and distress，行为福利）；⑤ 享有表达天性的自由（freedom to express normal behavior，心理福利）。

　　动物福利既保证了动物的生存状态，又保护了动物权利的存在。动物福利论主张在动物使用过程中遵守"3R"原则和"5F"理念，明确要求禁止肆意杀害动物、禁止肆意虐待动物，对人类行为加以约束，使动物得到充分的保护，免遭痛苦。

【练习题】

　　1. 实验动物伦理的"3R"原则不包括 ＿＿＿＿。

　　A. 保护　　　　　　　　B. 减少　　　　　　　C. 优化　　　　　　　D. 替代

　　2. 实验动物伦理的"5F"理念不包括 ＿＿＿＿。

　　A. 不受饥渴的自由　　　　　　　　B. 不受屠戮的自由

　　C. 生活舒适的自由　　　　　　　　D. 表达天性的自由

　　3. 关于动物福利说法不正确的是 ＿＿＿＿。

　　A. 满足动物维持生命的需要　　　　B. 绝对保护动物不受伤害

　　C. 动物福利受各国关注　　　　　　D. 尊重动物"内心感受"

【思考题】

　　（1）如何理解"安乐死"？

　　（2）你认为什么样的动物应予以保护？

【知识拓展】

致敬 "无名英雄"

　　每年的4月24日被定为"世界实验动物日"，是由英国反活体解剖协会（NAVS）于1979年发起的，受联合国认可的国际性纪念日，其前后一周则被称为"实验动物周"。世界实验动物日的设立旨在倡导科学、人道地开展动物实验，铭记实验动物为人类健康事业所作出的巨大贡献和牺牲，规范和合理地使用实验动物。

（成　敏）

第四节　磺胺嘧啶血浆半衰期的测定

【实验目的】

（1）学习磺胺嘧啶血药浓度和血浆半衰期的测定及计算方法。

（2）掌握药代动力学的计算方法及临床意义。

【实验原理】

血浆半衰期（half-life，$t_{1/2}$）指血浆药物浓度下降一半所需要的时间，以 $t_{1/2}$ 表示。临床常用药物中多数药物在体内按一级动力学消除，血药浓度与瞬时药物浓度成正比，即单位时间内药物浓度按照恒定比例消除，其血药浓度（对数值）–时间曲线为直线。按照零级动力学消除的药物，其血药浓度（对数值）–时间曲线为抛物线，属于非线性动力学消除；零级消除动力学是由体内消除药物的能力达到饱和所致，血药浓度–时间曲线为直线。

磺胺嘧啶（sulfadiazine，SD）为对氨基苯类化合物，在酸性环境下可使苯环上的氨基（-NH$_2$）离子化生成铵类化合物（-NH$_3^+$），可与亚硝酸钠起重氮反应，生成重氮盐（-N≡N$^+$-）。此重氮盐在碱性溶液中与酚类化合物（如麝香草酚）起偶联反应，生成橙红色的偶氮化合物（图 1-4-1）。偶氮化合物的显色深浅与磺胺嘧啶的浓度有关。采用分光光度计测定光密度，与标准品光密度比较，可对磺胺嘧啶的药物浓度进行定量分析。根据用药后不同时间血浆药物浓度的变化规律，可计算血浆半衰期等药代动力学参数。

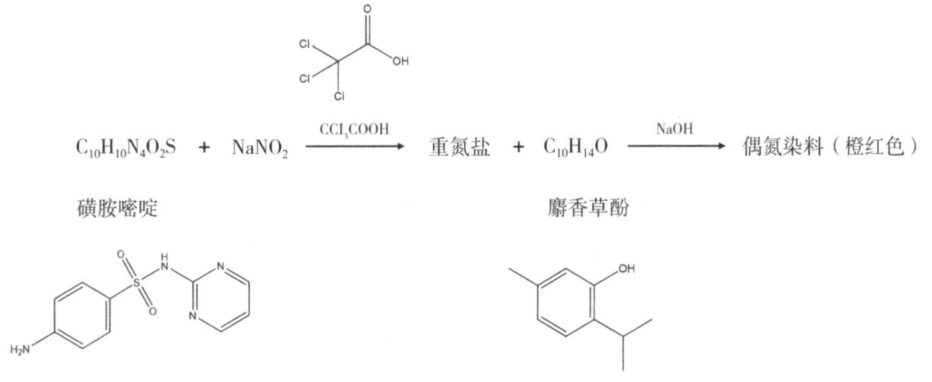

$$C_{10}H_{10}N_4O_2S \ + \ NaNO_2 \xrightarrow{\ CCl_3COOH\ } 重氮盐 \ + \ C_{10}H_{14}O \xrightarrow{\ NaOH\ } 偶氮染料（橙红色）$$

磺胺嘧啶　　　　　　　　　　　　　　　　　　　麝香草酚

图 1-4-1　磺胺嘧啶显色原理示意图

【实验器材】

721 分光光度计、离心机、兔固定器、手术器械一套、试管、离心管、烧杯、磅秤、注射器（1 mL、5 mL、10 mL）、移液枪、吸头、试管架、卫生纸、棉球、塑料盆。

【实验动物】

家兔，体重 2.0 ~ 3.0 kg，雌雄不拘。

【实验药品】

20% 磺胺嘧啶溶液、0.5% 肝素生理盐水、0.5% 亚硝酸钠溶液、0.02% 磺胺嘧啶钠标准液、7.5% 三氯乙酸溶液、0.5% 麝香草酚溶液（用 20% 氢氧化钠溶液配制）。

【实验方法】

实验操作步骤如下，见图 1-4-2。

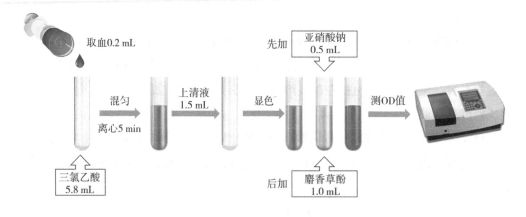

图 1-4-2　操作步骤示意图

1. **实验准备**　取试管 3 支，标记 A、B、C，各加入 7.5% 三氯乙酸溶液 5.8 mL。取另外 3 支试管，同样标记 A、B、C，备用。

2. **给药前取血**　取家兔 1 只，称重并记录体重，根据体重计算给药剂量，取药备用。取 1 mL 注射器 1 支，用 0.5% 肝素生理盐水润洗后，由家兔一侧耳缘静脉取血 0.2 mL，保留针头、取下注射器，将血液注入 A 管，摇匀备用。

3. **给药**　家兔第一次取血完成后，立即换上另一注射器（5 mL）自原针头注入 20% 的磺胺嘧啶溶液 2 mL/kg（根据给药剂量计算相应的给药体积）。记录注射完成的时间。

4. 给药后取血 在给药完成后 5 min 及 35 min，采用同样的方法自另外一侧的耳缘静脉各取血 0.2 mL，分别注入 B 管、C 管。准确记录取到血液样本的时间，计算两次取血的时间差。

5. 显色 将 A、B、C 3 支试管摇匀，以 1500 r/min 转速离心 5 min，用移液枪取离心后上清液 1.5 mL，加入对应标记的试管中，依次加入 0.5% 亚硝酸钠溶液 0.5 mL、0.5% 麝香草酚溶液 1.0 mL，混匀。

6. 比色 以给药前的样品管（A 管）调零点，校准。将反应后各管内溶液分别置于 721 分光光度计的 1.0 mL 比色杯内，在波长 525 nm 处比色，测出各样品管和标准管的光密度值。

7. 计算血药浓度 根据同一溶液浓度与光密度成正比的原理，可用无血液的标准管的浓度及其光密度值求出某一时间点血液中磺胺嘧啶的浓度。公式如下：

$$样品管浓度 / 标准管浓度 = 样品管光密度 / 标准管光密度$$

即

$$C_测 = OD_测 / OD_标 \times C_标$$

8. 计算血浆半衰期（$t_{1/2}$） 一室模型半衰期计算公式为：

$$t_{1/2}/T = \log(1/2)/\log R_T$$

式中 T 为间隔时间；R_T 为 T 时间段代谢后药物在体内的留存率（给药后两次取血的药物浓度比值），在本实验中为 35 min 对应的血药浓度与 5 min 对应的血药浓度的比值，可用 OD_C/OD_B 代替。

【实验记录与结果】

记录实验结果，根据公式计算出用药后 5 min 和用药后 35 min 时磺胺嘧啶的血药浓度、$t_{1/2}$。具体见表 1-4-1。

表 1-4-1 磺胺嘧啶血药浓度和血浆半衰期测定

取样时间	血样（mL）	三氯乙酸（mL）		上清液（mL）	NaNO₂（mL）	麝香草酚（mL）	光密度值（A）	浓度（mg/mL）
给药前	0.2	5.8		1.5	0.5	1.0		
给药后 5 min	0.2	5.8	离	1.5	0.5	1.0		
给药后 35 min	0.2	5.8	心	1.5	0.5	1.0		
标准品	（标准液）0.2	5.8		1.5	0.5	1.0		

【注意事项】

（1）取血液样本前注射器一定要用肝素生理盐水润洗。

（2）取血时每吸取一个血样，必须更换注射器，不能混用。

（3）各管每次加一种试剂后都必须充分混匀，加样顺序不能颠倒。

（4）各吸量管注意分开使用，比色杯要清洗干净，吸取药液要准确。

（5）离心时要注意离心管的配平。

（6）采血也可采用心脏取血法。

【练习题】

1. 耳缘静脉取血应从 _____ 开始取血。

A. 近心端　　　　　　B. 远心端　　　　　　C. 任何位置　　　　　　D. 耳背内缘

2. 有关一级消除动力学描述正确的是 _____。

A. 药物半衰期并非恒定值

B. 其消除速率表示单位时间内消除实际百分比

C. 其消除速率与体内药物量成正比

D. 为小部分药物的消除方式

3. 有关离心机的操作描述错误的是 _____。

A. 使用前预热 5 ~ 10 min

B. 离心管放置的位置必须相邻，不宜距离太远

C. 离心管不宜装得太满

D. 禁止超载

【思考题】

（1）药物的血浆半衰期是固定不变的吗？对临床用药有何指导意义？

（2）不同个体磺胺嘧啶的半衰期不同，除个体差异外还受什么因素影响？

【知识拓展】

"磺胺" 药物的发现

磺胺嘧啶是一种磺胺染料，1932 年由德国生物化学家格哈德·多马克（Gerhard Domagk）发现，是世界上第一个商用的抗菌化学治疗剂。最初叫"百浪多息"，

是一种工业染料，因被发现其中包含一些具有消毒作用的成分，曾被用于治疗丹毒等。然而，在实验中发现其在试管中却没有明显的杀菌作用，因而没有引起医学界的重视。多马克最早的患者是他年仅6岁的女儿，因不慎用未消毒的针刺伤造成感染，病情恶化，医生已经开始考虑截肢。绝望的多马克给女儿使用了百浪多息，这种药物还没有完成临床试验，幸运的是其女儿在2天后痊愈出院。多马克因发现百浪多息的抗菌作用获得了诺贝尔生理学或医学奖。研究发现，百浪多息只有在体内才能杀死链球菌，而在试管内则不能。它可以裂解为氨苯磺胺，将"磺胺"进行动物实验发现与百浪多息相同，磺胺的名字迅即在医学界广泛传播。

（赵春贞）

第五节　普鲁卡因半数致死量测定

【实验目的】

序贯法测定普鲁卡因的半数致死量。

【实验原理】

能引起50%的实验动物出现阳性反应时的药物剂量，若效应为死亡，则称为半数致死量（median lethal dose，LD_{50}）。LD_{50}是衡量药物毒性大小的指标之一，是申报新药过程中必须提供的药理学资料。半数有效量（median effective dose，ED_{50}）指在量反应中能引起50%最大反应强度的药量。LD_{50}和ED_{50}的比值称为治疗指数（therapeutic index，TI），用来评价药物的安全性。一般而言，治疗指数大的药物相对治疗指数小的药物安全，但并不完全可靠。

普鲁卡因（procaine）是一种局麻药，分子结构见图1-5-1，能暂时阻断神经纤维的传导而具有麻醉作用。当被大量吸收后会产生全身毒性反应，主要表现为中枢神经系统先兴奋后抑制，初期表现为眩晕、烦躁不安、肌肉震颤，进而发展为神经错乱、惊厥、昏迷、呼吸抑制等。患者可因呼吸衰竭而死亡。

LD_{50}的测定方法很多，如加权机率单位法（Bliss法）、寇氏法、序贯法等。Bliss法是目前推荐使用的方法，此法对剂量分组无严格要求，不需要剂量组有0%和100%死亡率，是目前公认最准确的测定方法。但本法计算烦琐，故现多采用计算机程序计算。我国卫生健康委员会规定，Bliss法是新药LD_{50}测定必须采用的方法。

序贯法又称序贯设计法或序贯检验法，是一种逐一进行试验、逐一进行分析的试验测定法。此法优点是节约受试动物，且易于观察实验结果，适用于用药后反应比较快的药物实验。

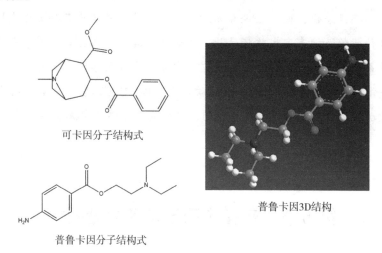

可卡因分子结构式

普鲁卡因3D结构

普鲁卡因分子结构式

图 1-5-1   普鲁卡因与可卡因的分子结构

【实验器材】

注射器、电子天平、鼠笼、函数型计算器。

【实验动物】

小鼠（18 ~ 22 g），雌雄各半。

【实验药品】

2% 普鲁卡因溶液、2% 苦味酸溶液。

【实验方法】

1. **确定给药剂量**   实验前预先拟定好药物剂量，相邻两剂量按照等比排列（对数差相等），如图 1-5-2 所示。

2. **抓取小鼠**   每实验组取小鼠 10 只，雌雄各半。小鼠称重后，用苦味酸标记。

3. **给药与结果记录**   先取小鼠 1 只，腹腔注射第一个剂量 2% 的普鲁卡因 0.1 mL/10 g，若出现死亡，下一只动物则用低一个剂量；若未出现死亡，下一只动物则用高一个剂量。将结果记录到表格中，动物死亡用"+"表示，未死亡用"–"表示。若在同一剂量中连续出现"−"两次，则下一次实验结束，最后一只动物不做实验，但需要在表格中标记"E"。

剂量	LogD	动物状态（死亡"+"或未死亡"-"）										R	R·logD
（mg/kg）		1	2	3	4	5	6	7	8	9	10		
125	2.097	+										1	2.097
87.5	1.942		+		+							2	3.884
61.3	1.787			−		+		+		E		4	7.148
42.9	1.632						−		−			2	3.264
合计												9	16.363

图 1-5-2　小鼠腹腔注射戊四氮的实验结果实例

4. 实验结果计算

$$LD_{50}=\log{-1}（C/N）\ mg/kg$$

式中：$C=\sum（R\cdot\log D）$；

　　　　$R=$ 剂量组的动物数；

　　　　$LogD=$ 剂量 D 的对数值；

　　　　$N=$ 实验动物总数 $=\sum R$。

【实验记录与结果】

实验结果记录表如表 1-5-1 所示。

表 1-5-1　小鼠腹腔注射普鲁卡因半数致死量实验结果

剂量	LogD	动物状态（死亡"+"或未死亡"−"）										R	R·logD
（mg/kg）		1	2	3	4	5	6	7	8	9	10		
222	2.347												
200	2.301												
180	2.255												
162	2.209												
145.8	2.163												
合计													

【注意事项】

（1）本实验为定量实验，注射剂量必须准确。

（2）给药后应仔细观察动物的反应，不能过多翻动小鼠，以免影响实验结果。

（3）因为体重对本药的死亡率影响较大，因此每组动物的体重分布应该一致。

【练习题】

1. 关于小鼠腹腔注射，下列说法不正确的是 _____。

A. 腹腔注射时动物头部向下不宜刺到内脏

B. 腹腔注射给药前要先排空注射器内的气泡

C. 注射针头应贴紧皮肤，尽量平行扎入

D. 当针尖穿过腹肌进入腹膜腔后抵抗感消失

2. LD_{50} 与毒性评价的关系是 _____。

A. LD_{50} 与毒性大小成正比 　　　　B. LD_{50} 与染毒剂量成正比

C. LD_{50} 与毒性大小成反比 　　　　D. LD_{50} 与急性阈剂量成反比

3. LD_{50} 测定最准确的方法是 _____。

A. 寇氏法 　　　　　　　　　　　　B. Bliss 法

C. 序贯法 　　　　　　　　　　　　D. 累计法

【思考题】

（1）LD_{50} 测定的意义是什么？

（2）在药物的安全性评价中，除了 LD_{50} 还需考虑哪些毒性指标？

【知识拓展】

普鲁卡因的经典"改造"历程

如果你去看过牙医，那十有八九用过普鲁卡因，一种局部麻醉药，而它的"亲戚"，则是"毒"名在外的可卡因。

可卡因，一种从南美古柯树叶中分离出来的一种生物碱，是最早使用的局部麻醉剂，于1884年用于临床。局麻效果非常有效，但毒性较大，易使人上瘾，甚至死亡。可卡因的化学结构是一种复杂的双环，1905年，德国慕尼黑大学的化学教授艾因霍恩（Alfred Einhorn）简化了可卡因的结构，合成出了只保留一个环且麻醉效果更好的化合物——普鲁卡因，而且它没有成瘾性、不会被滥用。这也是第一种可注射的局部麻醉剂。由此人们认识到，天然产物的复杂结构可以被简化，作用不变甚至会更好，新药的研发途径多了一条——简化天然产物结构。这是从天然化合物出发设计和发现新药的经典例子之一。

（赵春贞）

第六节 肝功能对药物作用的影响

【实验目的】

（1）观察肝功能对丙泊酚作用的影响。

（2）了解肝脏在药物代谢中的重要性。

（3）了解肝损害模型的制作方法。

视频 1

【实验原理】

肝脏是人体中是最大的实质性脏器，是药物代谢的主要器官。绝大部分药物经肝脏代谢后，代谢产物无活性；少数药物需经肝脏代谢转化成有活性的代谢产物发挥药理作用。当肝功能受损后，肝脏对药物的代谢功能减弱，引起原型药物浓度增加，$t_{1/2}$ 延长，使药物作用增强而不良反应增加。四氯化碳进入肝细胞后经细胞色素 P450 酶激活生成三氯甲基自由基（$.CCl_3$），后者与膜磷脂或蛋白分子发生共价结合，破坏膜组织结构和功能完整性，特别是损伤线粒体膜组织结构，影响代谢功能和能量合成，最终导致肝细胞变性甚至坏死。因此，四氯化碳中毒动物常被作为中毒性肝炎的动物模型用于观察肝脏功能状态对药物作用的影响，以及筛选和试验肝功能保护药。

丙泊酚（propofol，也称异丙酚）是一种起效迅速的短效全身静脉麻醉药，也用于加强监护患者接受机械通气时的镇静，以及用于麻醉下无痛人工流产手术等。丙泊酚的作用机制可能是激活中枢 γ- 氨基丁酸受体，并调节下丘脑睡眠通路。丙泊酚的脂溶性极高，血浆蛋白结合率 96% ~ 98%，由于药物被迅速代谢和清除，其麻醉时间很短，为 4 ~ 6 min。丙泊酚主要经肝脏代谢而消除，可能在肝中与葡糖醛酸结合代谢，代谢物由尿排出。肝脏功能状态直接影响其药理作用的强弱和维持时间的长短，如图 1-6-1 所示。

【实验器材】

电子天平、烧杯、注射器（1 mL）、鼠笼、蛙板、手术剪、镊子。

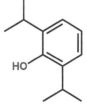

图 1-6-1 丙泊酚的化学结构式

【实验动物】

小鼠 4 只（18 ～ 22 g），雌雄不限。

【实验药品】

1% 丙泊酚溶液、10% 四氯化碳溶液、生理盐水、苦味酸溶液。

【实验方法】

实验操作步骤如下，见图 1-6-2。

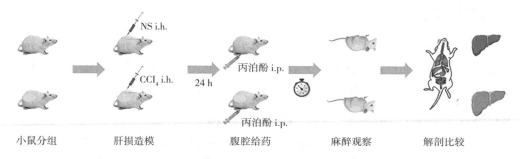

小鼠分组　　　　肝损造模　　　　腹腔给药　　　　麻醉观察　　　　解剖比较

图 1-6-2　操作步骤示意图

1. **实验动物分组编号**　取体重相近的小鼠 4 只，随机分为肝损组和正常组，称体重后用苦味酸标记编号，观察其正常活动。

2. **肝损模型**　肝损组小鼠在试验前 24 h 用 10% 四氯化碳按 0.1 mL/10 g 皮下注射，造成肝损伤，正常组小鼠注射生理盐水作为对照。

3. **给药前观察**　实验开始时对两组小鼠进行翻正反射（righting reflex，亦称复位反射，指动物体处于异常体位时所产生的恢复正常体位的反射）试验。将小鼠仰卧试验台上，若能恢复正常体位，为翻正反射存在，否则为翻正反射消失。

4. **给药**　两组小鼠分别腹腔注射 1% 溶液丙泊酚溶液 0.1 mL/10 g（剂量 100 mg/kg，即 1 mg/10 g），给药后立即记录时间，通过观察翻正反射消失作为麻醉起效标志，记录该时间段为麻醉开始时间。继续观察小鼠直至翻正反射恢复，记录该时间段为麻醉维持时间。其他观察指标包括小鼠活动情况、呼吸深浅及频率。比较小鼠麻醉作用维持时间有何差异。

5. **解剖观察**　小鼠苏醒后用颈椎脱臼法处死，剖视肝脏观察形态上差异，比较两组肝脏大小、颜色及充血程度，并注意肝脏形态改变与麻醉作用维持时间的关系。

【实验记录与结果】

记录实验结果,将各组小鼠的麻醉起效时间、维持时间及肝脏形态记录于表1-6-1。

表1-6-1　肝功能对丙泊酚作用的影响

组别	编号	体重 （g）	给药剂量 （mg/10 g）	麻醉开始时间 （min）	麻醉维持时间 （min）	解剖后肝脏形态
肝损组	1					
	2					
正常组	3					
	4					

【注意事项】

（1）室温最好保持在25℃左右,如在20℃以下应给麻醉中的小鼠保温,否则动物因体温下降,代谢减慢,不易苏醒。

（2）四氯化碳对人体有毒性,在使用时要注意安全,建议由教研室统一提前处理建立肝损伤模型。

（3）在建立肝损伤时应注意四氯化碳的剂量,避免剂量过大导致小鼠死亡。

（4）翻正反射消失指小鼠仰面朝上,1 min内不自主翻身为标准,如能自主翻身则判为清醒。

【练习题】

1. 四氯化碳中毒引起的肝细胞病变是 _____。

A. 玻璃样变性 　　　　　　　　　　B. 脂肪变性

C. 钙化 　　　　　　　　　　　　　D. 纤维素样坏死

2. 有关丙泊酚药理特点不正确的是 _____。

A. 起效迅速,诱导平稳

B. 可降低脑血流量、脑代谢率和颅内压

C. 没有呼吸抑制作用

D. 可引起注射部位疼痛和局部静脉炎

3. 肝功能受损患者在服用经肝代谢失活的药物时用药剂量应 _____。

A. 增加 　　　　　　　　　　　　　B. 减少

C. 不变 　　　　　　　　　　　　　D. 禁用

【思考题】

（1）肝脏损害的小鼠较正常小鼠注射丙泊酚后麻醉时间有何不同？为什么？

（2）肝脏功能状态对临床用药剂量有何指导意义？

【知识拓展】

中医理论下的肝脏

古人对肝脏的认识主要基于中医理论。肝脏被视为五脏之一，具有主疏泄、藏血和主筋等生理功能。在中医中，肝脏与情绪、眼睛和消化等方面有着密切的联系。古人认为肝脏是人体内重要的器官，对于维护身体健康起着至关重要的作用。同时，中医也提出了一些与肝脏相关的理论和治疗方法，用以调理身体和治疗疾病。

《黄帝内经》作为中医理论的奠基之作，对肝脏的功能和药物代谢有着深刻的论述。例如，《素问》中提到"肝者，将军之官，谋虑出焉"，形象地描述了肝脏在人体中的重要地位和作用。

在东汉张仲景所著的《伤寒杂病论》中，不仅包含了对多种疾病的治疗方剂，也隐含了中药在人体内代谢和转化的思想。

药物代谢实例：如中药柴胡，在中医理论中具有疏肝解郁、升举阳气的功效。现代研究也发现，柴胡中的有效成分在肝脏内经过代谢后，能够发挥抗炎、抗病毒等药理作用。

综上所述，我国中医关于肝脏和药物代谢的记载不仅体现了中医理论的博大精深，也为现代中医药研究提供了宝贵的参考和借鉴。

（童骏森）

第七节　不同剂量对药物作用的影响

【实验目的】

观察不同剂量的药物（戊巴比妥钠或水合氯醛）对小鼠作用的差异。

【实验原理】

药物的剂量与临床药理效应之间的关系较为复杂，因进入体内的药物产生的作用受到体内复杂的调节代偿机制的影响。在仔细控制的体外（*in vitro*）实验系统中，药物浓度与其效应间的关系称为量效关系。药物效应与剂量在一定范围内呈比例关系。

药物剂量的大小决定药物在体内血药浓度的高低和药物作用的强弱。药物剂量增加时，药物的效应也增加。但是，这一效应的增加不是无限制的，当效应增加到一定程度后，继续增加药物浓度或剂量而其效应不会再继续增强，维持恒定在一定的水平。当药物的剂量过大时，可导致中毒或死亡。

戊巴比妥钠、水合氯醛均为中枢抑制药（图1-7-1），其剂量不同则药理效应不同。翻正反射（righting reflex）为本实验的观察指标。翻正反射指正常小鼠轻轻用手将其侧卧或仰卧立即恢复正常姿势。翻正反射消失是小鼠产生睡眠作用的客观指标，用手将小鼠轻轻侧卧或仰卧超过1 min不能翻正即为翻正反射消失。

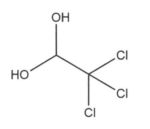
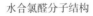
水合氯醛分子结构

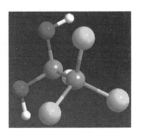
水合氯醛3D结构

图1-7-1　水合氯醛分子结构

【实验器材】

1 mL注射器、电子天平。

【实验动物】

小鼠，体重18 ~ 25 g，雌雄不拘。

【实验药品】

0.3%戊巴比妥钠溶液、2.5%水合氯醛溶液、4%水合氯醛溶液、2%苦味酸溶液、生理盐水。

【实验方法】

实验操作步骤如下，见图 1-7-2。

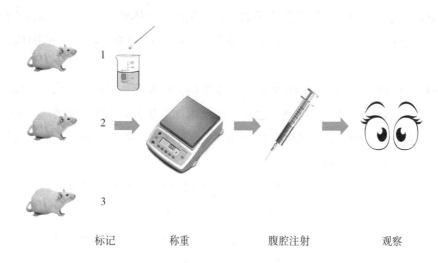

标记　　　　称重　　　　　　腹腔注射　　　　　观察

图 1-7-2　操作步骤示意图

1. 标记、称重　取小鼠 3 只，用苦味酸标记 1、2、3 鼠，观察小鼠的正常活动状态，如呼吸、活动度和运动协调程度。称重，记录体重。

2. 给药　根据小鼠体重计算给药剂量，并记录。鼠 1 腹腔注射生理盐水 0.1 mL/10 g，鼠 2 腹腔注射 2.5% 水合氯醛溶液 0.1 mL/10 g，鼠 3 腹腔注射 4% 水合氯醛溶液 0.1 mL/10 g。仔细观察小鼠给药后的反应，并记录翻正反射消失的时间和翻正反射恢复的时间。若注射药物为 0.3% 戊巴比妥钠溶液，给药方式如下：鼠 1 腹腔注射生理盐水 0.1 mL/10 g，鼠 2 腹腔注射 0.3% 戊巴比妥钠溶液 0.06 mL/10 g，鼠 3 腹腔注射 0.3% 戊巴比妥钠溶液 0.12 mL/10 g。

3. 观察、记录实验结果　仔细观察小鼠给药前后的反应，并如实记录。

【实验记录与结果】

将实验记录和结果填入表格中，具体见表 1-7-1。

表 1-7-1　剂量对药物作用的影响

鼠号	体重（g）	剂量体积（mL）	给药途径	翻正反射消失时间	翻正反射恢复时间
1					
2					
3					

【注意事项】

（1）实验动物的体重应均一，尽量减少误差。

（2）若室温低于 20℃，需给小鼠保暖，否则小鼠会因代谢减慢不易苏醒，影响实验观察。

（3）不同药物使用的注射器及针头应注意区分，每次注射前应将注射器清洗干净，以免影响实验结果。

【练习题】

1. 戊巴比妥钠 _____。

A. 半衰期超过 10 h　　　　　　　　B. 具有药品和毒品双重属性

C. 无须避光保存　　　　　　　　　D. 属于苯二氮卓类镇静催眠药

2. 效能是指 _____。

A. 极量产生的效应　　　　　　　　B. 治疗剂量下产生的效应

C. 最大效应　　　　　　　　　　　D. 药物的效价

3. 下列有关水合氯醛的描述正确的是 _____。

A. 不刺激胃黏膜　　　　　　　　　B. 可转化为作用更强的三氯乙醇

C. 无抗惊厥作用　　　　　　　　　D. 仅用于口服

【思考题】

（1）本实验对于药理学实验和临床用药有何启示？

（2）比较戊巴比妥钠 / 水合氯醛诱导小鼠睡眠的机理有何差异？

【知识拓展】

安乐死与戊巴比妥钠

　　目前世界上只有个别国家对积极的安乐死实行非犯罪化，在我国对安乐死持反对态度，禁止安乐死。国外进行安乐死时，选择口服或注射的药物为戊巴比妥钠。戊巴比妥钠的有效成分是戊巴比妥，戊巴比妥的钠盐形式，在化学上称为戊巴比妥钠。戊巴比妥钠具有麻醉、镇静和催眠作用，属于巴比妥类镇静催眠药。在我国，戊巴比妥为《精神药品品种目录》中列管的第二类精神药品。在国内可以对动物合法地使用安乐死，用高浓度的戊巴比妥钠快速静脉注射即可，若幼小动物静脉

注射困难时，可以用同等剂量施以腹腔注射，小鼠因深麻醉引起意识丧失，呼吸
中枢抑制及呼吸停止，导致心脏停止跳动。

（赵春贞）

第八节　不同给药途径对硫酸镁作用的影响

【实验目的】

观察不同给药途径对硫酸镁作用的影响。

【实验原理】

药物进入人体有多种途径，不同的治疗需求、药物的理化性质和生物学特点、患
者的安全性和依从性等因素决定了采用何种给药方法。

给药途径是影响药物作用的重要因素，不同的给药途径，导致药物的吸收、分布
等的速度也不同，会影响药物作用的强度和速度，甚至改变药物的作用性质。给药途
径不同可直接影响药物效应的快慢和强弱（图1-8-1），依据药效出现时间从快到慢，
顺序依次为：静脉注射、吸入给药、舌下给药、肌内注射、皮下注射、口服、皮肤给药。

本实验采用的硫酸镁在临床上有口服、静脉注射、肌内注射、外敷这四种给药途
径，不同给药途径对应不同的适应证及治疗效果。

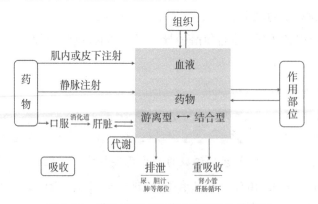

图 1-8-1　药物经不同给药途径在体内的代谢

【实验器材】

1 mL 注射器、电子天平、小鼠灌胃针头。

【实验动物】

小鼠，体重 18 ~ 25 g，体重相近。

【实验药品】

15% 硫酸镁溶液。

【实验方法】

实验操作步骤如下，见图 1-8-2。

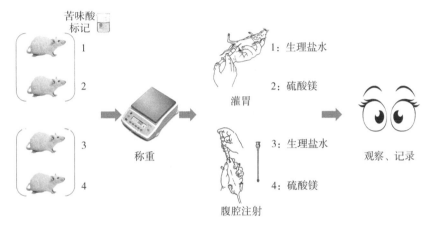

图 1-8-2　操作步骤示意图

1. **标记**　取小鼠 4 只，用苦味酸编号 1、2、3、4 鼠，观察小鼠的正常活动状态，如呼吸、活动度和运动协调程度。

2. **称重**　用电子天平称量体重，记录。

3. **给药**　根据小鼠体重计算给药剂量，并记录。鼠 1 腹腔注射生理盐水 0.2 mL/10 g，鼠 2 腹腔注射 15% 硫酸镁溶液 0.2 mL/10 g，鼠 3 以相同的剂量灌胃生理盐水 0.2 mL/10 g，鼠 4 以相同的剂量灌胃 15% 硫酸镁溶液（0.2 mL/10 g）。

4. **观察、记录**　将小鼠放置于鼠笼中，观察各组小鼠的表现，做好记录。

【实验记录与结果】

将实验记录和结果填入表格中，具体见表 1-8-1。

表 1-8-1 给药途径对硫酸镁作用的影响

鼠号	体重（g）	药物	剂量（mL）	给药途径	给药前表现	给药后表现
1						
2						
3						
4						

【注意事项】

（1）灌胃时注意不要误入气管或插破食管，否则容易出现动物窒息，甚至死亡。

（2）注射药物后作用较快，需留心观察。

（3）灌胃给药前动物一般应进行一段时间的禁食，不禁水。

【练习题】

1. 除血管给药外，吸收速度最快的给药方式是 _____。

A. 吸入   B. 舌下含服

C. 直肠给药   D. 皮下注射

2. 药瓶上要贴有明显的标识，一般口服药瓶外贴 _____。

A. 红色边   B. 黑色边

C. 蓝色边   D. 黄色边

3. 硫酸镁抗惊厥的机制是 _____。

A. 降低血钙的效应

B. 升高血镁的效应

C. 升高血镁和降低血钙的联合效应

D. 竞争性抑制钙作用，减少运动神经末梢释放乙酰胆碱

【思考题】

（1）硫酸镁灌胃给药和腹腔注射给药所产生的效应有何差异？

（2）试分析给药途径不同导致不同的药物作用的机制，这对于临床用药具有什么临床指导意义？

【知识拓展】

小儿热性惊厥知多少？

党的二十大报告指出，把保障人民健康放在优先发展的战略位置，完善人民健康促进政策。儿童是国家的未来、民族的希望，儿童健康是经济社会可持续发展的重要保障。热性惊厥是儿童时期常见的神经系统疾病之一，其发病率在各个国家地区之间有所差别，我国为 5% ~ 6%。热性惊厥首次发作多见于 6 月龄至 5 岁，为发热状态下（肛温 ≥ 38.5℃，腋温 ≥ 38℃）出现的惊厥发作，无中枢神经系统感染证据及导致惊厥的其他原因，无热惊厥病史。部分热性惊厥患儿以惊厥起病，发作前可能未察觉到发热，但发作时或发作后立即出现发热，临床上应注意避免误诊为癫痫首次发作。热性惊厥通常发生于发热后 24 h 内，如发热 > 3 d 才出现惊厥发作，注意寻找其他导致惊厥发作的原因。惊厥发作多为短暂的自限性发作，家长应镇定。然而，目前关于惊厥的共识，尚缺乏针对国内儿童的高质量的临床研究证据，随着各类热性惊厥儿童的临床证据的积累，其预防、诊断和治疗，以及健康教育与长期管理等将更科学化和规范化。

（赵春贞）

第九节　药物体外 IC_{50} 的测定

【实验目的】

（1）学习 MTT 法检测抗肿瘤药物对肿瘤生长抑制 IC_{50} 的检测方法。

（2）了解计算药物体外 IC_{50} 的意义。

【实验原理】

半抑制浓度（50% inhibitory concentration，IC_{50}）指"反应"被抑制 50% 时抑制剂的浓度，这里的反应可以是酶催化反应、抗原抗体反应或肿瘤细胞对抗肿瘤药物的凋亡反应等。在凋亡方面，可以理解为一定浓度的某种药物诱导肿瘤细胞凋亡 50%，该浓度称为 50% 抑制浓度，即凋亡细胞与全部细胞数之比等于 50% 时所对应的浓度。IC_{50} 值可以用来衡量药物诱导凋亡的能力，即诱导能力越强，该数值越低，当然也可以反向说明某种细胞对药物的耐受程度。

MTT（methyl thiazolyl tetrazolium，甲基噻唑基四唑）是一种黄色化合物，能够检测细胞存活和生长，其检测原理为活细胞线粒体中的琥珀酸脱氢酶能将外源性MTT还原为不溶于水的蓝紫色甲䐶结晶沉积在细胞中（图 1-9-1）。甲䐶结晶的生成量与活细胞的数目成正比（死细胞中琥珀酸脱氢酶消失，不能将 MTT 还原）。二甲基亚砜能溶解细胞中的甲䐶，用酶联免疫检测仪在 490 nm 波长处检测其光吸收值，可间接反映活细胞的数量，光吸收值越高，代表活细胞数量越多。

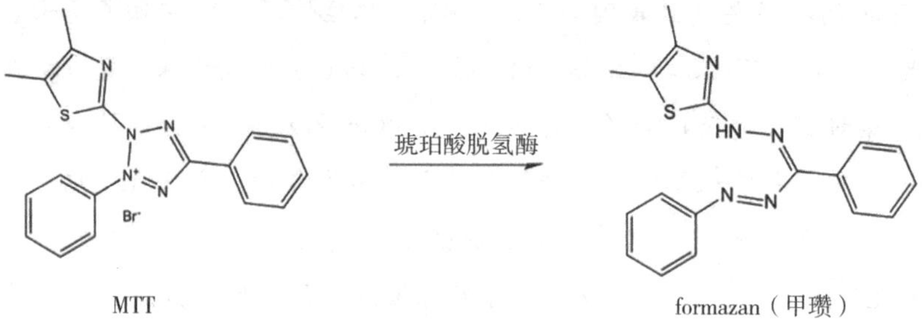

图 1-9-1 MTT 原理图

【实验器材】

二氧化碳细胞培养箱、超净工作台、台式离心机、酶联免疫检测仪、显微镜、25 cm² 无菌培养瓶、无菌 96 孔培养板、微量移液器、无菌枪头（1 mL、200 μL、10 μL）、试管架。

【细胞株】

人非小细胞肺癌细胞株 A549。

【实验药品】

紫杉醇、DMEM 培养基、胎牛血清、胰酶、100 U/mL 青霉素、100 U/mL 链霉素、5 mg/mL MTT 溶液、二甲基亚砜。

【实验方法】

1. **实验前准备** 使用 75% 的乙醇清洁超净台及实验所需的移液器、枪头、试管架、培养瓶及培养板的外包装。打开紫外灭菌灯照射至少 30 min 进行杀菌消毒处理。

2. **细胞培养** A549 细胞是肺癌研究常用的细胞系，具有上皮形态，呈多边形贴壁生长。实验选取指数生长的 A549 细胞，培养于含 10% 胎牛血清的 DMEM 培养基中，培养基中另添加青霉素及链霉素防止细菌感染。当培养瓶中的细胞密度达到 80%～90% 时，使用胰酶消化细胞，使其悬浮，收集细胞悬液，将密度调整至 5×10^4 个 /mL，接种于 96 孔培养板中，每孔体积 100 μL，将培养板培养在含 5% CO_2 的 37℃培养箱内。

3. **药物处理**　待 24 h 细胞完全贴壁后，将细胞进行分组，每组设置 6 个复孔。各组分别加入终浓度为 1nmol/L、2 nmol/L、4 nmol/L、8 nmol/L、16 nmol/L、32 nmol/L、64 nmol/L 的紫杉醇，每孔终体积为 100 μL。阴性对照组加入等量的 DMEM 培养基，将细胞继续培养 48 h。

4. **MTT 检测**　细胞培养 48 h 后，每孔加入 5 mg/mL 的 MTT 20 μL；继续放入培养箱培养 4 h，显微镜下可见紫色结晶沉积于细胞内。小心吸弃孔内的培养基，每孔内加入 100 μL 的二甲基亚砜，摇匀震荡 5 min，使紫色结晶完全溶解。

5. **吸光值检测**　使用酶标仪，波长设置为 490 nm，检测各孔的吸光值。

6. **计算 IC_{50}**　根据吸光值与细胞数量成正比的原理，可以得到不同浓度紫杉醇处理下细胞的相对数量，可以计算得到不同浓度紫杉醇对肺癌细胞生长的抑制率。公式如下：

$$GI（生长抑制率）=［1-（药物组 OD 值 / 阴性对照组 OD 值）］\times 100\%$$

根据各实验组的抑制率使用 SPSS 软件（logit 法）计算得到紫杉醇作用 A549 细胞 48 小时的 IC_{50} 值。

【实验记录与结果】

记录实验结果，根据公式计算出不同浓度紫杉醇对 A549 细胞活力的抑制率。具体见表 1-9-1。依据抑制率，计算出紫杉醇作用 A549 细胞 48 小时的 IC_{50} 值并作图。

表 1-9-1　不同浓度紫杉醇对 A549 细胞活力的抑制率

组别	阴性对照	1 nmol/L 紫杉醇	2 nmol/L 紫杉醇	4 nmol/L 紫杉醇	8 nmol/L 紫杉醇	16 nmol/L 紫杉醇	32 nmol/L 紫杉醇	64 nmol/L 紫杉醇
抑制率								

【注意事项】

（1）细胞培养时应注意无菌操作，细菌感染会影响细胞生长。

（2）加入药物的剂量应准确。

（3）MTT 对光敏感，加入 MTT 时应注意避光操作。

（4）MTT 试剂和二甲基亚砜试剂具有毒性，操作时请注意佩戴手套。

【练习题】

1. 紫杉醇抗癌作用机制为 _____。

A. 影响蛋白质的合成和功能   B. 直接破坏 DNA 结构

C. 干扰核酸生物合成   D. 干扰生物碱合成

2. 紫杉醇在细胞内的作用位点是 _____。

A. 微管   B. 线粒体   C. 细胞核   D. 端粒

【思考题】

药物的 IC_{50} 值是固定不变的吗？对临床用药有何指导意义？

【知识拓展】

紫杉醇的发现

紫杉醇是全球销量第一的天然抗肿瘤药物，具有高效、低毒、广谱等优点，来源于珍稀濒危裸子植物红豆杉。最早是从短叶红豆杉树皮中分离出来的，1971年通过 X 射线衍射和核磁共振确认其分子结构。但是紫杉醇的提取产率非常低，仅有 0.004%，同时珍稀保护植物短叶红豆杉数量稀少，生长缓慢，这大大地限制了紫杉醇的应用。2024 年 1 月，中国农业科学院深圳农业基因组研究所的研究团队，成功鉴定了紫杉醇生物合成途径中的关键缺失酶，揭示了植物细胞中氧杂环丁烷结构形成的全新机制，并建立了迄今为止最短的紫杉醇生物合成途径。这项研究标志着我国在紫杉醇合成生物学理论和技术上达到世界领先水平，代表着我国一批中青年科学家在合成生物学领域探索奋斗近二十年所达到的里程碑式的新高度。

（王琳琳）

第二章　传出神经系统药理

第一节　乙酰胆碱的量效关系实验

【实验目的】

（1）理解乙酰胆碱的量效关系。

（2）熟悉量效关系实验方法和量效曲线的绘制。

视频 2

【实验原理】

药理效应与剂量在一定范围内成比例，这就是剂量 - 效应关系（dose-effect relationship）。以效应强弱为纵坐标、药物剂量或浓度为横坐标作图得量 - 效曲线为直方双曲线。如将药物浓度改用对数值作图则呈典型的对称 S 形曲线，这就是我们通常所讲的量反应的量 - 效曲线。

乙酰胆碱作用于骨骼肌引起肌肉收缩，且在一定剂量范围内，药理效应与剂量成正相关。以乙酰胆碱浓度的对数值为横坐标，肌肉收缩效应为纵坐标作图，可获得 S 型量 - 效曲线。

【实验器材】

手术器械 1 套、蛙板、探针、缝合线、1 mL 注射器、平滑肌浴皿、通气钩、肌力换能器、空气球胆、BL-422 生物机能实验系统。

【实验标本】

蟾蜍离体腹直肌。

【实验药品】

乙酰胆碱溶液、任氏液。

【实验方法】

实验主要操作步骤如下，见图 2-1-1。

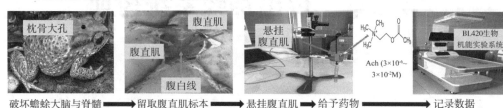

破坏蟾蜍大脑与脊髓 ➡ 留取腹直肌标本 ➡ 悬挂腹直肌 ➡ 给予药物 ➡ 记录数据

图 2-1-1　操作步骤示意图

1. 仪器准备　刷洗平滑肌浴皿，给空气球胆通气，打开 BL-422 生物机能实验系统软件并设置相关参数。

2. 制备离体腹直肌标本　用探针破坏蟾蜍大脑与脊髓，仰卧位固定于蛙板上。剪开腹部皮肤，暴露腹直肌，在腹白线一侧的耻骨端及胸骨端剥离一段长 2 ~ 3 cm、宽 0.5 ~ 0.8 cm 的腹直肌，两端用缝合线结扎后剪下。注意不可过度牵拉腹直肌。

3. 悬挂腹直肌　将腹直肌一端固定在通气钩上，浸入含 30 mL 任氏液的平滑肌浴皿中（调整线的长度，腹直肌完全浸入任氏液），并向任氏液中通入空气；另一端连接肌力换能器及 BL-422 生物机能实验系统。

4. 给药观察　腹直肌在平滑肌浴皿中稳定 10 min，描记其正常收缩曲线并记录此时的肌肉张力值，即可按表 2-1-1 所示剂量（浓度）依次加入乙酰胆碱溶液进行实验。采用累积给药法，按低浓度→高浓度加入乙酰胆碱溶液。信号记录速度要慢，每次加药后 2 ~ 3 min，待肌肉收缩反应不再继续增大，记录此张力值，再加入下一个剂量，依次进行直到出现最大效应并记录此时的张力值。

5. 计算数值　各剂量效应百分率＝各剂量的效应／最大效应 ×100%。

6. 绘制量效曲线　手绘或计算机自动绘图。

【实验记录与结果】

记录各剂量效应并计算效应反应百分率，见表 2-1-1。以反应百分率为纵坐标，以乙酰胆碱剂量的对数值为横坐标，绘制量效曲线。

【注意事项】

（1）实验前、后必须充分洗净浴皿。

（2）通入空气 1 ~ 2 气泡 /s。

（3）任氏液应保持在 26±0.5℃。

（4）离体腹直肌标本与换能器的连线不要触及浴皿管壁。

（5）每次加药剂量要准确，加药时勿滴在线及浴皿管壁上，否则影响实验结果。

表 2-1-1　乙酰胆碱溶液剂量与效应

原始记录				整理后记录	
Ach（M）	用量（mL）	浴槽浓度	效应（g）	LgC	效应（g）
3×10^{-6}	0.1	1×10^{-8}		-8	
	0.2	3×10^{-8}		-7.5	
3×10^{-5}	0.1	1×10^{-7}		-7	
	0.2	3×10^{-7}		-6.5	
3×10^{-4}	0.1	1×10^{-6}		-6	
	0.2	3×10^{-6}		-5.5	
3×10^{-3}	0.1	1×10^{-5}		-5	
	0.2	3×10^{-5}		-4.5	
3×10^{-2}	0.1	1×10^{-4}		-4	
	0.2	3×10^{-4}		-3.5	

【练习题】

1. 乙酰胆碱激动的受体类型包括 _____。

A. α 受体　　　　　　　　　　　　B. $β_1$ 受体

C. M、N 受体　　　　　　　　　　D. α、β 受体

2. 下列关于量效曲线的意义，不正确的是 _____。

A. 比较药效强弱　　　　　　　　　B. 反映药物的吸收范围

C. 提供临床用药剂量的参考值　　　D. 评价药物安全性

3. 从量反应的量效曲线，无法观察到的参数是 _____。

A. 最小有效剂量　　　　　　　　　B. 最大效应

C. 效价强度　　　　　　　　　　　D. 半数致死量

【思考题】

（1）根据实验结果，分析药物的剂量和效应间的关系，这种量效关系有何规律？说明药物应用过程中应注意哪些问题？

（2）量效曲线与药物受体间的亲和力和内在活性有什么关系，如何从量效曲线

比较药物与受体的内在活性和亲和力？

【知识拓展】

乙酰胆碱的发现

乙酰胆碱是人类发现的第一个神经递质，作用部位为全部交感神经和副交感神经的节前纤维，运动神经、全部副交感神经的节后纤维和极少数交感神经的节后纤维。乙酰胆碱具有舒张血管、减弱心肌收缩力、兴奋胃肠道平滑肌、引起骨骼肌收缩等作用。

乙酰胆碱的发现可追溯到德国科学家Otto Loewi开展的经典双蛙心灌流实验。通过该实验，Loewi推测迷走神经兴奋时会释放某种化学物质，这种物质通过液体传递，能够影响另一只青蛙的心脏活动。Loewi在1926年初步将这种化学物质确定为乙酰胆碱。随后的研究，特别是1930年，英国科学家Dale进一步确认了这一化学物质，将这一物质正式命名为乙酰胆碱，并和Loewi共同获得了1936年的诺贝尔生理学或医学奖。我国现代生理学主要奠基者人张锡钧教授首次在哺乳动物的脾脏中测得乙酰胆碱结晶，为研究乙酰胆碱的生理机制开辟了途径。乙酰胆碱的发现进一步揭开了神经递质的神秘面纱，它的发现告诉我们只要孜孜不倦地思考和探求，成功就会属于我们。

（潘瑞艳）

第二节　传出神经系统药物对离体肠管平滑肌的作用

【实验目的】

（1）了解乙酰胆碱对肠道平滑肌M胆碱受体的激动作用，以及它们的受体阻断药阿托品的阻断作用。

（2）学习离体小肠平滑肌的制备。

【实验原理】

消化道平滑肌与骨骼肌、心肌一样，具有肌肉组织共有的特性，如兴奋性、传导性和收缩性等。但消化道平滑肌兴奋性较低，收缩缓慢，富有伸展性，具有紧张性、自动节律性，对化学、温度和机械牵张刺激较敏感等特点。给予离体肠肌接近于在体内情况的适宜环境，消化道平滑肌仍可保持良好的生理特性。

胃肠道、膀胱等平滑肌以胆碱能神经占优势，小剂量或低浓度的乙酰胆碱能激动M胆碱受体，产生与兴奋胆碱能神经节后纤维相似的作用，兴奋胃肠道平滑肌。阿托品与胆碱受体结合而本身不产生或较少产生拟胆碱作用，却能阻断胆碱能递质或拟胆碱药物与受体的结合，从而产生抗胆碱作用。

【实验器材】

麦式浴槽、张力换能器、BL-422 生物机能实验系统、HW-200S 离体肠管及热板试验恒温装置、空气球胆、培养皿、1 mL 注射器、手术器械一套、缝合线、木槌。

【实验动物】

豚鼠，体重 200 ~ 250 g，雌雄不限。

【实验药品】

10^{-2} g/L 乙酰胆碱溶液、1 g/L 阿托品溶液、台式液。

【实验方法】

实验主要操作步骤如下，见图 2-2-1。

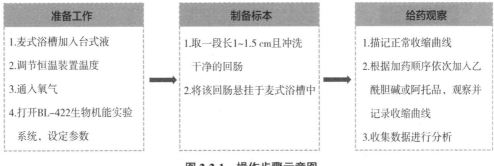

准备工作	制备标本	给药观察
1.麦式浴槽加入台式液	1.取一段长1~1.5 cm且冲洗干净的回肠	1.描记正常收缩曲线
2.调节恒温装置温度	2.将该回肠悬挂于麦式浴槽中	2.根据加药顺序依次加入乙酰胆碱或阿托品，观察并记录收缩曲线
3.通入氧气		3.收集数据进行分析
4.打开BL-422生物机能实验系统，设定参数		

图 2-2-1 操作步骤示意图

1. 准备工作 麦氏浴槽中加固定量的台氏液，调节 HW-200S 离体肠管及热板试验恒温装置的温度，使麦氏浴槽内温度稳定在 37 ± 0.5℃。充入氧气，用螺丝夹调节气体管道的气体流量，调节至浴槽中气泡一个个逸出为止。张力换能器固定于铁支柱上，换能器输出线接计算机生物信号处理系统。打开 BL-422 生物机能实验系统，设定实验相关参数。

2. 制备标本

（1）取豚鼠一只，用木槌猛击其后枕部致死，立即剖开腹腔，找到回盲部，在离回盲部 1 cm 处剪断，取出回肠（约 10 cm）一段，置于盛有预热台氏液的培养皿中，并持续通氧。沿肠壁分离掉肠系膜，用台氏液将肠内容物冲洗干净，然后将回肠剪成数小段（每段 1 ~ 1.5 cm），换以新鲜台氏液备用。注意操作时勿牵拉肠段以免影响收缩功能。

（2）取上述处理好的回肠一段，在其两端对角壁处，分别用缝针穿线，并打结。注意保持肠管通畅，勿使其封闭。肠管一端连线系于浴槽固定钩上，然后放入 37 ℃ 麦氏浴槽中，肠管的另一端系于张力换能器的悬臂梁上，调节肌张力至 2 g。

3. 给药观察

待离体回肠稳定 10 min 后，记录一段正常收缩曲线后，再依次向麦氏浴槽中滴加下列药物。加入一种药液后，待药物与肠管接触 2 ~ 3 min，观察记录其肠管收缩幅度变化，然后用台氏液连续冲洗三次，待基线恢复到用药前的水平，随后记录一段基线，再加入第二种药液。注意浴槽液体的容量应相等。

（1）加入 10^{-2} g/L 乙酰胆碱 0.2 mL，观察并记录其收缩曲线，换液。

（2）加入 10^{-2} g/L 乙酰胆碱 0.2 mL，待作用明显或收缩达最高点时，加入 1 g/L 阿托品 0.2 mL，观察收缩曲线，此时不换液，待曲线降至基线或基本稳定后，再加入相同量的乙酰胆碱，观察并记录其收缩曲线。

【实验记录与结果】

将实验结果记录于实验报告纸上，作好给药标记，供分析。

【注意事项】

（1）动物在实验前 24 h 禁食，不禁水，以保持肠道无粪便。

（2）制作离体肠管标本时动作要轻柔敏捷，避免反复牵拉。

（3）向麦式浴槽内加药时，不要触碰连接线，也不要把药滴到管壁上。

（4）肠管与换能器连线不宜太紧，也不能与管壁接触。

（5）整个实验过程中，注意持续供氧、保持温度恒定。

【练习题】

1. 阿托品对以下哪种平滑肌作用最强？

A. 胃肠道平滑肌　　　　　　　　　　B. 支气管平滑肌

C. 胆道平滑肌　　　　　　　　　　　D. 子宫平滑肌

2. 肌注阿托品治疗肠绞痛，引起口干作用称为 _____。

A. 治疗作用 B. 变态反应

C. 副作用 D. 后遗效应

3. 治疗量的阿托品能引起 _____。

A. 胃肠平滑肌痉挛 B. 中枢抑制

C. 唾液腺分泌减少 D. 瞳孔散大，眼内压降低

【思考题】

（1）胃肠道平滑肌上存在哪些受体？激动、阻断它们分别产生什么效应？

（2）阿托品对不同内脏平滑肌的作用有何不同？

【知识拓展】

阿托品药物发现及作用

　　阿托品是一种 M 受体阻断剂，是从茄科植物颠茄、曼陀罗、洋金花或莨菪等提取的一种白色结晶状的消旋莨菪碱，目前也可人工合成。阿托品的发现可追溯到公元前 4 世纪，古希腊科学家泰奥弗拉斯曾记录曼陀罗可以治疗疼痛、痛风、失眠。德国化学家费迪南德伦哥首先研究了阿托品的散瞳效用。1831 年，德国药剂师梅因成功从植物中提纯得到有毒的阿托品纯结晶，直到 1894 年，德国有机化学家理查德·威尔斯特阐明了阿托品的化学结构，并在 1901 年首次人工合成了阿托品。阿托品除了具有抑制胃肠道平滑肌痉挛外，还具有抗心律失常、抑制腺体分泌、扩瞳、升高眼内压、抗休克、抢救急性有机磷农药中毒等作用，是临床常用的药物之一。

（潘瑞艳）

第三节　传出神经药物对家兔瞳孔的影响

【实验目的】

（1）观察抗胆碱药（阿托品）及拟肾上腺素药（去氧肾上腺素）对家兔瞳孔的作用并分析其作用机制。

（2）学习家兔滴眼及瞳孔测量方法。

视频 3

【实验原理】

视觉是人们从外部世界获得信息的最主要的途径，眼是引起视觉的外周感觉器官，包括眼球、视路和眼附属器。眼球由眼球壁及内容物组成，其中眼球壁包括外膜、中膜和内膜三层。虹膜是中膜的最前部，为圆盘状薄膜，中央有圆孔，称为瞳孔，瞳孔的功能包括调节到达视网膜的光线数量、减少角膜和晶状体光学系统周围性不完整引起的色差和球差、增加视野等。正常人眼的瞳孔直径在 1.5 ~ 8.0 mm 之间，瞳孔的大小与视觉质量密切相关。瞳孔在强光照射时缩小而在光线变弱时散大的反射，称为瞳孔的对光反射。它是眼的一种适应功能，其意义在于调节进入眼内的光线量，避免视网膜因光量过强而受到损伤，也不会因光线过弱而影响视觉。

瞳孔的大小受瞳孔括约肌和瞳孔开大肌的双重影响，瞳孔括约肌上主要分布有胆碱能 M 受体，瞳孔开大肌上主要分布有肾上腺素能 α 受体。胆碱受体激动药滴眼后可激动瞳孔括约肌上 M 受体使瞳孔缩小；M 胆碱受体阻断药滴眼后可阻断瞳孔括约肌上 M 受体，致瞳孔括约肌松弛，而肾上腺素能神经支配的瞳孔开大肌功能占优，导致瞳孔扩大。去氧肾上腺素滴眼后可直接激动瞳孔开大肌上 α 受体，使瞳孔扩大（图 2-3-1）。

对光反射的过程是当强（或弱）光照射视网膜时产生的冲动沿视神经传到中脑的顶盖前区更换神经元，然后到达双侧的动眼神经缩瞳核，再沿动眼神经中的副交感纤维传向睫状神经节，最后经睫状神经支配瞳孔括约肌，使瞳孔缩小（或扩大）。瞳孔对光反射的中枢位于中脑，在临床上常将对光反射用作判断麻醉深度和病情危重程度的一个指标。此外，临床利用它评价视网膜、视神经和随之的前视路的视觉传入性输入，有助于视觉传出系统疾病的诊断和监测。

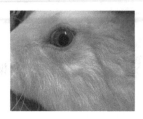
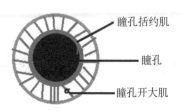

瞳孔括约肌

瞳孔

瞳孔开大肌

图 2-3-1 家兔瞳孔及瞳孔大小调节示意图

【实验器材】

手术剪、滴管、兔箱、直尺、手电筒。

【实验动物】

家兔。

【实验药品】

1% 硫酸阿托品溶液、1% 盐酸去氧肾上腺素。

【实验方法】

（1）取健康家兔 1 只，标记后放入兔固定箱内，剪去眼睫毛，在自然光线下测量并记录两侧正常瞳孔直径（mm）及对光反射，然后按下列顺序给药各 4 ~ 5 滴：①左眼 1% 硫酸阿托品；②右眼 1% 去氧肾上腺素。

滴药时将下眼睑拉成杯状，并用手指按住鼻泪管，使药物在眼睑内保留 1 min，然后将手轻轻放开，任其自然溢出。

（2）滴药 15 min 后，在同样强度的光线下，再分别测量并记录各眼瞳孔大小和对光反射。

【实验记录与结果】

记录实验结果，将实验结果整理记入表 2-3-1 内。

表 2-3-1 传出神经药物对家兔瞳孔的影响

眼	药物	瞳孔直径（mm）		对光反射	
		用药前	用药后	用药前	用药后
左	硫酸阿托品				
右	去氧肾上腺素				

【注意事项】

（1）测量瞳孔勿刺激角膜，否则会影响瞳孔大小。

（2）滴药时应按压内眦部的鼻泪管，以防药液进入鼻腔，经鼻黏膜吸收。

（3）各眼滴药量要准确，在眼内停留时间要一致，以确保药液充分作用。

（4）测量瞳孔条件务求给药前后一致，如光线的强度、光源的角度等。

（5）观察对光反射时周围环境光线不能太强也不能太弱。

【练习题】

1. 测量瞳孔时，以下说法错误的是 _____。

A. 测量前需剪去睫毛

B. 测量时直尺要紧贴家兔角膜

C. 给药前后的光线强度要相同

D. 给药前后的光源角度要一致

2. 滴眼后，按压家兔鼻泪管的目的是 _____。

A. 防止药物经鼻泪管吸收　　　　　　B. 减少药物对瞳孔的刺激

C. 增加角膜对药物的吸收　　　　　　D. 增加房水的生成

3. 阿托品对眼睛的药理作用不包括 _____。

A. 扩瞳　　　　　B. 调节痉挛　　　　　C. 升高眼内压　　　　　D. 调节麻痹

【思考题】

（1）什么是瞳孔对光反射？临床检测患者的对光反射有什么意义？

（2）试述本实验用药对瞳孔的影响是什么？有什么临床应用？

（3）青光眼可以用哪些药物进行治疗？

【知识拓展】

慎用低浓度阿托品滴眼液

2024 年 3 月 5 日，国家市场监督管理总局批准 0.01% 硫酸阿托品滴眼液上市，用于缓解 6 ~ 12 岁青少年近视加深。该药是国内首款批准上市用于延缓儿童近视进展的药物。

阿托品是 M 胆碱受体阻断药，能阻断 ACh 或胆碱受体激动药与受体结合，拮抗其对 M 受体的激动效应。阿托品能阻断瞳孔括约肌上的 M 受体，导致瞳孔括约肌松弛，使肾上腺素能神经支配的瞳孔开大肌功能占优势，瞳孔扩大。同时由于瞳孔扩大，虹膜退向四周边缘，阻碍了房水的回流，导致眼内压升高。此外，还能阻断睫状肌的 M 受体，使晶状体呈扁平状态，屈光度下降，导致看近物模糊，视远物清晰（即调节麻痹）。早期研究发现，高浓度阿托品能明显抑制眼球前后径的增长，减慢近视度数的加深，其对近视的控制效率在 60% ~ 96%。但高浓度阿托品又会导致畏光、面部发红、心跳加快、视力下降等不良反应及停药后反弹效应。临床研究发现，0.01%硫酸阿托品（低浓度）具有明显延缓近视进展的效果，其近视防控效率在27%～83%，且具有累积效应，但是尚未发现其严重的全身不良反应，具有较小的不良反应和停药后反弹效应。但是，该药既不能预防近视，更不能治疗近视，只是延缓儿童近视进展，且不同个体的控制效果也不同。因此，青少年儿童近视防控，还应从用眼卫生习惯和生活学习环境等方面加以重视。

（李成檀）

第四节　阿托品对小鼠平滑肌的抑制作用

【实验目的】

（1）观察阿托品对小鼠平滑肌蠕动的抑制作用。

（2）了解胃肠道平滑肌运动的神经调节机制。

【实验原理】

肠道是人体消化系统中重要的组成部分，指胃幽门至肛门的消化管道，是消化系统中最长的一段，也是功能最重要的一段。哺乳动物的消化道包括小肠和大肠。小肠盘曲于腹腔内，上连胃幽门，下接盲肠；盲肠呈囊袋状，属于大肠始端；盲肠后至肛门部分为大肠。肠道外包裹肠系膜，起到悬吊、固定肠管的作用。小肠壁厚度较薄，表面光滑（图2-4-1）。

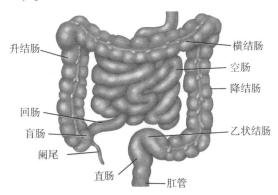

图 2-4-1　肠道结构示意图

消化道平滑肌具有肌肉组织的共同特点，具有兴奋性、传导性和收缩性，还具有自身的功能特点如兴奋性较低、收缩缓慢、拥有自动节律性，具有一定的紧张性和较大的伸展性，并能产生推进性运动。肠道平滑肌对电刺激、切割和灼烧不敏感，但对机械牵张、温度变化和化学刺激特别敏感，其活动还受神经、体液因素的调节。消化道平滑肌受副交感神经和交感神经双重支配：副交感神经兴奋时，其末梢释放的神经递质乙酰胆碱作用于平滑肌上的 M 受体产生兴奋效应，引起肠肌收缩；交感神经兴奋时，绝大多数节后纤维释放去甲肾上腺素，与平滑肌细胞膜上 α、β 受体结合，产生抑制作用，使胃肠运动减弱。某些药物如肾上腺素、新斯的明、阿托品等可以改变消化道平滑肌的收缩活动，表现为收缩的节律、强度、速度及紧张性收缩等方面的改变。

阿托品（atropine）是乙酰胆碱 M 受体阻断药，能结合 M 胆碱受体从而竞争性拮抗 ACh 的作用。受到阿托品抑制后，胃肠道平滑肌变松弛，蠕动的幅度和频率降低。因此阿托品在解除胃肠道平滑肌痉挛和缓解胃肠绞痛疗效显著。除了用于各种内脏绞痛外，大剂量阿托品可解除小血管痉挛，改善微循环，同时抑制腺体分泌，解除迷走神经对心脏的抑制，使心搏加快，瞳孔散大、眼压升高，兴奋呼吸中枢，解除呼吸抑制，也可用于窦性心动过缓、房室传导阻滞等心律失常，感染性休克及有机磷中毒解救。

【实验器材】

电子天平、烧杯、注射器（1 mL）、鼠笼、蛙板、手术剪、镊子、直尺。

【实验动物】

小鼠 2 只（18 ~ 22 g），雌雄不限。

【实验药品】

0.05% 硫酸阿托品溶液、生理盐水、墨汁。

【实验方法】

实验操作步骤如下，见图 2-4-2。

1. **饥饿处理**　取体重相近的小鼠 2 只，称重后用苦味酸标记编号，禁食不禁水 12 ~ 24 h。

2. **灌胃给药**　对已饥饿处理的小鼠给药，甲鼠以 0.05% 硫酸阿托品溶液 0.1 mL/ 10 g（剂量 5 mg/kg，即 0.05 mg/10 g）灌胃，乙鼠以 0.2 mL 生理盐水灌胃。

3. **灌墨汁**　15 min 后，甲、乙两鼠各给予 0.2 mL 墨汁灌胃。

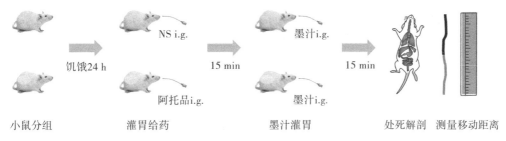

图 2-4-2 操作步骤示意图

4. **解剖** 经 15 min 后，分别将两鼠以颈椎脱臼法处死，立即剖腹。将小肠一端从胃幽门处切除，另一端从盲肠切除，分离出完整小肠放置于蛙板上，用少量生理盐水浸润。用镊子和手术剪剥离肠系膜，将肠管不加牵拉地轻轻平铺在蛙板上呈直线。

5. **测量墨汁移动距离** 以胃幽门为起点，盲肠端为终点，用直尺测量小肠全长并记录。同时测量自幽门开始，墨汁在肠管内移动的距离。

6. **计算胃肠推进率** 以墨汁流动距离除以小肠总长度 ×100%，计算小鼠体内墨汁移动距离占小肠全长的百分率为胃肠推进率。

【实验记录与结果】

记录实验结果，根据公式计算出墨汁在不同小鼠肠道内的推进率，具体见表 2-4-1。

表 2-4-1 阿托品对小鼠平滑肌的抑制作用

编号	体重（g）	药物	给药体积（mL）	小肠总长度（cm）	墨汁流动距离（cm）	胃肠推进率（%）
甲		硫酸阿托品				
乙		生理盐水				

【注意事项】

（1）墨汁灌胃体积必须准确。

（2）灌墨和处死的时间间隔必须准确。

（3）本试验中墨汁可改用 1% 卡红溶液。

（4）在取出胃肠道或测量小肠时，要避免牵拉肠管，以免影响测量长度的准确性。取出肠道后要保持湿润，可以加一些生理盐水，以免肠道与实验台粘连。

【练习题】

1. 新斯的明对肠道平滑肌运动的作用应该是 _____。

A.增强运动　　　　　B.减弱运动　　　　　C.无作用　　　　　D.引起痉挛

2. 对实验小鼠进行饥饿处理的目的是 _____ 。

A.增强消化道蠕动　　　　　　　　B.使小鼠丧失力气

C.排空肠道　　　　　　　　　　　D.增强药效

3. 下列哪项不属于阿托品的临床应用 _____ 。

A.解救有机磷酸酯类中毒　　　　　B.治疗晕动病

C.解除内脏痉挛　　　　　　　　　D.眼科散瞳检查

【思考题】

（1）肠道平滑肌上存在哪些受体？其激动后对肠平滑肌的运动产生何种影响？

（2）新斯的明对肠平滑肌的作用如何？与乙酰胆碱比较有何差异？

（3）肾上腺素对肠平滑肌活动有何影响？普萘洛尔和酚妥拉明对肾上腺素所致的小肠平滑肌收缩变化有何影响？为什么？

【知识拓展】

中国的抗胆碱药 "654-2"

　　654-2 为消旋山莨菪碱，与阿托品作用机制相似属于抗胆碱药，具有明显的外周抗胆碱作用。山莨菪碱是我国科学家首先从茄科植物山莨菪（Anisodus tanguticus）中提取的生物碱，而这一成果完成于 1965 年 4 月，故代号为 654。山莨菪是我国特有植物，别名樟柳、唐川那保、唐古特莨菪等，主要分布于甘肃、云南、青海等地，其天然品名称为 "654-1"，为右旋体；而用人工合成方法制得的产品为消旋体，称为 "654-2"。两者作用机制相同，而后者产生的效力更高，目前广泛用于临床。654-2 能解除乙酰胆碱所致平滑肌痉挛，对胃肠道平滑肌有松弛作用，并抑制其蠕动，作用较阿托品稍弱。还能解除微血管痉挛，改善微循环，其抑制唾液腺分泌及扩瞳作用较弱，为阿托品的 1/20 ～ 1/10。因不易通过血 - 脑脊液屏障，故中枢作用亦弱于阿托品，很少引起中枢兴奋症状。临床上多用于解痉止痛治疗，适应证包括感染中毒性休克、平滑肌痉挛、血管痉挛和栓塞引起的循环障碍、眼底疾病、各种神经痛、有机磷中毒、突发性耳聋、眩晕病等疾病。

（童骏森）

第五节 有机磷农药的中毒及解救

【实验目的】

（1）观察有机磷农药中毒时出现的 M 样症状、N 样症状及中枢症状。

（2）观察 M 受体阻断剂阿托品对 M 样症状的缓解作用及胆碱酯酶复活药解磷定对 N 样症状和中枢症状的缓解作用。

视频 4

【实验原理】

有机磷农药是一类不可逆的胆碱酯酶抑制剂，其脂溶性高，易经消化道、呼吸道甚至皮肤吸收引起中毒。有机磷农药中所含的磷酰基能够与胆碱酯酶（acetylcholinesterase，AChE）发生不可逆的结合，生成磷酰化 AChE，使 AChE 失去水解乙酰胆碱（acetylcholine，ACh）的活性，造成 ACh 在突触间隙或神经肌接头处大量积聚，引起胆碱样中毒症状（图 2-5-1）。有机磷农药中毒后可表现为 M 受体的激动效应（如心脏抑制、浅表腺分泌增加、内脏平滑肌收缩痉挛等）及 N 受体的激动效应（如肌张力增加甚至出现肌震颤），重度中毒时还会表现为中枢先兴奋后抑制的毒性反应。

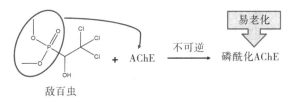

图 2-5-1 有机磷农药中毒机制

M 受体阻断剂阿托品能够选择性地阻断胆碱能 M 受体，有效地解除 M 样中毒症状；胆碱酯酶复活药解磷定（pralidoxime，PAM）能够与磷酰化 AChE 争夺磷酰基，生成磷酰化 PAM 并复活 AChE，快速解除有机磷酸酯类农药急性中毒时的肌肉震颤症状和中枢症状（图 2-5-2）。

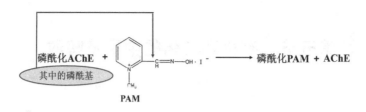

图 2-5-2　解磷定复活胆碱酯酶机制

【实验器材】

兔固定器、磅秤、注射器（1 mL、2.5 mL、5 mL、10 mL）、测瞳尺。

【实验动物】

家兔，体重 1.5 ~ 2.5 kg，雌雄不拘。

【实验药品】

5% 精制敌百虫溶液、0.2% 硫酸阿托品溶液、2.5% 碘解磷定溶液。

【实验方法】

1. **实验准备**　取家兔 1 只，称重并记录，根据体重计算给药剂量，取药备用。

2. **给药前观察**　将家兔置于实验台上，观察其活动、呼吸、唾液分泌、大小便及肌张力等情况，并用测瞳尺测量其瞳孔直径。

3. **给予有机磷农药观察中毒症状**　腹腔注射给予家兔 5% 精制敌百虫溶液 4 mL/kg，随后密切观察家兔的活动、呼吸、唾液分泌、大小便、瞳孔大小及肌张力（有无肌震颤）等指标变化，并注意观察家兔有无惊厥表现。同时，按家兔体重将解救药物抽好备用。

4. **给予阿托品观察 M 样症状的缓解**　在观察到家兔中毒的明显症状（瞳孔缩至绿豆大小、肌震颤明显）后，立即耳缘静脉注射 0.2% 硫酸阿托品溶液 1 mL/kg，随后密切观察家兔各项中毒症状的变化（注意观察哪些症状得到缓解，哪些症状还未缓解）。

5. **给予解磷定观察 N 样症状和中枢症状的缓解**　待家兔的 M 样症状缓解（瞳孔基本恢复至中毒前）后，继续耳缘静脉注射 2.5% 碘解磷定溶液 2 mL/kg，随后密切观察家兔各项中毒症状的变化（给予阿托品后未缓解的症状是否得到缓解）。

【实验记录与结果】

在表格中记录给药前后的家兔各项指标变化。具体见表 2-5-1。

表 2-5-1 有机磷农药的中毒及解救情况观察

	活动情况	呼吸情况	瞳孔大小	唾液分泌	大小便	肌张力	有无肌震颤	有无惊厥
给药前								
给敌百虫后								
给阿托品后								
给解磷定后								

【注意事项】

（1）给予家兔敌百虫溶液后应密切观察各中毒症状变化，如果家兔出现明显的肌震颤或中枢兴奋的症状，即使此时 M 样症状还未达到重度中毒的标准，也应立即耳缘静脉注射阿托品溶液进行解救，否则易致家兔死亡。

（2）敌百虫溶液为有机磷农药，有剧毒，抽取及使用时应注意防护。如皮肤接触到敌百虫溶液，不能用碱性物清洗。

（3）给敌百虫前后及解救后的瞳孔测量须在同侧同方位进行，以免不同侧眼睛及不同光线对瞳孔自身调节的影响造成实验误差。

（4）如腹腔注射敌百虫经 15 ~ 20 min 尚未出现明显中毒症状，可追加 1/3 量。

【练习题】

1. 患者呼吸中有何种气味时考虑有机磷农药中毒？

A. 烂苹果气味　　　　B. 大蒜味　　　　　C. 氨味　　　　　　D. 腥味

2. 有机磷农药中毒的症状不包括 _____。

A. 视物模糊　　　　　　　　　　　B. 大小便失禁

C. 呼吸频率减慢　　　　　　　　　D. 多汗、流涎

3. 有机磷农药中毒时的烟碱样症状是 _____。

A. 多汗　　　　　　B. 流涎　　　　　　C. 恶心呕吐　　　　D. 肌震颤

【思考题】

（1）有机磷农药中毒时为何需及时解救？

（2）阿托品和解磷定在临床上用于解救有机磷农药中毒时的使用原则有哪些？为什么？

【知识拓展】

环保的农药

农药品种繁多，按化学结构可分为有机氯、有机磷、有机氮、有机硫、氨基甲酸酯、拟除虫菊酯、酰胺类化合物等。有机氯类杀虫剂氯苯结构稳定，不易为生物所降解，在生物体内消除缓慢；在水中的半衰期可以达到20年之久，在土壤中半衰期大多在1～12年，对生态环境影响显著，早已列为禁用农药。有机磷类杀虫剂在农作物中产生不同程度的残留，各品种的毒性差异大，多数中高毒，少数为低毒，对人体的危害以急性毒性为主，多发生于大剂量或反复接触之后出现一系列神经毒性，如出汗、流涎、视物模糊、震颤、精神错乱、语言失常等，严重者会出现呼吸麻痹，甚至死亡。有机磷类杀虫剂在我国农业上曾经大量使用，但不利于生态文明建设，目前一些品种已经禁用（如对硫磷、甲胺磷、甲基对硫磷、磷胺、久效磷）。拟除虫菊酯类对人类低毒，主要有氯氰菊酯（灭百可）、溴氰菊酯（敌杀死）、杀灭菊酯（速灭杀丁）等，杀虫谱广、效果好，但对水生生物毒性高，不利于生态环境。二酰胺类杀虫剂是最新型的杀虫剂种类，优势突出，对人类高度安全，已成为目前杀虫剂研究开发的热点。杀虫剂的发展是向着高效、低毒、对环境和生态友好的方向，这也符合党中央提出的大力推进生态文明建设的战略决策，反映了党中央关于生态文明建设决策的科学性。

（王舒舒）

第三章　中枢神经系统药理

第一节　药物的镇痛作用实验

【实验目的】

（1）观察哌替啶、罗通定的镇痛效应。

（2）了解常用的镇痛实验方法，掌握扭体法的镇痛实验方法。

视频 5

【实验原理】

疼痛是临床常见的病症之一，是一种因实际或潜在的组织损伤而产生的痛苦感觉。剧烈疼痛不仅给患者带来痛苦和紧张不安等情绪反应，还可引起机体生理功能紊乱，甚至诱发休克。

制作疼痛动物模型的方式包括化学刺激法、机械刺激法、电刺激法等。化学刺激法是通过向动物体内注射或皮下注入化学物质，引起动物的疼痛反应，如向小鼠腹腔注射醋酸溶液或酒石酸锑钾溶液可以引起小鼠扭体反应。机械刺激法指通过施加压力或机械力作用于动物的身体部位引起疼痛反应，例如通过对大鼠尾尖施加一定的压力，使大鼠因疼痛而产生嘶叫反应，以大鼠嘶叫反应发生的压力大小作为疼痛阈值，疼痛阈值越小，药物的产生镇痛作用越弱。电刺激法指通过对动物身体部位进行电刺激而产生疼痛作用，例如通过电刺激大鼠尾部产生疼痛，以大鼠嘶叫反应作为疼痛指标，以大鼠嘶叫反应发生的电刺激大小作为疼痛阈值，疼痛阈值越小，药物的产生镇痛作用越弱。另外，疼痛模型的构建方法还有热板法，通过将小鼠置于热板之上，以小鼠出现跳跃或舔爪的行为对应的热板温度作为疼痛阈值，疼痛阈值越小，药物的产生镇痛作用越弱。

本次实验采取的实验方法为扭体法。小鼠腹膜有广泛的感觉神经分布，把冰醋酸注入腹腔，可使小鼠很快产生疼痛反应，表现为腹部内凹、躯干和后腿伸张，臀部高起，称为扭体反应。通常以扭体反应发生的次数作为疼痛指标，扭体反应发生次数越多，表示小鼠感受的疼痛越强。

【实验器材】

1 mL 注射器、鼠笼、电子天平。

【实验动物】

小鼠，体重 18 ~ 22 g，雌雄不拘。

【实验药品】

0.6% 冰醋酸溶液、生理盐水、0.2% 哌替啶溶液、0.2% 罗通定溶液、苦味酸溶液。

【实验方法】

实验操作步骤如下，见图 3-1-1。

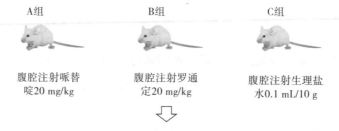

A组	B组	C组
腹腔注射哌替啶20 mg/kg	腹腔注射罗通定20 mg/kg	腹腔注射生理盐水0.1 mL/10 g

30 min后，各组小鼠同时腹腔注射冰醋酸0.2 mL/只

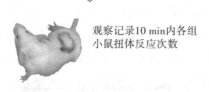

观察记录10 min内各组小鼠扭体反应次数

图 3-1-1　操作步骤示意图

1. **小鼠称量、标记**　取体重为 18 ~ 22 g 的健康小鼠 3 只，随机分为 3 组。称重，并记录体重，使用苦味酸进行标记。

2. **给药**　A 组小鼠腹腔注射 0.2% 哌替啶 20 mg/kg，B 组小鼠腹腔注射 0.2% 罗通定 20 mg/kg，C 组小鼠腹腔注射生理盐水 0.1 mL/10g。

3. **疼痛模型构建**　给药 30 min 后，A、B、C 三组小鼠同时腹腔注射 0.6% 冰醋酸 0.2 mL/ 只构建疼痛模型。冰醋酸能够刺激小鼠腹膜，产生痛感。

4. **观察记录**　注射完冰醋酸后，观察并记录 10 min 内各组出现的扭体反应次数。

扭体反应具体表现为腹部内凹、后腿伸张、臀部抬起。

5. **计算** 综合全班的实验结果，计算药物抑制扭体百分率，具体计算公式如下：

$$抑制扭体百分率 = \frac{对照组扭体反应均数 - 实验组扭体反应均数}{对照组扭体反应均数} \times 100\%$$

【实验记录与结果】

记录实验结果，根据公式计算出药物抑制扭体百分率。具体见表 3-1-1。

表 3-1-1　哌替啶、罗通定的镇痛作用

组别	药物	扭体反应次数								抑制扭体百分率（%）
		1	2	3	4	5	6	7	8	
甲	哌替啶									
乙	罗通定									
丙	生理盐水									

【注意事项】

（1）0.6% 冰醋酸溶液在临用时新配为宜，存放过久可使作用减弱。

（2）小鼠体重轻，"扭体反应"次数较低，因此各组小鼠体重差异不宜过大。

（3）室温以 20℃为宜，低温时小白鼠扭体次数减少。

（4）动物的疼痛反应个体差异较大，因此实验用动物数越多结果越可靠。

【练习题】

1. 哌替啶的作用是 _____。

A. 镇痛、镇静、镇咳　　　　　　　　B. 镇痛、呼吸兴奋

C. 镇痛、欣快、镇吐　　　　　　　　D. 镇痛、安定、散瞳

2. 对慢性钝痛不宜使用吗啡的主要理由为 _____。

A. 对钝痛效果差　　　　　　　　　　B. 成瘾

C. 可导致便秘　　　　　　　　　　　D. 引起直位性低血压

3. 哌替啶较吗啡应用较多的原因是 _____。

A. 镇痛作用强　　　　　　　　　　　B. 胃肠平滑肌作用强

C. 成瘾性较吗啡轻　　　　　　　　　D. 作用缓慢，维持时间长

4. 哌替啶的主要临床应用不包括下列哪一项？

A. 镇痛   B. 心源性哮喘

C. 恶心、呕吐、便秘   D. 麻醉前给药

【思考题】

（1）哌替啶与罗通定镇痛作用特点有何不同？其主要的临床用途有哪些？

（2）哌替啶和罗通定的作用机制有何不同？

【知识拓展】

吗啡的"功"与"过"

吗啡来源于植物罂粟，将罂粟未成熟的果实切开，伤口处会渗出白色汁液，将汁液收集起来，干燥后就形成了褐色的胶状物，这就是阿片，在国内也被称为"鸦片"。自公元前，阿片已经作为麻醉药使用，明代的《医林集要》中记载了中国最早制作使用鸦片的方法，当时鸦片通常被称作"阿芙蓉"。1803 年，德国药剂师泽尔蒂纳从阿片中分离提取了吗啡，提高了阿片的镇痛作用，在二战期间，吗啡成功缓解了伤员的痛苦，成为重要的医疗物资。同时，由于吗啡在镇痛的同时会产生欣快感，使大量伤员在战后对吗啡成瘾。吗啡成瘾后，对健康产生巨大的危害，使吸食者丧失劳动能力，同时因成瘾导致家庭破产、妻离子散甚至违法犯罪，危害很大。我们应该明确毒品与药物的界定，合理使用吗啡等中枢镇痛药品，加强医德医风教育，依法依规行医。

（王琳琳）

第二节　氯丙嗪对电刺激小鼠激怒反应的影响

【实验目的】

观察氯丙嗪对抗电刺激小鼠激怒反应的作用。

【实验原理】

氯丙嗪为抗精神分裂症药，主要通过阻断中脑 - 边缘通路和中脑 - 皮质通路的 D_2

受体，对中枢神经系统有较强的抑制作用，也称为神经安定作用。

小鼠足部持续受到弱电流或低电压刺激后，可出现激怒行为，表现为逃避、格斗、互相撕咬等。氯丙嗪对抗小鼠受到电刺激引起的激怒反应。

【实验器材】

YLS-9A 药理生理多用仪、电刺激激怒盒、1 mL 注射器、天平。

【实验动物】

小白鼠，18 ~ 22 g，雌雄不拘。

【实验药品】

0.1% 氯丙嗪溶液、生理盐水、苦味酸。

【实验方法】

实验操作步骤如下，见图 3-2-1。

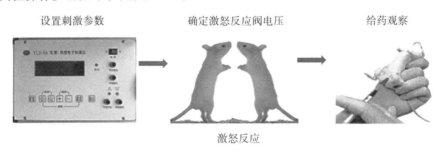

图 3-2-1　操作步骤示意图

1. **设置刺激参数**　YLS-9A 药理生理多用仪，选择"连续波输出"的刺激方式。

2. **确定激怒反应阈电压**　取小鼠 4 只，称重、标记，每两只一组。每次取 2 只放入电刺激激怒盒中，接通药理生理多用仪电源开关，由低到高调节刺激电压，直至小鼠出现电激怒反应（小鼠前肢离地，竖立、对峙，甚至互相撕咬）。此时电压即为该组小鼠出现电激怒反应所需的阈电压。

3. **给药观察**　一组小鼠分别按剂量 0.15 mL/10 g 腹腔注射 0.1% 氯丙嗪，另一组小鼠分别按剂量 0.15 mL/10 g 腹腔注射生理盐水作对照。给药 20 min 后，分别以各组给药前阈电压刺激小鼠，观察两组小鼠给药前后的对电刺激反应有何不同。

【实验记录与结果】

记录实验结果，具体见表 3-2-1。

表 3-2-1 氯丙嗪对电刺激小鼠激怒反应的影响

鼠号	药物	体重（g）	剂量（mg/kg）	阈电压（V）	激怒反应	
					药前	药后
1	0.1% 氯丙嗪溶液					
2	0.1% 氯丙嗪溶液					
3	生理盐水					
4	生理盐水					

【注意事项】

（1）刺激电压设置应从小到大，过低不易引起小鼠激怒反应，过高易导致小鼠逃避。

（2）给药前和给药后应用同等大小的阈电压刺激小鼠，对比小鼠反应的异同。

（3）应随时清除导电铜丝板上的小鼠大小便，以免短路。

【练习题】

1. 氯丙嗪在正常人引起的作用是 _____。

A. 烦躁不安　　　　B. 情绪高涨　　　　C. 紧张失眠　　　　D. 感情淡漠

2. 氯丙嗪抗精神分裂症作用的主要机制是 _____。

A. 阻断 α 受体

B. 阻断 M 受体

C. 阻断结节 - 漏斗系统的 D_2 受体

D. 阻断中脑 - 边缘系统和中脑 - 皮层系统的 D_2 受体

3. 胆碱受体阻断药可加重氯丙嗪的哪些反应？

A. 帕金森综合征　　　　　　　　B. 迟发性运动障碍

C. 静坐不能　　　　　　　　　　D. 直立性低血压

【思考题】

（1）中枢神经系统中多巴胺神经通路有哪些？氯丙嗪是如何影响多巴胺神经通路的？

（2）本研究是如何证明氯丙嗪具有安定作用的？

【知识拓展】

中国自主研发的抗精神分裂症新药——瑞欣妥获批上市

　　精神分裂症是一种反复发作的慢性迁延性疾病，因患者中断治疗或自行减药而导致的病情反复是当下精神分裂症治疗的主要难点。数据统计显示，首次发作的患者有 60% 服药依从性差，5 年内的复发率超过 80%。多次复发导致病程迁延，增加治疗难度和治疗负担。

　　2021 年，我国自主研发的抗精神分裂症新药——瑞欣妥正式上市。这是中国首个具有自主知识产权并开展全球注册的创新微球制剂，也是国内首个自主研发的第二代抗精神病长效针剂，为我国约 1000 万名精神分裂症患者重返社会带来新希望。目前，瑞欣妥已纳入国家医保药品目录。

（房春燕）

第三节　阿司匹林与氯丙嗪对体温的影响

【实验目的】

视频 6

　　（1）观察阿司匹林和氯丙嗪在不同环境中的降温作用。

　　（2）掌握阿司匹林和氯丙嗪降温作用特点，并比较其异同点。

【实验原理】

　　恒温动物具有完善的体温调节机制。当外界环境温度变化时，体温调节中枢通过调节产热和散热过程维持体温的相对恒定。氯丙嗪，又名冬眠灵，是中脑 - 边缘系统和中脑 - 皮质通路多巴胺 D_2 受体的阻断剂，因此临床上一般用作中枢神经抑制剂，发挥抗精神病的药理作用。氯丙嗪对下丘脑体温调节中枢有很强的抑制作用，机体的体温随环境温度而改变，在物理降温的配合下，还可使正常体温降至正常水平以下。

　　阿司匹林，又名乙酰水杨酸，是非甾体抗炎药中的典型代表。非甾体抗炎药的作用机理是通过抑制前列腺素合成酶，使花生四烯酸转化为前列腺素的能力降低，进而使得发热者的体温下降或恢复至正常水平。阿司匹林对正常人的体温没有影响。

【实验器材】

电子秤、肛温表、1 mL 注射器、制冰机或冰箱（冰块）、烧杯。

【实验动物】

小鼠，体重 22 ~ 25 g，雌雄不限。

【实验药品】

0.08% 盐酸氯丙嗪溶液、1% 阿司匹林溶液、生理盐水、10% 酵母悬液、液状石蜡。

【实验方法】

1. **实验准备**　小鼠随机分组，称重、编号。本实验包括解热实验和低温实验两部分，每个实验 6 只小鼠。每个实验中的小鼠分为甲、乙、丙三组，每个小组 2 只小鼠，实验前观察小鼠的活动情况。

2. **体温测定**　一只手固定小鼠，另一只手将测温探头末端涂有液体石蜡的肛温表轻轻插入小鼠肛门约 1 cm 处，3 min 后取出，读取数值，作为小鼠正常体温。

3. **解热实验**　干酵母致小鼠发热：皮下注射 10% 酵母悬液，3 h 后测试小鼠体温。当体温升高 0.8℃ 以上时开始实验，将甲、乙、丙三组小鼠分别腹腔注射 0.08% 盐酸氯丙嗪溶液、1% 阿司匹林溶液和生理盐水（0.1 mL/10 g），30 min 和 60 min 后各测体温一次，观察小鼠活动情况并记录（图 3-3-1）。

4. **低温实验**　将甲、乙、丙三组小鼠分别腹腔注射 0.08% 盐酸氯丙嗪溶液、1% 阿司匹林溶液和生理盐水（0.1 mL/10 g）；用药后，将甲 1、乙 1、丙 1 三只小鼠放入烧杯中，将烧杯置于冰箱或冰浴中；甲 2、乙 2、丙 2 三只小鼠则置于常温下。30 min 和 60 min 分别再次检测各组小鼠肛温，记录并观察小鼠的活动情况（图 3-3-2）。

【实验记录与结果】

解热实验，将结果记录至表 3-3-1；低温实验，将结果记录至表 3-3-2。

【注意事项】

（1）室温影响实验结果，最好在 20 ~ 25℃ 室温进行实验，并保持室温恒定。

（2）将烧杯放在冰浴中进行实验。

（3）温度计头端涂少许液体石蜡，测肛温时减少阻力。

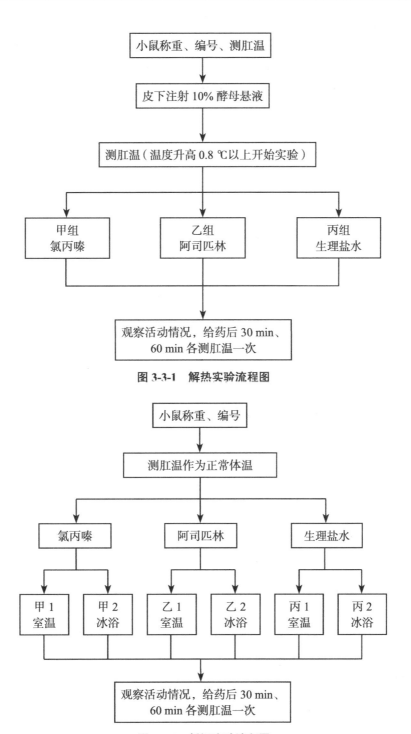

图 3-3-1　解热实验流程图

图 3-3-2　低温实验流程图

（4）测体温时，固定好小鼠，勿使小鼠过度躁动。每次温度计插入的深度和时间保持一致，并且保证每只动物固定使用同一支温度计。

表 3-3-1　氯丙嗪与阿司匹林对小鼠体温的影响（解热实验）

组别	药物	环境	体温			活动情况	
			用药前	用药后 30 min	用药后 60 min	用药前	用药后
甲	氯丙嗪	室温					
乙	阿司匹林	室温					
丙	生理盐水	室温					

表 3-3-2　氯丙嗪与阿司匹林对小鼠体温的影响（低温实验）

组别	药物	环境	体温			活动情况	
			用药前	用药后 30 min	用药后 60 min	用药前	用药后
甲 1	氯丙嗪	室温					
甲 2	氯丙嗪	冰浴					
乙 1	阿司匹林	室温					
乙 2	阿司匹林	冰浴					
丙 1	生理盐水	室温					
丙 2	生理盐水	冰浴					

【练习题】

1. 有关氯丙嗪的药理作用描述错误的是 _____。

A. 抗精神病　　　　B. 催吐作用　　　　C. 镇静作用　　　　D. 降温作用

2. 有关阿司匹林的药理作用描述错误的是 _____。

A. 镇痛作用　　　　B. 抗炎作用　　　　C. 解热作用　　　　D. 镇静作用

3. 抗精神病药物作用的主要作用通路是 _____。

A. 结节 - 漏斗系统　　　　　　　　B. 网状上行系统

C. 黑质 - 纹状体系统　　　　　　　D. 中脑 - 边缘系统

【思考题】

（1）氯丙嗪降温作用与阿司匹林的解热作用有何不同？

（2）根据阿司匹林和氯丙嗪的作用特点，阐述其临床应用。

【知识拓展】

精神科的良药

在氯丙嗪发现之前，对于精神病患者的治疗可谓"无药可用"，先后经历了中世纪的驱魔治疗、热疗法、精神外科治疗、电休克治疗等阶段，但是都收效甚微。直到1950年，罗纳·普朗克公司原本是希望从抗组胺类药物中找出抗疟疾药物，合成了氯丙嗪等产品，当时公司将其中一种以"异丙嗪"的药名出售。同年，巴黎的外科医生亨利·拉伯里特发现，患者应用了异丙嗪之后情绪显得十分平静、放松。基于此，拉伯里特发表了一篇没有数据的临床记录观察，十分巧合的是，这篇论文很快就被罗纳·普朗克公司看到，公司立即着手将抗组胺药物转向开发作用于中枢神经系统的药物。1952年拉伯里特建议氯丙嗪可以用于精神病的治疗，临床发现氯丙嗪可以明显减轻精神病患者的幻想和错觉，这一结果在医学界引起轰动。氯丙嗪的发现诞生了"抗精神病药"这个崭新的药物品种，无数的精神病患者得到解放，实现了精神病医学史上的革命，因此，有人把氯丙嗪称为精神科的"青霉素"。

（韩　雪）

第四节　泮库溴铵和琥珀胆碱对家兔肌松作用的比较

【实验目的】

（1）学习肌松药的家兔垂头实验法。

（2）观察除极化和非除极化型肌松药作用的区别。

【实验原理】

骨骼肌松弛药作用于神经肌肉接头，与 N_M 胆碱受体结合，阻断神经肌肉间的兴奋传递，产生肌肉松弛作用。可分为除极化型肌松药和非除极化型肌松药两大类。两类药均可产生神经肌肉接头阻滞作用，但阻滞方式不同，作用特点也不相同。

琥珀胆碱是除极化型肌松药的代表，又称非竞争型肌松药，特点为：①与 N_2 受体结合后产生持久除极化，使受体不再对 ACh 起反应而使骨骼肌松弛。②不易被胆碱酯酶水解，抗胆碱酯酶药不但不能拮抗琥珀胆碱的作用，反而可以加重其肌肉松弛作用，因此过量时不能用新斯的明解救。

泮库溴铵是非除极化型肌松药，此类药物又称竞争型肌松药，特点为：①可与乙酰胆碱竞争神经肌肉接头的N_2受体，但不激动受体，能竞争性阻断ACh的除极化作用，使骨骼肌松弛。②抗胆碱酯酶药可拮抗其肌松作用，故过量可用适量的新斯的明解救。

【实验器材】

2 mL 注射器、婴儿秤。

【实验动物】

家兔，体重 2.0 ~ 3.0 kg，雌雄不拘。

【实验药品】

0.008% 泮库溴铵溶液、0.05% 琥珀胆碱溶液、0.05% 硫酸新斯的明溶液、0.05% 阿托品溶液。

【实验方法】

实验操作步骤如下，见图 3-4-1。

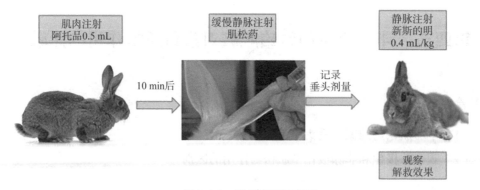

图 3-4-1　操作步骤示意图

1. 取家兔2只，称重、标号　观察家兔呼吸、体位、颈部及四肢肌张力等情况，分别肌注射阿托品溶液 0.5 mL/ 只，等待 10 min。

2. 甲兔　按照 0.5 mL/min 的速度，缓慢静脉注射 0.008% 泮库溴铵溶液（方式：推 - 停 - 推 - 停 - 推……），剂量为 0.5 mL/kg。出现肌松要暂停并密切观察，注意肌松情况。如发现家兔有垂头倾向，应立即暂停注射，并轻叩其头，若此时该兔仍不能抬头，记录已经注入的药量，即为该兔的垂头剂量（约半量）。稍后继续缓慢注射约1倍量泮库溴铵溶液，观察家兔四肢肌张力、呼吸和体位的变化，并立即静脉注射 0.05% 硫酸新斯的明溶液 0.4 mL/kg，观察家兔的变化。

3. 乙兔　如上方法，缓慢静脉注射 0.05% 琥珀胆碱溶液 0.5 mL/kg，观察家兔是否有肌肉震颤、垂头或全身瘫痪等表现。出现肌松现象后，立即静脉注射 0.05% 硫酸新斯的明溶液 0.4 mL/kg，观察家兔的变化，并与甲兔的变化进行比较。

【实验记录与结果】

记录实验结果，具体见表 3-4-1。

表 3-4-1　泮库溴胺和琥珀胆碱对家兔肌松作用的比较

兔号	体重（kg）	给药	剂量	药后表现
甲		泮库溴铵		
		新斯的明		
乙		琥珀胆碱		
		新斯的明		

【注意事项】

（1）缓慢恒速注射肌松药，速度约 0.5 mL/min，以便准确测出垂头剂量，观察肌松药对家兔的作用。

（2）家兔出现肌松表现后，要快速注射新斯的明，以防不易解救。如果解救效果不好，可加大新斯的明的用量。

【练习题】

1. 下列哪种药物可加重琥珀胆碱的肌松作用？

A. 阿托品　　　　　　　　　　　　B. 肾上腺素

C. 新斯的明　　　　　　　　　　　D. 毛果芸香碱

2. 琥珀胆碱松弛骨骼肌的作用机制是 _____。

A. 引起骨骼肌运动终板持久除极化　　B. 阻断 N_2 受体

C. 阻断 N_1 受体　　　　　　　　　D. 阻断 M 受体

3. 下列哪种药物中毒可用新斯的明来解救？

A. 泮库溴铵　　　　　　　　　　　B. 毛果芸香碱

C. 琥珀胆碱　　　　　　　　　　　D. 毒扁豆碱

【思考题】

（1）除极化型肌松药和非除极化型肌松药的区别有哪些？

（2）本实验中新斯的明用于解救两类药物过量中毒时，对家兔的作用有何不同？为什么？

【知识拓展】

琥珀胆碱在临床中的应用

在医学的浩瀚星空中，骨骼肌松弛药如同璀璨星辰，照亮了外科手术与急救的道路。其中，琥珀胆碱作为最早被发现的去极化型肌松药，以其独特的药理作用和广泛的应用领域，成为医学史上不可忽视的一笔。

琥珀胆碱自1942年被发现以来，迅速成为麻醉师手中的重要工具。它能在极短的时间内（通常几秒钟内）引起全身骨骼肌松弛，为气管插管、机械通气及复杂外科手术提供了有力支持。这一发现，不仅是麻醉学领域的一次重大突破，也是医学科技进步的生动体现。琥珀胆碱的研发与应用，是科研人员勇于探索、敢于创新的结果。它启示我们，在科技日新月异的今天，只有不断创新，才能推动医学事业的持续发展。

在手术室中，琥珀胆碱的应用不仅仅是技术的展现，更是人文关怀的体现。它让原本因肌肉紧张而难以进行的手术操作变得轻松可行，为患者争取了宝贵的治疗时间。同时，在急救领域，琥珀胆碱也是挽救生命的重要武器。在紧急情况下，它能迅速缓解患者的呼吸肌紧张，为后续的救治赢得时间。在医疗实践中，医护人员始终将患者的生命安全和健康放在首位。琥珀胆碱的应用，正是这一理念的生动体现，它要求我们在工作中时刻关注患者的需求和感受，以患者为中心开展诊疗活动。

尽管琥珀胆碱在医疗领域发挥了重要作用，但其使用也伴随着一定的风险。如使用不当可能导致高钾血症、心律失常等严重并发症。因此，医护人员在使用琥珀胆碱时，必须严格遵守操作规程和用药原则，确保患者的安全。医疗工作是一项高度专业化的工作，需要医护人员具备严谨的工作态度和高度的责任心，在使用骨骼肌松弛药等高风险药物时，更要时刻保持警惕和谨慎。

（房春燕）

第五节　苯巴比妥钠的抗惊厥作用

【实验目的】

（1）学习小鼠电刺激惊厥法和药物致惊厥法模型制作。

（2）观察苯巴比妥钠的抗惊厥作用，掌握其作用机制。

【实验原理】

惊厥（convulsion）是由于脑组织中部分神经元发生不同程度异常放电而导致的全身或局部骨骼肌不自主地收缩运动。常用的惊厥动物模型有小鼠电惊厥模型和小鼠药物性惊厥模型等。小鼠电刺激惊厥法是用仪器产生电流，通过夹于小鼠两耳的电极，兴奋大脑，产生全身强直性惊厥，表现为前肢屈曲、后肢伸直。小鼠药物致惊厥法则常采用戊四氮、尼可刹米等药物作为惊厥诱导剂，通过大剂量腹腔注射或皮下注射，直接兴奋中枢，诱导小鼠出现惊厥发作，表现为全身肌肉的强直 - 阵挛性收缩。上述两种模型，均可用于抗惊厥药物的药效评价以及具有潜在抗惊厥活性化合物的筛选。

苯巴比妥钠为巴比妥类化合物，其作用机制主要是通过激动 $GABA_A$ 受体，延长 Cl^- 通道开放的时间，增加 GABA 介导的 Cl^- 内流，引起超级化抑制性突触效应，从而对中枢神经系统产生明显的抑制作用。随着其剂量的增加，中枢抑制逐渐增强，大于催眠剂量时可产生抗惊厥作用（图 3-5-1）。

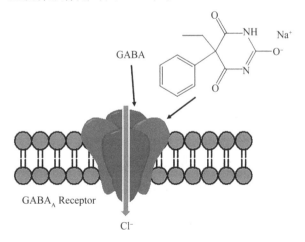

图 3-5-1　苯巴比妥钠结构及其与 $GABA_A$ 受体结合位点示意图

【实验器材】

YSD-4G 药理生理多用仪（或电刺激仪）、导线和鳄鱼夹、小鼠实验笼具、棉球、注射器（1 mL）、天平。

【实验动物】

小鼠，体重 22 ~ 25 g，雌雄不拘。

【实验药品】

0.5% 苯巴比妥钠溶液、生理盐水、0.5% 戊四唑溶液。

【实验方法】

1. 电刺激惊厥法

1）阈值刺激法

（1）将输出导线前端的鳄鱼夹尖端用生理盐水浸湿的棉球包绕，分别夹于小鼠双耳根部。将 YSD-4G 药理生理多用仪（或电刺激仪）参数设置为刺激方式"单次正弦脉冲"，刺激频率"50 Hz"，刺激时长"0.2 s"。刺激电流强度从 7 mA 开始，每隔 1 min 提高 1 mA，直至小鼠后肢出现强直反应为止，记录该电流强度为该小鼠电惊厥阈值。用上述方法测定 6 只小鼠电惊厥阈值。

（2）将 6 只小鼠称重，标记，随机分为甲、乙两组，每组 3 只。甲组小鼠腹腔注射 0.5% 苯巴比妥钠溶液 15 mg/kg，乙组小鼠注射等量的生理盐水作为对照。

（3）给药 30 min 后，使用每只小鼠此前测得的阈值，作为刺激电流，再次电刺激小鼠，其余参数同上。记录小鼠惊厥等级，无反应记为 0 级，出现前后肢阵挛记为 1 级，出现前肢强直记为 2 级，出现后肢强直记为 3 级。

（4）将各组小鼠实验结果记录在表 3-5-1 中。

2）固定电流强度刺激法

（1）将 6 只小鼠称重，标记，随机分为甲、乙两组，每组 3 只。甲组小鼠腹腔注射 0.5% 苯巴比妥钠溶液 50 mg/kg，乙组小鼠注射等量的生理盐水作为对照。给药 30 min 后，进行电惊厥刺激测试。

（2）将输出导线前端的鳄鱼夹尖端用生理盐水浸湿的棉球包绕，分别夹于小鼠双耳根部。将 YSD-4G 药理生理多用仪（或电刺激仪）参数设置为"单次正弦脉冲"，刺激频率"50 Hz"，刺激时长"0.2 s"，刺激电流强度"25 mA"。刺激每只小鼠，并记录小鼠的惊厥等级。无反应记为 0 级，出现前后肢阵挛记为 1 级，出现前肢强直记为 2 级，出现后肢强直记为 3 级。

（3）将各组小鼠实验结果记录在表 3-5-2 中。

2. 药物致惊厥法

（1）取小鼠 2 只，称重，标记，分别腹腔注射 0.5% 苯巴比妥钠溶液 10 mL/kg 和等量生理盐水。

（2）10 min 后，两鼠均皮下注射 0.5% 戊四唑溶液 50 mg/kg，注射完成后立即开始观察有无惊厥反应，并记录惊厥发作的潜伏期（给予戊四唑后出现第一次阵挛性惊厥发作的时间）和小鼠是否死亡。实验观察时间为 30 min。

（3）将各小鼠实验结果记录在表 3-5-3 中。

【实验记录与结果】

根据所用诱导惊厥的方法不同，将实验结果记录在对应的表格内。具体见表 3-5-1 至表 3-5-3。

表 3-5-1 苯巴比妥钠对电刺激致惊厥小鼠的抗惊厥作用（阈值刺激法）

组别	编号	体重	用药前阈值	所给药物及给药体积	用药后惊厥等级
甲					
甲					
甲					
乙					
乙					
乙					

表 3-5-2 苯巴比妥钠对电刺激致惊厥小鼠的抗惊厥作用（固定电流强度法）

组别	编号	体重	所给药物及给药体积	用药后惊厥等级
甲				
甲				
甲				
乙				
乙				
乙				

表 3-5-3 苯巴比妥钠对药物致惊厥小鼠的抗惊厥作用

组别	编号	体重	所给药物及给药体积	惊厥潜伏期	是否惊厥	是否死亡
甲						
乙						

【注意事项】

（1）小鼠对电刺激的反应存在个体差异，为避免电流过大引起大量小鼠死亡，因此采用电刺激惊厥法诱导小鼠惊厥模型时，推荐采用阈值刺激法。

（2）采用电刺激惊厥法时，应注意在设备通电的情况下，实验者的手不可接触鳄鱼夹的金属部分或金属导线，两鳄鱼夹也不可相互接触。

（3）给药剂量要准确，观察结果要及时仔细。

（4）本实验可用 0.1% 地西泮溶液替代 0.5% 苯巴比妥钠溶液；药物致惊厥法中，亦可用 5% 尼可刹米溶液替代 0.5% 戊四唑溶液。

【练习题】

1. 巴比妥类镇静催眠药的结合位点位于 _____。

A. NMDA 受体　　　　　　　　　　　B. GABA 受体

C. 5-HT 受体　　　　　　　　　　　D. DA 受体

2. 下列有关巴比妥类的作用和应用的叙述，错误的是 _____。

A. 随剂量增加其对中枢神经系统抑制作用程度逐渐加深

B. 大于催眠剂量时可产生抗惊厥作用

C. 该类药物目前仍作为临床镇静催眠一线药使用

D. 药物起效快慢与脂溶性有关

3. 有关小鼠皮下注射操作描述正确的是 _____。

A. 只能单人操作，不能两人配合

B. 注射部位一般是小鼠颈背部皮下

C. 小鼠皮下注射吸收快于静脉注射

D. 小鼠皮下注射体积没有限制

【思考题】

（1）具有抗惊厥作用的药物有哪些？其抗惊厥机制有何不同？

（2）引起惊厥的原因有哪些？

【知识拓展】

药物非治疗作用与治疗作用的转化

　　苯巴比妥是一种巴比妥类镇静催眠药，1912年开始上市销售并使用，一直应用到20世纪60年代。苯巴比妥具有明显的后遗效应，易产生耐受性和依赖性，急性中毒也较易发生。此外，该药还是一种较强的肝药酶诱导剂，能诱导多种肝药酶活性升高或数量增加，导致与其合用的药物代谢加快，作用下降。由于以上不良反应，该药的使用受到了限制，逐渐被后来上市的苯二氮䓬类药物取代，已不再作为镇静催眠药常规使用。然而其肝药酶诱导作用被发现具有新的临床应用价值，其原理是苯巴比妥诱导的肝药酶中有一种葡萄糖醛酸转移酶，后者能促进葡萄糖醛酸与血中胆红素的结合，从而加快胆红素的代谢。因此苯巴比妥能通过其肝药酶诱导作用，降低胆红素浓度，治疗高胆红素血症和胆汁淤积性黄疸。这一"老药新用"的例子说明，药物的作用往往有利有弊，但又是对立统一的，药物的非治疗作用在一定条件下可以转化为治疗作用。这就提示我们要全面掌握药物的各项作用，这不仅有助于我们深入理解药物作用的复杂性，也能为我们在临床实践中制定科学合理的治疗方案提供有益的指导。

（钟　恺）

第六节　药物抗尼可刹米惊厥的作用

【实验目的】

　　（1）观察地西泮预防性对抗由尼可刹米引起小鼠的惊厥作用。

　　（2）学习应用药物制备动物惊厥模型的实验方法。

【实验原理】

　　惊厥是由多种原因所引起的中枢神经系统过度兴奋的一种症状，表现为全身或局部肌肉不由自主地抽搐。惊厥发生的机制是脑内抑制性和兴奋性神经递质失衡，导致大脑运动神经元异常放电。惊厥发作时间多在 3 ~ 5 min 之间，有时可反复发作，呈持续状态。常见症状包括四肢和面部肌肉抽动、眼球上翻、口吐白沫、面色发紫发青、神志不清、呼吸暂停等。

呼吸兴奋剂尼可刹米（nikethamide），又名可拉明（coramine），在治疗剂量时既可直接兴奋延脑呼吸中枢，也可通过刺激颈动脉体和主动脉体的化学感受器反射性兴奋呼吸中枢。达到中毒剂量时可导致整个中枢神经系统兴奋性显著升高而引发机体惊厥症状，甚至可由惊厥转为难以恢复的中枢抑制，最终可导致动物死亡。

地西泮（diazepam，药名"安定"）为长效苯二氮䓬类药物，能够增强脑主要的抑制性神经递质 γ- 氨基丁酸（GABA）的效能，具有镇静、催眠、抗焦虑、抗惊厥和中枢性骨骼肌松弛的作用，还可用于治疗酒精戒断症状以及麻醉前给药等。对各种原因引起的惊厥，如子痫、破伤风、小儿高烧惊厥等都有作用。与巴比妥类催眠药相比，它具有治疗指数高、对呼吸影响小、对快波睡眠（REM）几无影响、对肝药酶无影响，以及大剂量时亦不引起麻醉等特点，是目前临床上最常用的催眠药之一。地西泮抗惊厥作用很强，为氯氮䓬的 10 倍。血浆半衰期为 20 ～ 50 h，属长效药。

尼可刹米和地西泮的分子结构，见图 3-6-1。

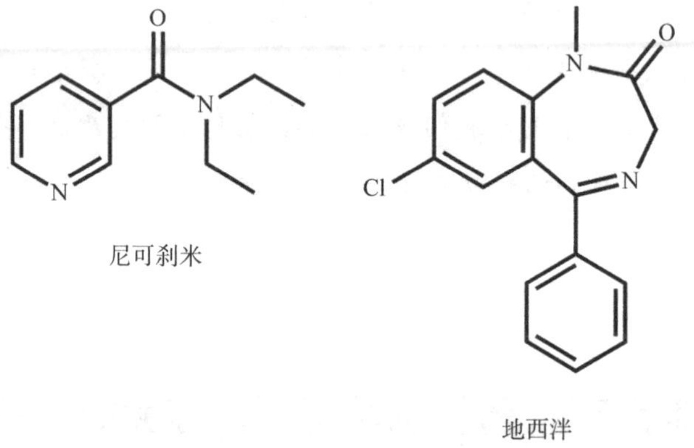

尼可刹米

地西泮

图 3-6-1　尼可刹米和地西泮的分子结构

【实验器材】

鼠笼、电子天平、烧杯、注射器（0.25 mL）。

【实验动物】

小鼠 2 只（18 ～ 22 g），雌雄不限。

【实验药品】

0.5% 地西泮、2% 尼可刹米、生理盐水、苦味酸。

【实验方法】

实验操作步骤如下，见图 3-6-2。

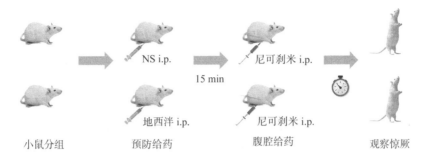

小鼠分组　　　　预防给药　　　　　腹腔给药　　　　观察惊厥

图 3-6-2　操作步骤示意图

1. 动物分组　取小鼠 2 只，称重、苦味酸标记编号。

2. 给药　甲鼠 0.5% 地西泮腹腔注射 0.017 mL/10 g（剂量 8.5 mg/kg），乙鼠腹腔注射生理盐水 0.017 mL/10 g。

3. 药物致惊厥　15 min 后，两鼠均腹腔注射 2% 尼可刹米 0.1 mL/10 g（剂量 200 mg/kg）。

4. 观察惊厥现象　观察两鼠有无惊厥（以阵挛性惊厥或异常跳跃为指标）发生，记录惊厥发生情况、惊厥强度和死亡情况。

【实验记录与结果】

记录实验结果，记录小鼠有无发生惊厥、惊厥强度和死亡情况。具体见表 3-6-1。

表 3-6-1　药物抗尼可刹米惊厥的作用

编号	体重（g）	预防药物	给药体积（mL）	尼可刹米剂量（mg/10 g）	发生惊厥时间（min）	惊厥强度及现象	是否死亡
甲		地西泮					
乙		生理盐水					

【注意事项】

（1）注射尼可刹米后，惊厥先兆可表现为竖尾、尖叫、咬齿等，出现异常跳跃可判定为发生惊厥。

（2）腹腔注射时应注意规范操作，避免伤及内脏。

【练习题】

1. 小鼠腹腔注射时小鼠与注射器角度应为 _____。

A. 0°   B. 15°   C. 45°   D. 90°

2. 下列哪项关于地西泮的描述是不正确的？

A. 是第二类精神药品，是处方药

B. 能产生镇静、催眠效果

C. 没有成瘾性

D. 作用于大脑皮层，抑制中枢神经系统兴奋

3. 下列哪项不是尼可刹米适应证？

A. 一氧化碳中毒   B. 哮喘   C. 吗啡中毒   D. 心力衰竭

【思考题】

（1）地西泮抗尼可刹米引起小鼠惊厥作用的机制？

（2）常用抗惊厥药物有哪几类？其主要作用和用途有何异同？

（3）尼可刹米过量引起惊厥的发生机理是什么？

【知识拓展】

"常青树"药物——地西泮

青霉素、阿司匹林、地西泮是公认的医药史上的三种常青树药物，在人类历史上留下浓重的一笔，其中的地西泮开启了镇静催眠药物的新篇章。地西泮是20世纪50年代末，由现代药理学奠基人之一的瑞典化学家 Leo Sternbach 博士研发的，商品名"安定"。在1959年，就有2000名内科医师用它治疗了2万名患者，效果显著。目前地西泮广泛应用于焦虑症、癫痫、惊厥、失眠和急性酒精戒断综合征等症状的治疗。该药物的显著药效使它成为首个销售额超过10亿美元的"重磅炸弹"药物，彰显了其在医药史上的重要地位。它的研发开创了苯二氮䓬类镇静催眠药的黄金时期。尽管地西泮在临床上具有显著疗效，但其也存在一定的药物依赖性，长期使用地西泮可能会导致患者产生心理和身体上的依赖性反应，停用可能发生戒断反应。地西泮及同类药品，如氯硝西泮、阿普唑仑等均列为第二类精神药品，是国家严格管制的药品。第二类精神药品处方一般不得超过7日用量，处方至少保存2年。因此，临床上应该合理、规范、安全地使用该药物，切勿自

行使用或者随意加大剂量或者延长疗程。

（童骏森）

第七节　地西泮的抗焦虑作用

【实验目的】

（1）学习利用高架十字迷宫实验评价小鼠的焦虑样行为。

（2）观察地西泮的抗焦虑作用，分析其作用机制和临床意义。

【实验原理】

焦虑症是一种以持续性紧张、担忧、恐惧或发作性惊恐为特征的神经精神类疾病，严重影响患者的正常生活，且容易引发众多身心疾病及社会问题。焦虑症的研究目前广泛采用动物行为学评价方法，此类方法具有资源相对易得、操作性强、涉及伦理道德问题较少等特点，已成为抗焦虑药物研究中的重要药效评价方法。

高架十字迷宫（the elevated plus maze，EPM）实验是应用广泛且最为有效的焦虑症行为评价方法之一，具有设计简单、经济实用、无需长期训练、对药物具有双向敏感性等优点。EPM 由对称的 2 个开臂、2 个闭臂和 1 个中央区组成，高于地面约 0.5 m。EPM 的开臂对动物来说同时具有新奇性和威胁性，动物在产生探究好奇心的同时会产生焦虑性反应。将动物置于 EPM 的中央区，观察一定时间内动物的行为活动，记录其运动轨迹以及分别进入开臂和闭臂的时间及次数。若动物主要退缩至闭臂中活动，则说明其焦虑水平高；反之，则说明其焦虑水平低。

目前焦虑症的治疗药物主要有苯二氮䓬类、选择性 5- 羟色胺再摄取抑制剂、选择性 5- 羟色胺和去甲肾上腺素再摄取抑制剂等，其中地西泮为苯二氮䓬类，其作用机制主要是与 $GABA_A$ 受体复合物上的苯二氮䓬结合位点结合，诱导受体构象改变，促进 GABA 与 $GABA_A$ 受体结合，增加 Cl^- 通道开放的频率，增强 GABA 介导的 Cl^- 内流，从而产生明显的中枢抑制效应，小剂量地西泮即可产生抗焦虑作用（图 3-7-1）。

【实验器材】

高架十字迷宫、摄像头、视频分析软件、鼠笼、天平、注射器（1 mL）。

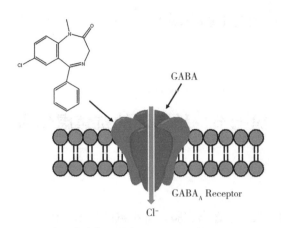

图 3-7-1　地西泮结构及其与 GABA$_A$ 受体结合位点示意图

【实验动物】

小鼠，体重 22 ~ 25 g，雌雄不拘。

【实验药品】

0.1% 地西泮溶液、生理盐水。

【实验方法】

（1）实验开始前，先将小鼠放到高架十字迷宫所在实验室适应环境 1 h。

（2）取适应环境结束的小鼠 2 只，称重、编号，分别编入甲、乙两组，甲组小鼠腹腔注射 0.1% 地西泮溶液 10 mL/kg，乙组小鼠腹腔注射等量生理盐水作为对照。

（3）30 min 后，分别将小鼠置于迷宫中央区，头朝向开臂区，通过摄像头垂直拍摄记录小鼠 5 min 内的活动情况。采用视频分析软件，分析小鼠的运动轨迹，计算小鼠进入开臂次数、开臂内滞留时间、开臂内运动距离等指标，以及相应的百分比指标，记录在表 3-7-1 中。

（4）收集全班各组的原始数据，列表进行统计处理，求出甲、乙两组各项指标的均数、标准差，并对各项指标的差异作统计检验。

【实验记录与结果】

记录实验结果，其中小鼠进入开臂次数、开臂内滞留时间、开臂内运动距离等指标一般由软件直接得出，百分比指标计算公式如下：进入开臂次数百分比 = 进入开臂次数 /（进入开臂次数 + 进入闭臂次数）× 100%，开臂内滞留时间百分比 = 开臂内

滞留时间 /（开臂内滞留时间 + 闭臂内滞留时间）× 100%，开臂内运动距离百分比 =
开臂内运动距离 / 小鼠在迷宫内运动总距离 × 100%。具体见表 3-7-1。

表 3-7-1 地西泮对小鼠高架十字迷宫实验的抗焦虑作用

组别	体重	所给药物及给药体积	进入开臂次数	进入开臂次数百分比	开臂内滞留时间	开臂内滞留时间百分比	开臂内运动距离	开臂内运动距离百分比
甲								
乙								

【注意事项】

（1）实验前 3 天，实验人员可每天将小鼠放到手上抚触 5 min 以消除小鼠的紧张恐惧感。

（2）实验宜在安静环境下进行，实验室内光线强度应适中（以 1.5 m 距离处能区分小鼠细微活动的最低亮度为准）且保持稳定，尽量减少无关应激刺激。

（3）每只小鼠测试结束后，应及时清除高架十字迷宫内的排泄物，并使用 75% 酒精擦拭迷宫以消除异味，减少这些因素对后续实验小鼠的影响。

（4）本实验可用 1.25% 丁螺环酮溶液替代 0.1% 地西泮溶液。

【练习题】

1. 苯二氮䓬类药物引起中枢抑制的作用机制是 _____。

A. 增加 Na^+ 通道开放　　　　　　　　B. 增加 K^+ 通道开放

C. 增加 Ca^{2+} 通道开放　　　　　　　D. 增加 Cl^- 通道开放

2. 下列有关地西泮的叙述中，错误的是 _____。

A. 对地西泮急性中毒进行急救时，无可用的特异性拮抗剂

B. 癫痫持续状态可用大剂量地西泮治疗

C. 地西泮小剂量有抗焦虑作用，中等剂量有镇静催眠作用

D. 随剂量增加其对中枢神经系统抑制作用逐渐增强

3. 有关高架十字迷宫描述正确的是 _____。

A. 高架十字迷宫离地需 1.5 m 以上

B. 当小鼠主要在闭臂活动时，说明其焦虑水平低

C. 当小鼠主要在开臂活动时，说明其焦虑水平低

D. 当小鼠主要在开臂活动时，说明其焦虑水平高

【思考题】

（1）抗焦虑药物的动物行为学评价方法还有哪些？

（2）目前临床为何较少使用地西泮治疗焦虑症？

【知识拓展】

实验失误造就的经典药物——地西泮

20世纪50年代，当时市场上主流的镇静催眠药还是巴比妥类，但其在临床应用中已经表现出了一系列令人难以忍受的不良反应。因此，许多制药公司和研究所均成立了专门的研究小组，开始了新型镇静催眠药的研发尝试。罗氏公司研究员莱奥·斯特恩巴赫（Leo Sternbach）领导的研究小组也是其中之一。然而，该小组先后合成的40种新化合物，经药理检测均未发现明显的镇静催眠活性，罗氏公司因而决定放弃和解散斯特恩巴赫的团队。就在他们清理实验室时，有人发现了一个此前因为投料错误而意外合成的化合物Ro-50690，该化合物当时被认为是实验失误而没有进行药理活性检测。斯特恩巴赫得知后，虽然觉得有效的可能性不大，但考虑到该化合物是本组解散前能送检的最后一个化合物了，便还是送去做了检测。结果几天后，药理部主任就打来了电话，说测试结果非常惊人，该化合物不仅具有镇静、抗焦虑和松弛肌肉的作用，而且比当时市售的巴比妥等药物效果都好。于是，罗氏公司决定以Ro-50690为先导化合物重启研究，又先后合成了3000个相关化合物，最终在1959年得到了地西泮，并于1963年成功上市。上市后地西泮因其疗效确切，不良反应较小，很快成为药物史上最畅销的药物之一，被誉为医药史上三大经典药物之一。

（钟 恺）

第八节　尼可刹米对吗啡呼吸抑制的解救作用

【实验目的】

（1）观察吗啡过量对呼吸的影响。

（2）观察尼可刹米对吗啡呼吸抑制的解救作用。

（3）学习并掌握家兔的呼吸频率测定及观察方法。

【实验原理】

尼可刹米是一种呼吸兴奋剂，能选择性地兴奋延髓呼吸中枢，可通过颈动脉体和主动脉体化学感受器反射性地兴奋呼吸中枢，使呼吸加深加快。当呼吸中枢被抑制时，其兴奋作用更为明显。吗啡是一种强效镇痛药，但同时具有抑制呼吸的不良反应。本实验通过向家兔注射吗啡造成呼吸抑制，然后注射尼可刹米观察其对呼吸抑制的解救作用。

【实验器材】

注射器、马利氏气鼓、鼻插管、计时器、实验台、电子秤、铁支架、兔固定箱、胶布、呼吸频率监测仪。

【实验动物】

家兔。

【实验药品】

1% 盐酸吗啡溶液、5% 尼可刹米溶液、0.5% 地西泮溶液。

视频 7

【实验方法】

（1）将家兔称重后置于实验台上，固定好头部和四肢，连接呼吸频率监测仪。

（2）记录家兔的正常呼吸频率。

（3）耳缘静脉缓慢注射 1% 盐酸吗啡溶液（根据家兔体重计算剂量，0.5 ~ 1.0 mL/kg），观察家兔呼吸频率和瞳孔的变化。

（4）当家兔呼吸频率显著降低时（如降至正常值的 50% 以下），立即耳缘静脉注射 5% 尼可刹米溶液（根据家兔体重计算剂量，0.5 mL/kg），观察呼吸频率的恢复情况以及瞳孔变化。

（5）如家兔出现惊厥反应（如面部肌肉痉挛、肢体抽动等），立即耳缘静脉注射 0.5% 地西泮溶液进行解救。

（6）记录实验过程中的呼吸频率变化、注射时间、解救时间等数据（图 3-8-1）。

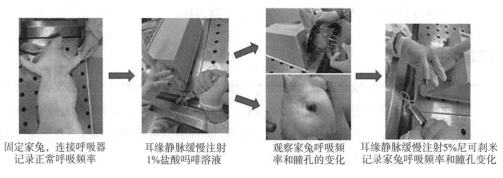

固定家兔，连接呼吸器　　　耳缘静脉缓慢注射　　　观察家兔呼吸频　　　耳缘静脉缓慢注射5%尼可刹米
记录正常呼吸频率　　　　　1%盐酸吗啡溶液　　　率和瞳孔的变化　　　记录家兔呼吸频率和瞳孔变化

图 3-8-1　实验步骤示意图

【实验记录与结果】

（1）记录实验过程中家兔呼吸频率的变化情况，绘制呼吸频率变化曲线图。

（2）记录家兔注射吗啡后和注射尼可刹米后的瞳孔变化情况。

（3）记录实验过程中的呼吸频率变化、解救时间等数值填入表 3-8-1。

表 3-8-1　尼可刹米对抗吗啡呼吸抑制的作用

记录项目	正常对照	注射吗啡后	注射尼可刹米后
瞳眬变化			
呼吸频率（次 /min）			
解救时间			

【思考题】

（1）分析尼可刹米对吗啡呼吸抑制的解救作用，以及可能出现的不良反应（如惊厥）。

（2）讨论尼可刹米作为呼吸兴奋剂的药理作用机制，以及在实际应用中可能遇到的问题和注意事项。

（3）分析实验中出现的惊厥反应的原因及解救措施。

【注意事项】

（1）实验过程中应确保家兔处于安静状态，避免外界干扰。

（2）注射药品时应准确计算剂量，避免过量或不足。

（3）注射药品时应缓慢且稳定，避免药液外漏或注射过快。

（4）实验中应密切关注家兔的呼吸变化及可能出现的不良反应，及时采取解救措施。

（5）实验结束后应对家兔进行妥善处理，避免伤害实验动物。

【练习题】

1.尼可刹米主要用于解救哪种药物引起的呼吸抑制？

A.哌替啶　　　　　B.吗啡　　　　　　C.苯巴比妥　　　　　D.氯丙嗪

2.在本实验中，家兔注射吗啡后呼吸频率和幅度如何变化？

A.呼吸频率加快，幅度增大　　　　C.呼吸频率和幅度均无明显变化

B.呼吸频率减慢，幅度减小　　　　D.呼吸频率加快，幅度减小

3.尼可刹米对抗吗啡引起的呼吸抑制的机制是什么？

A.抑制阿片受体　　　　　　　　B.兴奋延髓中枢受体

C.抑制多巴胺受体　　　　　　　D.兴奋多巴胺受体

【思考题】

尼可刹米在解救吗啡呼吸抑制时可能出现的并发症及相应的处理措施有哪些？

【知识拓展】

可拉明——提神醒脑的兴奋剂

尼可刹米，也叫可拉明，是比较少见的呼吸兴奋剂。可拉明是由北美洲山梗菜科植物山梗菜中提取出山梗菜碱的盐酸盐，现已多为化学合成。山梗菜遍布北美大陆，是一种草本植物，印第安人曾用来治疗哮喘。少量摄入这种物质是安全的，但吸食过量会导致呕吐、痉挛、高血压、癫痫等，甚至可能致命。

研究表明，可拉明对睡眠、情感、情绪等生理活动有重要影响，曾被称为苏醒药。1972年慕尼黑奥运会上两名分别来自荷兰和西班牙的自行车运动员，在公路团体和公路个人赛上均获得铜牌，然而，赛后兴奋剂检查为可拉明阳性而取消奖牌。

（周　倩）

第九节　普鲁卡因的局部作用及全身作用

【实验目的】

（1）了解药物的兴奋作用和抑制作用；局部作用和全身作用等。

（2）观察硫喷妥钠的抗惊厥作用。

【实验原理】

普鲁卡因是一种常用的局麻药，其局部注射后能够阻滞神经细胞膜钠离子内流，阻断动作电位的产生和传导，暂时阻断痛觉和运动功能的传导。普鲁卡因自用药部位进入血液循环则会发生吸收作用，阻滞心血管系统的细胞膜钠离子内流，抑制心血管的兴奋性，导致循环抑制的毒性反应。此外，普鲁卡因吸收后还会对中枢神经系统产生影响，导致中枢先兴奋后抑制的毒性反应。

本实验通过普鲁卡因注射入家兔坐骨神经周围产生同侧后肢痛觉和运动障碍，观察其局部作用，即为阻断痛觉和运动功能的作用；并进一步通过普鲁卡因肌内注射观察其吸收作用，实验可观察到中枢的先兴奋后抑制的毒性反应，即为先出现惊厥，如解救不及时可出现死亡。硫喷妥钠为中枢神经系统的抑制药物，可对抗肌注普鲁卡因导致的惊厥。

【实验器材】

兔固定器、磅秤、注射器（2.5 mL、5 mL、10 mL）、医用纱布。

【实验动物】

家兔，体重 1.5 ~ 3.0 kg，雌雄不拘。

【实验药品】

5% 普鲁卡因溶液、2.5% 的硫喷妥钠溶液。

【实验方法】

1. **实验准备**　取家兔一只，称重，先观察正常活动情况，如四肢站立和行走姿态；并用针刺其后肢，测其有无痛觉反射。

2.**局部作用观察** 于一侧坐骨神经周围（使家兔做自然俯卧式，在尾部坐骨嵴与股骨头间摸到一凹陷处）（图 3-9-1）注入 5% 普鲁卡因溶液 1 mL/kg（50 mg/kg），观察同侧后肢有无运动和感觉障碍。

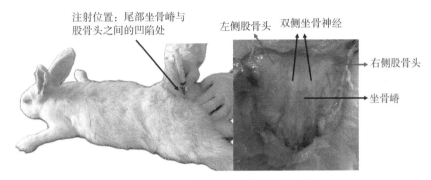

注射位置：尾部坐骨嵴与股骨头之间的凹陷处　　左侧股骨头　双侧坐骨神经　　右侧股骨头　　坐骨嵴

图 3-9-1　坐骨神经周围注射示意图

3.**全身作用观察** 待局部作用明显后（2 ~ 3 min），于家兔另一侧后肢肌内注射 5% 普鲁卡因溶液 1 mL/kg，并按家兔体重准备好相应剂量的硫喷妥钠，密切观察家兔反应至出现中毒症状（惊厥）。

4.**中毒解救** 观察到家兔惊厥后，立即由耳缘静脉缓慢注射 2.5% 的硫喷妥钠溶液至肌肉松弛为止（约 0.5 mL/kg）。

【实验记录与结果】

观察记录实验结果，填入表 3-9-1 中。

表 3-9-1　普鲁卡因的局部作用和吸收作用

动物	体重（kg）	观察阶段	家兔活动情况及表现
家兔		给药前	
		坐骨神经周围注射普鲁卡因后	
		肌内注射普鲁卡因后	
		静脉注射硫喷妥钠后	

【注意事项】

（1）测试痛觉反射针刺后肢踝关节处，轻度适中。

（2）确定坐骨神经部位时后肢拉直，在坐骨嵴与股骨头间摸到一凹陷处即是。注射部位尽量靠近股骨头，针尖插到髂骨稍回退一点。

（3）普鲁卡因注于坐骨神经周围，可产生传导阻滞，剂量过大或误入血管可致中毒，主要表现有中枢先兴奋后抑制，如不安、惊厥、昏迷、呼吸抑制等。

【练习题】

1. 普鲁卡因一般不用于 _____。

A. 表面麻醉　　　　　B. 浸润麻醉　　　　　C. 传导麻醉　　　　　D. 腰麻

2. 腰麻时使用麻黄碱的目的是 _____。

A. 防止过敏性休克　　　　　　　　　B. 防止血管扩张

C. 防止麻醉过程中血压降低　　　　　D. 延长局麻药作用时间

3. 家兔坐骨神经周围注射普鲁卡因属于何种局麻方法？

A. 浸润麻醉　　　　　B. 传导麻醉　　　　　C. 表面麻醉　　　　　D. 腰麻

【思考题】

（1）局麻药吸收入血后会对患者产生哪些不良反应？临床上如何减少或避免局麻药的吸收？

（2）普鲁卡因的选择作用表现在哪些方面？哪些有治疗作用？哪些是不良反应？

【知识拓展】

中药麻醉剂

根据文献记载，世界上最早的麻醉药是我国东汉末年著名的医学家华佗所发明的麻沸散，他的发明比美国的牙科医生摩尔顿（1846 年）发明乙醚麻醉要早1600 多年。不过，华佗晚年因遭曹操怀疑，下狱被拷问致死，他的医书自此失传，麻沸散自然也被湮没在历史中。据考证，麻沸散的主要成分可能是曼陀罗花（洋金花）、莨菪子。根据日本外科学家的考证，麻沸散的组成是曼陀罗花一升，生草乌、全当归、香白芷、川芎各四钱，炒南星一钱，其中曼陀罗花中含有的阿托品类物质，具有定喘、祛风、麻醉止痛的效果，可作外科手术麻醉剂；草乌为祛风湿药，可治疗风寒湿痹、心腹冷痛，也可用于跌打损伤和麻醉止痛，其中含有的乌头碱有明显的抗炎、镇痛作用，有大毒；白芷具有祛风止痛之功效，川芎具有活血止痛之功效。继华佗之后，医生们也研制出了不同的麻醉药：宋朝《扁鹊心书》有用曼陀罗花和大麻花制作的"睡圣散"；明初年间，明朝《普济方》问世后，"草乌散"成了最常见的麻醉药，书中规定了用药时的严格剂量，这时的麻醉药已经比较安全；明代医生王肯堂以酒混合麻醉药物成功完成了局部麻醉；

在吴谦的《医宗金鉴》里，也大量记载了以局部麻醉的方式成功完成的各类外科手术。麻醉药的研发每一步都具有相当大的风险性，这突飞猛进的麻醉技术背后，是一代代名医们以身试药，几乎用生命在践行的心血。中国医学先贤们在留下了精湛的医术，实用、安全的医书方药的同时，也留给了我们上下求索的倔强身影和不畏艰难、精益求精的探索精神。

（王舒舒）

第四章　心血管系统药理

第一节　传出神经系统药物对家兔血压的影响

【实验目的】

（1）观察肾上腺素、去甲肾上腺素及酚妥拉明对家兔血压的影响，并分析药物作用的相互影响及机制。

（2）熟练掌握家兔实验的基本操作。

视频 8

【实验原理】

血压与心室射血、血管阻力和循环血量三个基本因素有关，通过神经 - 体液调节机制维持正常血压。传出神经系统药物通过激动或阻断分布于心血管的肾上腺素受体和乙酰胆碱受体，影响心肌收缩性、血管的舒张与收缩程度，从而使血压升高或降低。

肾上腺素用于因支气管痉挛所致严重呼吸困难，可迅速缓解药物等引起的过敏性休克，亦可用于延长浸润麻醉用药的作用时间等。具有 α 受体和 β 受体激动作用：α 受体激动引起皮肤、黏膜、内脏血管收缩；β 受体激动引起冠状血管扩张、骨骼肌血管扩张、心肌兴奋、心率增快、支气管平滑肌扩张。肾上腺素对血压的影响与剂量有关，常用剂量使收缩压上升而舒张压不升或略降，大剂量使收缩压、舒张压均升高。口服后有明显的首过效应。

去甲肾上腺素为 α 肾上腺素受体激动药，作为急救时补充血容量的辅助治疗药物，使血压回升；也可用于椎管内阻滞时的低血压及心脏骤停复苏后血压维持等。去甲肾上腺素对 α 受体具有明显的激动作用，但较肾上腺素稍弱，对 α_1 和 α_2 受体无选择性。本品主要作用于 α 受体，使血管收缩，导致收缩压和舒张压上升，伴随反射性心率减慢。临床上一般采用静脉滴注，静脉给药后起效迅速，停止滴注后作用时效维持 1 ~ 2 min。

酚妥拉明为 α 肾上腺素受体阻断药，能拮抗血液循环中肾上腺素和去甲肾上腺素的作用，使血管扩张而降低周围血管阻力，拮抗儿茶酚胺效应，用于诊治肾上腺嗜铬细胞瘤，但对正常人或原发性高血压患者的血压影响甚少。酚妥拉明能降低外周血管阻力，使心脏后负荷降低，左心室舒张末压和肺动脉压下降，心搏出量增加，可用于治疗心力衰竭。

【实验器材】

兔台，动脉夹，组织剪，止血钳，动脉套管，压力换能器，眼科剪，镊子，玻璃分针，BL-422 生物机能实验系统，1 mL、10 mL 注射器，丝线。

【实验动物】

家兔，体重 2.0 ~ 3.0 kg。

【实验药品】

0.002% 肾上腺素溶液，0.002% 去甲肾上腺素溶液，2.5% 酚妥拉明溶液，生理盐水，25% 乌拉坦溶液，肝素溶液。

【实验方法】

实验操作步骤示意图见图 4-1-1。

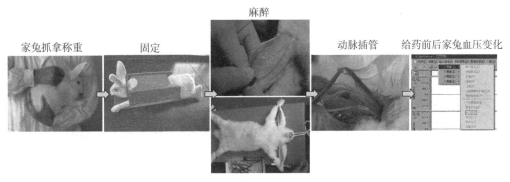

图 4-1-1　操作步骤示意图

1. **称重、固定和麻醉**　家兔一只，称重（捉持方法，提背托臀），记录体重计算给药剂量，固定后以 25% 乌拉坦 4 mL/kg 耳缘静脉注射麻醉。慢推 2/3 量，观察呼吸、心跳、肌张力、角膜反射。

2. **动脉插管**　仰位固定，在颈部正中作一 4 cm 切口，分离肌肉，暴露气管，喉头下第二环作"T"切口插入气管插管，结扎固定。分离颈总动脉、远心端结扎，近心端动脉夹阻断血流，靠近结扎线处剪一"V"形小口。动脉插管内充满肝素生理盐水溶液，朝向心方向插入颈总动脉，结扎固定，动脉插管的另一端与压力换能器相连。

3. 给药并记录 打开动脉夹，记录正常血压曲线（BL-422 生物机能实验系统 - 输入信号 - 通道 1- 压力，走纸速度调到最慢）。耳缘静脉分别按下列顺序给药，立即记录血压曲线，每次给药后待血压恢复正常后再加入下一个药物。

（1）第一组药：

目的是分别仔细观察肾上腺素、去甲肾上腺素对家兔血压的影响有何不同，重点观察酚妥拉明对去甲肾上腺素作用的影响。

① 生理盐水 0.5 mL；

② 0.002% 肾上腺素 0.25 mL/kg；（待血压稳定后加③）

③ 0.002% 去甲肾上腺素 0.25 mL/kg；（待血压稳定后加④）

④ 2.5% 酚妥拉明 0.3 mL/kg；（观察血压变化，5 ~ 10 min 后加⑤）

⑤ 0.002% 去甲肾上腺素 0.25 mL/kg。（观察血压变化）

（2）第二组药：

目的是分别仔细观察去甲肾上腺素、肾上腺素对家兔血压的影响有何不同，重点观察酚妥拉明对肾上腺素作用的影响。

① 生理盐水 0.5 mL；

② 0.002% 去甲肾上腺素 0.25 mL/kg；（待血压稳定后加③）

③ 0.002% 肾上腺素 0.25 mL/kg；（待血压稳定后加④）

④ 2.5% 酚妥拉明 0.3 mL/kg；（观察血压变化，5 ~ 10 min 后加⑤）

⑤ 0.002% 肾上腺素 0.25 mL/kg。（观察血压变化）

【实验记录与结果】

记录实验结果，描绘给药前后家兔血压变化曲线，分析血压变化的机制，如表 4-1-1 所示，以第一组为例。

表 4-1-1 家兔动脉血压的影响

药物处理分组	绘制家兔动脉血压曲线
肾上腺素 0.25 mL/kg	
去甲肾上腺素 0.25 mL/kg	
酚妥拉明 0.3 mL/kg	
去甲肾上腺素 0.25 mL/kg	

【注意事项】

（1）采取保温措施，防止家兔麻醉后体温下降。

（2）皮肤、皮下、肌肉，依次有层次分开。

（3）操作过程中，勿污染、挤压、损伤和用力牵拉。

（4）药液临用现配，准确把握给药剂量。

（5）麻醉不宜过深。

（6）实验结束后空气栓塞处死家兔。

【练习题】

1. 在药物对家兔血压调节实验中，注射肝素生理盐水的目的是 _____。

A. 抗凝，防止动脉插管堵塞　　　　　B. 补充血容量

C. 升高血压　　　　　　　　　　　　D. 降低血压

2. 在药物对家兔血压调节实验中，说法错误的是 _____。

A. 麻醉动物应掌握宁浅勿深，宁慢勿快的原则

B. 分离血管神经应避免过度牵扯

C. 颈动脉切口应以靠近心端为宜

D. 压力换能器与兔心脏位置处于同一水平面

3. 去甲肾上腺素与肾上腺素对心血管的作用，不同的是 _____。

A. 正性肌力作用　　　　　　　　　　B. 升高血压

C. 舒张冠状血管　　　　　　　　　　D. 负性频率作用

【思考题】

（1）肾上腺素、去甲肾上腺素和酚妥拉明分别对家兔血压有何影响？

（2）酚妥拉明对肾上腺素、去甲肾上腺素的作用有何影响？有无不同？试以受体学说分析。

【知识拓展】

中医与现代医疗 - 共筑健康防线

《黄帝内经》中的"治未病"思想，提醒我们预防胜于治疗。面对高血压这一全球性健康问题，中医与现代医学的结合显得尤为重要。高血压，作为心血管

综合征的一种表现，其预防和治疗同等重要。中医视高血压为身体失衡的信号，强调适时调整，恢复平衡。正如放下重物后，身体自然恢复常态，血压亦然。然而，现代生活的压力往往使人们忽视了这一自然规律。长期紧张导致血压恢复时间延长，最终可能形成高血压。这时，现代医学的检测和治疗手段就显得尤为重要，结合中医的生活方式调整和现代医学的科学治疗，我们可以有效预防和控制高血压。合理饮食、适量运动、心情舒畅，这些都是中医推荐的预防措施。同时，现代医学提供的药物和治疗，帮助患者稳定血压，减少并发症。通过中医的智慧和现代医学的科学，我们共同构建起一道健康防线，不仅守护个人健康，也为社会公共卫生作出贡献。让我们携手，用智慧和科学守护健康，共创和谐社会。

（方　辉）

第二节　利多卡因对抗电刺激诱发心律失常的作用

【实验目的】

（1）观察利多卡因对电刺激引起的心律失常的对抗作用。

（2）学习电刺激诱发心律失常的方法。

【实验原理】

电刺激法指应用电刺激动物的迷走神经，增加乙酰胆碱的释放。乙酰胆碱作用于M胆碱能受体，能够减慢心率、减慢传导、心肌收缩力下降，抑制窦房结和房室结的传导。电刺激诱发动物模型难度相对较低，操作简单、可控性强，并具有一定的可逆性。利多卡因是 I b 类抗心律失常药物，能够抑制浦肯野纤维和心室肌细胞的 Na^+ 内流，促进 K^+ 外流，降低自律性，缩短动作电位时程和有效不应期，从而发挥抗心律失常作用。

【实验器材】

BL-422 生物机能实验系统，刺激电极，1 mL 注射器，普通剪刀，手术剪，镊子，蛙板，图钉，蛙心夹，铁架台等。

【实验动物】

蟾蜍 1 只。

【实验药品】

0.2% 利多卡因，任氏液。

【实验方法】

1. **样本准备**　取蟾蜍 1 只，破坏脑及脊髓后，用图钉仰位固定于蛙板上，然后沿着腹壁两侧剪开腹壁，在胆囊附近找到回流到肝脏的腹壁浅静脉，用线结扎并在结线下方剪断。将腹壁向下翻转，然后沿胸骨打开胸腔，用镊子提起心包膜，小心剪破心包膜，暴露心脏。用一端系有长线的蛙心夹夹住心尖，将线连于记录仪的换能器上。

2. **记录正常心电图**　启动生物信号采集系统，描记一段正常心脏的舒缩曲线。

3. **诱发心律失常**　将刺激电极置于接近房室间隔的心室肌表面。参数设置：粗电压，连续单刺激，刺激频率 10 次 /s，电压强度 1 ~ 10 V，刺激时间 30 s，观察和记录蟾蜍心电图的变化。

4. **给药**　待心律出现显著不规则（室颤）后，立即从腹壁浅静脉缓慢注入 0.2% 利多卡因溶液 0.4 ~ 0.6 mL。用药 3 ~ 4 min 后以同样的刺激强度和频率再刺激 30 s，观察心电图的变化并记录（图 4-2-1）。

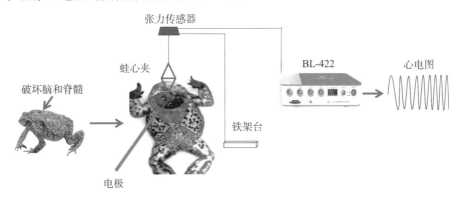

图 4-2-1　实验操作流程示意图

【实验记录与结果】

观察并记录给予利多卡因前后蟾蜍心脏心电图的变化。描记曲线图。

【注意事项】

（1）室温宜保持在 25 ℃左右，温度太低影响实验结果。

（2）暴露的心脏要经常滴加任氏液保持湿润。

（3）电极放在心室肌上不要靠得太紧，以免影响心脏的跳动。

【练习题】

1. 利多卡因抗心律失常的作用机制是 _____。

A. 提高心肌自律　　　　　　　　　　C. β 受体阻断作用

C. 抑制 K^+ 外流　　　　　　　　　　D. 改变病变区传导速度

2. 下列哪项不属于利多卡因的临床应用？

A. 急性心肌梗死所致室性心律失常

B. 心导管检查所致室性心律失常

C. 洋地黄中毒所致室性心律失常

D. 阵发性快速房颤

3. 任氏液的成分不包括 _____。

A. 氯化钠　　　　　B. 氯化钾　　　　　C. 氯化钙　　　　　D. 氢氧化钠

4. 电极应放置在 _____。

A. 心房　　　　　　B. 心室　　　　　　C. 房室间隔　　　　D. 心尖

【思考题】

（1）诱导心律失常的方法有哪些？

（2）快速型心律失常选择哪些药物治疗？

【知识拓展】

利多卡因的历史

利多卡因作为Ⅰ类抗心律失常药物二十年前曾广泛应用于室性心律失常的治疗和预防。1989 年心律失常抑制试验 CAST 试验及其后的 CAST2 实验结果显示，Ⅰ类抗心律失常药物恩卡尼、氟卡尼及乙马噻嗪对心肌梗死后室性早搏治疗有效，但增加患者总病死率，自此所有Ⅰ类抗心律失常药物应用迅速减少。

（孙志朋）

第三节　抗心律失常药物对氯化钡诱导心律失常的治疗作用

【实验目的】

（1）学习用氯化钡诱发家兔心律失常的方法。

（2）观察利多卡因的抗心律失常作用。

【实验原理】

氯化钡可促进浦肯野纤维的 Na^+ 内流，抑制 K^+ 外流，促进 4 相自动除极，从而增强自律性，诱发室性心律失常；此外还可抑制 Na^+-K^+-ATP 酶，使细胞内 K^+ 减少，导致最大舒张电位减少，细胞内 Na^+ 增加，通过 Na^+-Ca^{2+} 交换使细胞内 Ca^{2+} 增加，导致震荡后电位及触发活动而使自律性增加，使心肌交感神经兴奋性增加，导致异位节律，表现为室性期前收缩、二联律、三联律、心室纤颤等，常用于制作各种室性心律失常模型。该心律失常模型制作方法较简单，稳定性好，成功率高。该模型与人类相关疾病的发生存在差异性，但是对心律失常机制及相关指标表达调控研究更为客观。氯化钡致心律失常模型是目前常用的快速性心律失常模型之一。

利多卡因（lidocaine）属于 Ⅰ b 类抗心律失常药，可阻滞钠通道的激活状态和失活状态，通道恢复至静息态时阻滞作用迅速解除，因此利多卡因对除极化组织作用强，对缺血或强心苷中毒所致的除极化型心律失常有较强的抑制作用。该药抑制参与动作电位复极 2 期的少量 Na^+ 内流，缩短或不影响浦肯野纤维和心室肌的动作电位时程。减少动作电位 4 相去极斜率，提高兴奋阈值，降低自律性而发挥抗快速型室性心律失常的作用。

【实验器材】

BL-422 生物机能实验系统、手术剪、兔手术台、注射器、静脉注射针头、棉球、体重秤。

【实验动物】

家兔 1 只，体重 2 ~ 3 kg。

【实验药品】

0.4% 氯化钡溶液、0.5% 利多卡因注射液、20% 乌拉坦，生理盐水

【实验方法】

（1）取家兔 1 只，称重，耳缘静脉注射 20% 乌拉坦 4 ～ 5 ml/kg 麻醉，固定于兔手术台上。

（2）将针形电极插入家兔的四肢远端皮下，连接 BL-422 生物机能实验系统，选择标准 II 导联，描记正常心电图（标准电压 1 mV 相对于 10 mm，纸速 25 mm/s）（图 4-3-1）。

（3）耳缘静脉注射 0.4% 氯化钡溶液 0.5 mL/kg，再推入生理盐水 0.5 mL/kg，立即描记心电图观察是否出现心律失常。

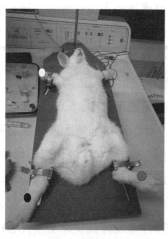

图 4-3-1　家兔 II 导心电图电极连接示意图

（4）出现心律失常的心电图后，立即由耳缘静脉注入 0.5% 利多卡因注射液 1 mL/kg（即 5 mg/kg），描记心电图，观察药物能否立即制止心律失常，以及心电图维持正常的持续时间。

【实验记录与结果】

记录实验结果，包括利多卡因起效时间及治疗维持时间，并选择正常心电图、氯化钡引起的心律失常典型心电图、利多卡因治疗后的典型心电图，打印。

【注意事项】

（1）用利多卡因拮抗氯化钡的诱发心律失常作用，奏效极快。因而在推注利多卡因期间即可开始描记心电图，以便观察其转变过程。

（2）导联线必须接触良好，以减少交流干扰。针头电极不能刺入四肢肌肉，以免肌电干扰。

（3）室温较低时注意动物的保暖，以免肌肉颤动而影响记录。

（4）家兔麻醉程度适当，避免麻醉太浅或太深甚至导致死亡。

【练习题】

1.在正常心电图中，P 波代表了 _____。

A.心房除极
B.房室传导时间

C.心室除极
D.心室复极

2.利多卡因对抗氯化钡诱发的心律失常时，记录心电图时应 _____。

A.注射利多卡因的同时记录家兔心电图

B.待注射完利多卡因后再记录家兔心电图

C.待注射完利多卡因 1 ~ 2 min 后再记录家兔心电图

D.待注射完利多卡因 5 min 后再记录家兔心电图

3.氯化钡通常引起的心律失常是 _____。

A.缓慢型心律失常
B.快速型室性心律失常

C.快速型房性心律失常
D.房室传导阻滞

【思考题】

（1）利多卡因抗心律失常的特点是什么？临床用途是什么？

（2）临床常用的抗心律失常药物有哪几类？治疗快速型心律失常应如何选择药物？

【知识拓展】

利多卡因的药理学作用

利多卡因是 1948 年上市的一种氨基酰胺类局部麻醉药，通过阻断 Na^+ 通道而发挥作用。利多卡因是临床常用的局麻药，因其起效快、作用强而持久、穿透力强及安全范围较大，对组织几乎无刺激性，用于多种形式的局部麻醉，有"全能麻醉药"之称。此外，该药还用于心律失常的治疗，主要用于各种室性心律失常的治疗，如急性心肌梗死或强心苷中毒所致心动过速或心室纤颤。近年来研究发现，利多卡因对疼痛具有一定的疗效。在带状疱疹引起的后神经痛治疗中，5%利多卡因凝胶贴膏是一线镇痛药，推荐用于无破损皮肤，覆盖疼痛最严重区域。糖尿病引起的周围神经痛也可用该剂型进行治疗。而静脉注射利多卡因，可减少围术期阿片类药物的用量，减少围术期炎性细胞因子（如 IL-6、IL-8、IL-1、TNF-a）的释放，促进抗炎因子（如 IL-10）释放。此外，利多卡因还可通过抑制肿瘤细胞增殖，激活细胞凋亡通路而发挥抗肿瘤作用。利多卡因不但可抑制乳腺癌细胞的转移，而且能增加顺铂的抗瘤效应。

（李成檀）

第四节　强心苷对离体蛙心舒缩作用的影响

【实验目的】

（1）学习离体蛙心的制作方法。

（2）观察药物对离体蛙心收缩强度和节律的影响。

【实验原理】

强心苷类药物可与心肌细胞膜上的钠钾 ATP 酶（sodium-potassium ATP enzyme，Na^+-K^+-ATPase）结合，抑制 Na^+-K^+-ATP 酶的活性，从而抑制 Na^+-K^+ 的转运。细胞内 Na^+ 逐渐增加，K^+ 逐渐减少。细胞膜上的 Na^+-Ca^{2+} 交换系统将 Na^+ 与 Ca^{2+} 交换，增加 Na^+ 流出和 Ca^{2+} 流入，从而增加细胞内 Ca^{2+}。Ca^{2+} 作用于心脏收缩蛋白，增加心肌收缩性，其正性肌力作用和负性频率作用在缺钙引起的心力衰竭中更为明显。

【实验器材】

手术器械一套、蛙板、探针、斯氏蛙心插管、蛙心夹、铁支架、烧杯、滴管、图钉、棉线、BL-422 生物机能实验系统、张力换能器等。

【实验药品】

西地兰注射液（或 5% 洋地黄溶液、0.1% 毒毛旋花苷 G 溶液）、林格液（pH7.0）、低钙林格液（其中 $CaCl_2$ 含量为常规林格液的 25%）或无钙林格液，1% 氯化钙溶液。

【实验动物】

青蛙或蟾蜍 1 只。

【实验方法】

1. **制备蛙心**　取蛙 1 只，用探针从枕骨大孔处插入，破坏大脑和脊髓，用图针仰位固定于蛙板上。剪开胸部皮肤及胸骨，暴露心脏（图 4-4-1）。

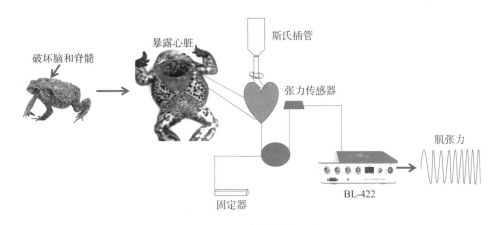

图 4-4-1　实验操作流程示意图

2. **斯氏蛙心插管**　在左主动脉下穿一条线，打一个活结。左手提起主动脉上的结扎线，右手用眼科剪刀在结扎线下方的动脉沿向心方向切一斜切口。选择合适大小的蛙心套管针，并将少量复方氯化钠注射（林格氏）液插入细长蛙心套管的开口中。当套管针的尖端到达动脉锥的底部时，应稍微缩回套管针，将尖端推向动脉锥的后部和下部以及心尖的方向。通过主动脉瓣将其插入心室腔，不要太深，以避免心室壁堵塞套管针开口。此时，可看到血液涌入套管针，导致液位随着心跳上下移动。用滴管从套筒中抽血，并用新鲜的林格溶液替换。鞘管稳定后，轻轻提起备用线，用双线将左右主动脉与插入的鞘管紧紧地绑在一起。然后将结固定在鞘管的小玻璃钩上，切断结扎线上方的血管。轻轻提起导管和心脏，清楚地看到静脉窦的位置，切除静脉窦下方的受累组织，只保留静脉窦和心脏之间的连接，让心脏分离。用复方氯化钠注射液反复冲洗心室中的残余血液，以确保套管针内的灌注液中没有残余血液，并在进行实验前保持套管针内相同的液位。

3. **连接生物信号采集系统**　将蛙心套管用试管夹固定于铁架台上，用蛙心夹在心舒期夹住心尖部，连接于换能器并与生物信号采集系统相连，待收缩稳定后开始记录。

给药及给药后的记录

记录正常的心脏活动曲线，然后按以下顺序加药物试剂，记录收缩幅度和心率变化。①换入低钙复方氯化钠注射液；②当心脏收缩显著减弱时，向套管里面加入西地兰注射液，或者 5% 洋地黄溶液，或者 0.1% 毒毛花苷 G 溶液 0.2 mL。

【实验记录与结果】

本实验主要观察给药前后心脏的收缩幅度和心率变化。将观察数据记录，并将实验组的结果计算后填入表 4-4-1 中。

表 4-4-1　强心苷对蛙心的强心作用（$\bar{x} \pm s$）

组别	例数（n）	心脏频率（次/min）	振幅（mm）
正常对照组			
低钙林格液组			
强心苷组			

【注意事项】

（1）本实验用蛙心为好，因为蟾蜍的心脏对强心苷药物敏感性低。

（2）青蛙质量最好在 50 ～ 200 g，如果过大，插管容易从心室脱离。

（3）在整个实验过程中应保持套管内液面高度不变，以保证心脏固定的负荷。

（4）为防止血液凝固堵塞蛙心管口，可在复方氯化钠注射液中加入适量的肝素抗凝血。一般用量为 1000 mL 复方氯化钠注射液中加入 2 mL 肝素注射液。

（5）结扎的时候避开静脉。

【练习题】

1. 强心苷所致心律失常最为常见的是 _____。

A. 室性早搏 　　　　　　　　　　　B. 窦性心动过缓

C. 室性心动过速 　　　　　　　　　D. 房室传导阻滞

2. 强心苷的不良反应不包括 _____。

A. 胃肠道反应 　　　　　　　　　　B. 内分泌系统反应

C. 房室传导阻滞 　　　　　　　　　D. 窦性心动过缓

3. 强心苷引起心脏房室传导阻滞时，除停用强心苷及排钾药外，最好选用 _____。

A. 阿托品 　　　　　　　　　　　　B. 氯化钾

C. 利多卡因 　　　　　　　　　　　D. 普萘洛尔

【思考题】

（1）强心苷增强心肌收缩力的特点有哪些？

（2）实验过程中，灌流量对心脏活动有何影响？

【知识拓展】

心肌细胞的动作电位时程

1. 去极化过程（0 期）　当心肌细胞接受一个阈上刺激时，膜内电位由静息状态时的 -90 mV 去极化并反极化到 +20 ～ +30 mV，构成动作电位的上升相，称为 0 期。当心室肌细胞受到刺激产生兴奋时，首先引起少量 Na^+ 离子内流，膜局部去极化。当去极化到阈电位水平（-65 mV）时，Na^+ 离子内流，使膜进一步去极化。

2. 复极化过程　当心室肌细胞去极化达到顶峰后，开始复极化过程。根据膜电位变化曲线的形状及其形成的离子机制不同，可将其可分为 4 个时期：

（1）快速复极化初期（1 期）：膜电位由 +30 mV 迅速下降至 0 mV 左右。K^+ 离子瞬时外流，引起膜电位初期的快速复极化。

（2）平台期（2 期）：表现为膜电位变化较小，电位接近于 0 mV 水平，持续 100 ～ 150 ms。Ca^{2+} 离子的内流和 K^+ 离子的外流导致。

（3）快速复极化末期（3 期）：继平台期之后，细胞膜复极化速度加快，膜内电位由 0 mv 逐渐下降到 -90 mV 的静息电位水平。历时 100 ～ 150 ms，外向 K^+ 离子流逐渐增强，超过内流的 Ca^{2+} 离子。

（4）静息期（4 期）：膜复极化完毕，膜电位恢复并稳定在 -90 mV 的静息电位水平。通过 Na^+-K^+ 泵和 Na^+-Ca^{2+} 交换作用，将内流的 Na^+ 和 Ca^{2+} 离子排出膜外，将外流的 K 离子转运入膜内，使细胞内外离子分布恢复到静息状态水平，从而保持心肌细胞正常的兴奋性。

（孙志朋）

第五节　普萘洛尔对小鼠缺氧耐受力的影响

【实验目的】

（1）学习制作缺氧动物模型的方法。

（2）评价异丙肾上腺素和普萘洛尔对小鼠缺氧耐受力的影响，并分析其作用机制。

【实验原理】

异丙肾上腺素为 β 肾上腺素受体激动药，通过激动心肌细胞上的 $β_1$ 受体使心率加快、心肌收缩力增强、心脏传导加快、心肌耗氧量增加。普萘洛尔为非选择性 β 受体阻断药，能够阻断异丙肾上腺素对心脏的作用，使心率减慢、心肌收缩力减弱、心脏传导减慢、心肌耗氧量减少，从而增强小鼠对缺氧的耐受力。使用异丙肾上腺素可制作高耗氧小鼠模型，进而观察普萘洛尔对提高缺氧耐受力的影响。

【实验器材】

电子天平、缺氧装置、秒表、鼠笼、注射器（1 mL）。

【实验动物】

小鼠，体重 22 ~ 25 g，雌雄不限。

【实验药品】

0.05% 异丙肾上腺素溶液、0.1% 普萘洛尔溶液、生理盐水、凡士林（可选）。

【实验方法】

（1）实验开始前，先将小鼠放到实验室适应环境 1 h。

（2）取适应环境结束的小鼠 3 只，称重、编号，观察小鼠正常表现后，分别随机分为甲、乙、丙三组，给药途径、剂量和给药时间见表 4-5-1。

表 4-5-1　给药途径、剂量和给药时间表

分组	第一次给药剂量（0.2 mL/10 g）	15 min 后第二次给药剂量（0.2 mL/10 g）
甲	0.05% 异丙肾上腺素溶液，皮下注射	0.1% 普萘洛尔溶液，腹腔注射
乙	0.05% 异丙肾上腺素溶液，皮下注射	生理盐水，腹腔注射
丙	生理盐水，皮下注射	生理盐水，腹腔注射

（3）第二次给药 3 min 后将小鼠分别放入 100 mL 缺氧瓶中，每瓶放 1 只，迅速塞紧瓶塞后开始计时，观察小鼠活动状态，以呼吸停止作为判断小鼠死亡的标志，确定小鼠死亡即停止计时，记录小鼠存活时间（min）。缺氧瓶装置见图 4-5-1。

（4）收集全班各组的原始数据，列表进行统计处理，计算甲、乙、丙三组小鼠平均存活时间，并对平均存活时间的差异作统计检验（表 4-5-2）。

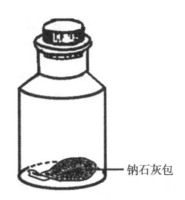

　钠石灰包

图 4-5-1　缺氧装置示意图

【实验记录与结果】

表 4-5-2　普萘洛尔对小鼠缺氧耐受力的影响实验记录表

分组	体重（g）	第一次给药		第二次给药		平均存活时间（min）
		药物	给药体积（mL）	药物	给药体积（mL）	
甲						
乙						
丙						

【注意事项】

（1）缺氧瓶必须完全密闭，必要时可用凡士林涂在瓶口增加密闭性。

（2）正确掌握小鼠腹腔注射和皮下注射的部位和方法，以免对药物吸收产生影响。

（3）观察小鼠存活时间时禁止晃动缺氧瓶，以免造成小鼠增加额外耗氧。

【练习题】

1. 异丙肾上腺素属于 _____。

A. α_1 受体激动药　　　　　　　　B. α、β 受体激动药

C. β_1 受体激动药　　　　　　　　D. β 受体激动药

2. 普萘洛尔主要通过 _____ 提高小鼠对缺氧的耐受力？

A. 阻断 β_1 受体对心脏产生抑制作用，心肌耗氧量降低

B. 阻断 β_2 受体使冠状血管收缩，机体耗氧量降低

C. 阻断 β_2 受体使支气管收缩，机体耗氧量降低

D. 阻断 M 受体使胃肠平滑肌舒张，机体耗氧量降低

3. 缺氧装置中钠石灰的主要作用是 _____。

A. 吸水　　　　　　　　　　　B. 吸收产生的 CO_2，使整个环境处于缺氧状态

C. 除去缺氧瓶中的异味　　　　D. 吸收 O_2，防止小鼠吸入过多的 O_2

【思考题】

（1）异丙肾上腺素增加心肌耗氧量的作用机制是什么？

（2）简述普萘洛尔在增强机体对缺氧耐受力作用时的利弊？

【知识拓展】

心得安——β 受体阻断药普萘洛尔的发现

　　二战结束不久，格拉斯哥大学的年轻讲师布莱克（James Black, 1924—2010）受聘成为英国帝国化学工业集团（ICI）的首批药物研究员。他对美国佐治亚州医学院的 R. 阿尔奎斯特（Raymond P Alqvist）提出的假说——体内存在 α 受体和 β 受体两种肾上腺素受体的观点深信不疑，并从 1952 年开始着手寻找 β 受体阻断剂。他花了整整十年时间探索肾上腺素和去甲肾上腺素如何与受体结合，结合之后又如何进行化学信息传递。1962 年，布莱克和他的同事成功合成第一个 β 受体阻断剂——丙萘洛尔，然而遗憾的是丙洛萘尔会使小鼠产生胸腺瘤，不能用于临床。但布莱克毫不气馁，最终合成出了不仅比丙萘洛尔更为有效且可避免致癌作用及不存在"内在拟交感活性"的药物心得安——普萘洛尔。使用普萘洛尔后，可使心率减慢，心肌收缩力和心排出量降低，冠脉血流量下降，心肌耗氧量明显减少，血压下降。如今，普萘洛尔已广泛应用于高血压、心绞痛和心肌梗死、心律失常、慢性心力衰竭及甲亢等疾病的治疗。但是，由于其可以有效减慢心率，并产生缓解焦虑的作用，1986 年已经被国际奥委会列为运动员禁药。

（叶夷露）

第五章　激素内脏药理

第一节　硫酸鱼精蛋白对肝素抗凝活性的拮抗作用

【实验目的】

（1）观察硫酸鱼精蛋白对肝素抗凝活性的拮抗作用。

（2）学习小白鼠球后静脉取血方法。

（3）学习用毛细玻管法测定凝血时间的方法。

视频 9

【实验原理】

　　肝素呈强酸性，带有大量负电荷。肝素能增强抗凝血酶Ⅲ（AT-Ⅲ）与凝血因子的亲和力，可使多种凝血因子灭活，产生迅速而强大的体内、体外抗凝作用，从而延长凝血时间。当血液接触毛细玻管后，外源性凝血系统启动，在一定时间毛细玻管折断处会出现丝状物。

　　硫酸鱼精蛋白呈强碱性，带有大量正电荷，在体内可与肝素结合成稳定的复合物，使肝素失去抗凝血能力，每 1.0 ~ 1.5 mg 鱼精蛋白可中和 100 U 肝素。

【实验器材】

　　1 mL 注射器、内径 1 mm 的毛细玻璃管、天平、小鼠笼、秒表。

【实验动物】

　　小鼠，18 ~ 22 g，雌雄不拘。

【实验药品】

　　0.0025% 肝素溶液、0.0125% 硫酸鱼精蛋白溶液、生理盐水、苦味酸。

【实验方法】

毛细玻管法

实验操作步骤如下，见图 5-1-1。

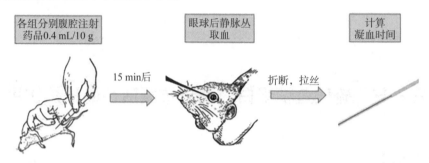

图 5-1-1　操作步骤示意图

1. **注射药物**　取小鼠 3 只，称重编号后，以苦味酸标记。腹腔注射各药品 0.4 mL/
10 g，如下所示：甲鼠注射生理盐水，乙鼠注射 0.0025% 肝素溶液，丙鼠注射 0.0025%
肝素溶液。过 15 min 后再给丙鼠腹腔注射 0.0125% 硫酸鱼精蛋白溶液 0.4 mL/10 g。

2. **取血、计算凝血时间**　各组给药 15 min 后，将各鼠分别用毛细玻璃管刺入眼
内眦部，进行一侧球后静脉丛取血，血液注满毛细玻璃管后取出，平放于桌面上，并
启动秒表计时。此后每隔 30 s ～ 1 min 将毛细玻璃管折断约 0.5 cm，并轻轻向左右方
向拉开，注意观察折断处有无丝状物出现。计算从毛细玻璃管取血到折断毛细玻璃管
出现凝血丝的时间，即为小鼠的毛细玻管法凝血时间。

【实验记录与结果】

汇集全实验室结果，计算三组小鼠所得平均凝血时间，填入表 5-1-1 中。

表 5-1-1　硫酸鱼精蛋白对肝素抗凝活性的拮抗作用

组别	药物	组别						平均凝血时间
		1组	2组	3组	4组	5组	6组	
甲	生理盐水							
乙	0.0025% 肝素							
丙	0.0025% 肝素 +0.0125% 硫酸鱼精蛋白							

【注意事项】

（1）严格控制药物注射速度，避免太快或太慢，速度力求一致，尤其鱼精蛋白注射时速度要慢。

（2）注射肝素和鱼精蛋白的注射器不能混用，以免出现沉淀。

（3）毛细玻璃管内径需均匀一致，清洁干燥。

（4）凝血时间受室温影响，实验时室温在15℃左右较为适宜。采血后的毛细玻管不宜长时间拿在手中，以免影响实验结果。

（5）毛细玻璃管插入眼内眦后，如无血液流出，可将毛细玻管轻轻旋转。

【练习题】

1. 治疗肝素过量引起出血应选用 _____。

A. VitK　　　　　　B. 鱼精蛋白　　　　　C. 阿司匹林　　　　　D. 氨甲苯酸

2. 肝素体内抗凝最常用的给药途径为 _____。

A. 口服　　　　　　B. 肌内注射　　　　　C. 皮下注射　　　　　D. 静脉注射

3. 有关肝素的抗凝血机制，下列说法正确的是 _____。

A. 直接灭活凝血因子Ⅱa、Ⅶa、Ⅸa、Ⅹa

B. 直接与凝血酶结合，抑制其活性

C. 增强抗凝血酶Ⅲ的活性

D. 拮抗 VitK

【思考题】

鱼精蛋白对肝素的抗凝活性有什么影响？两者相互影响的机制是什么？有何临床意义？

【知识拓展】

肝素的发现

1916年，Jay McLean 在寻找促凝血物质时意外发现了具有抗凝血作用的肝素。这一发现起初被导师视为"错误"，但 McLean 坚持自己的发现，并在导师的鼓励下发表了论文，从而开启了肝素在医学领域的广泛应用。这一故事告诉我们，在科学探索中，坚持与勇气是取得突破的关键。面对未知和质疑，只有坚持不懈，勇于探索，才能发现新的科学真理。

（房春燕）

第二节　胰岛素的过量反应及解救

【实验目的】

（1）观察小鼠注射过量胰岛素导致的低血糖反应，解救低血糖反应小鼠。

（2）熟练操作腹腔注射小鼠的实验方法。

【实验原理】

胰岛素是由胰岛 β 细胞分泌的一种蛋白质激素，受内源性或外源性物质如葡萄糖、乳糖、核糖、精氨酸、胰高血糖素等的刺激而分泌。胰岛素的主要生理功能是调节代谢。药用胰岛素多从猪、牛等家畜的胰腺中提取。目前也可以通过 DNA 重组技术人工合成胰岛素。胰岛素口服无效，注射给药，皮下注射吸收快。有速效、中效、长效胰岛素制剂之分。胰岛素是机体内降低血糖唯一的激素，同时又促进糖原、脂肪、蛋白质的合成。给小鼠注射过量胰岛素之后，血糖快速降低引起低血糖性休克，发生精神不安、惊厥等现象。

【实验器材】

普通天平或电子秤、1 mL 注射器、大烧杯、小鼠笼。

【实验动物】

小鼠，18 ～ 22 g。

【实验药品】

酸性生理盐水、50% 葡萄糖注射液、胰岛素溶液（2 U/mL）。

【实验方法】

实验示意图如下，见图 5-2-1。

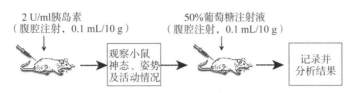

图 5-2-1　实验操作流程示意图

（1）取小鼠 3 只，编号为Ⅰ、Ⅱ、Ⅲ并进行标记，称重，Ⅰ、Ⅱ为实验组，Ⅲ为对照组。

（2）给实验组Ⅰ、Ⅱ两只小鼠腹腔注射 2 U/mL 胰岛素溶液 0.1 mL/10 g，给对照组小鼠Ⅲ注射酸性生理盐水 0.1 mL/10 g。

（3）将小鼠均置于 30 ~ 37℃ 环境下，记录下时间，注意观察并比较两组小鼠的神态、姿势及活动情况。当实验组小鼠出现明显反应时，给Ⅰ鼠腹腔注射 50% 葡萄糖注射液 0.1 mL/10 g 进行解救，Ⅱ鼠不进行解救处理。

（4）比较Ⅰ、Ⅱ、Ⅲ鼠的活动情况，进行记录并分析结果。

【实验记录与结果】

将上述结果记录于表 5-2-1 中，并进行分析。

表 5-2-1　胰岛素的过量反应观察及解救

标号	体重（g）	药物及剂量	用药后反应

【注意事项】

（1）小鼠在实验前 18 ~ 24 h 禁食。

（2）酸性生理盐水配置：将 10 mL 0.1 mol/L 盐酸溶液加入 300 mL 生理盐水中，调节其 pH 值在 2.5 ~ 3.5。

（3）2 U/mL 胰岛素溶液配置：宜使用普通胰岛素，因普通胰岛素显效快实验现象明显；并应使用酸性生理盐水进行稀释至所需浓度，因胰岛素在酸性环境下才有效应。

（4）实验温度：夏季可为室温，冬季最好将注射胰岛素的小鼠放在 30 ~ 37℃ 环境中保温，因温度过低，低血糖反应出现较慢。

【练习题】

1. 胰腺主要是由 _____ 和血管共同组成，共同调节着营养的平衡。

A. 外分泌细胞、内分泌细胞、导管细胞

B. 外分泌细胞、内分泌细胞、腺细胞

C. 泡心细胞、β 细胞、导管细胞

D. 泡心细胞、β 细胞、腺细胞

2. 静脉胰岛素输注或重症监护 ICU 患者，住院期间血糖应如何监测？

A. 三餐前 + 睡前监测

B. 每 4 h 监测一次

C. 全天 7 点监测

D. 每 1 ~ 2 h 监测一次

3. 腹腔注射的正确顺序是 _____。

①抓取小鼠，使其腹部朝上头部略向下垂

②抓紧背部皮肤使腹部皮肤紧绷，于两大腿根连线与腹中线交叉点一侧约 1 cm 位置刺入皮下

③针尖通过腹肌后，抵抗力消失，回抽无回流物，缓慢推入药物

④在皮下平行腹中线推进针头 3 ~ 5 mm，再以 45° 角向腹腔内刺入

A. ①②③④   B. ①②④③   C. ①③②④   D. ①④②③

【思考题】

（1）胰岛素的药理作用和临床用途有哪些？

（2）胰岛素过量会引起什么不良反应？如何抢救？

【知识拓展】

人工合成胰岛素的诞生

1965 年 9 月 17 日，中国科学家人工合成了具有生物活力的结晶牛胰岛素，它是第一个在实验室中用人工方法合成的蛋白质，稍后美国和联邦德国的科学家也完成了类似的工作。1956 年初，党中央发出了"向科学进军"的号召，随后，中华人民共和国第一个中长期科技发展规划《1956—1967 年科学技术发展远景规划》正式出炉。1958 年 6 月，中国科学院上海生物化学研究所的会议室里，在所

长王应睐的主持下，九位科学家一起讨论所里下一步要研究的重大课题。有人提出了一个大胆的设想——要"合成一个蛋白质"。1958 年底，人工合成胰岛素项目被列入 1959 年国家科研计划，并获得国家机密研究计划代号"601"，也就是"60 年代第一大任务"。然而，在此之前，除了制造味精之外，我国还从未制造过任何形式的氨基酸，而氨基酸正是蛋白质合成的基本材料。在如此极端困难的条件下，一切都要从零开始。在科研基础十分薄弱、设备极其简陋的年代，历经七年的不懈攻关，这项凝聚着中国科学院生化所、有机所和北京大学三家单位百名科研人员心血的项目，终于获得成功。中国科学家成功合成胰岛素，标志着人类在探索生命奥秘的征途中迈出了关键的一步，它开辟了人工合成蛋白质的时代，在生命科学发展史上产生了重大影响，也为我国生命科学研究奠定了基础。

（方　辉）

第三节　阿司匹林拮抗血栓形成的作用

【实验目的】

（1）熟练掌握动静脉旁路血栓形成的实验方法。

（2）分析血栓形成的原因以及阿司匹林抗血栓的作用机制。

（3）评价阿司匹林对血栓形成的拮抗作用。

【实验原理】

细胞中的花生四烯酸以磷脂的形式存在于细胞膜中。多种刺激因素均可激活磷脂酶 A，使花生四烯酸从膜磷脂中释放出来。游离的花生四烯酸在环加氧酶（cyclooxygenase，COX）的作用下转变成前列腺素 G_2（PGG_2）和前列腺素 H_2（PGH_2）。在环氧酶体内有两种同工酶：COX-1 与 COX-2，两者都作用于花生四烯酸产生相同的代谢产物 PGG_2 和 PGH_2。血小板内有血栓素 A_2（TXA_2）合成酶，可将 COX 的代谢产物 PGH_2 转变为 TXA_2，有强烈的促血小板聚集作用。血管内皮细胞含有前列环素（PGI_2）合成酶，能将 COX 的代谢产物 PGH_2 转变为 PGI_2，它是至今发现的活性最强的内源性血小板抑制剂，能抑制 ADP、胶原等诱导的血小板聚集和释放。

阿司匹林使血小板内环氧化酶第 530 位丝氨酸残基乙酰化，破坏酶的活性中心，阻止血栓素（TXA_2）的合成。由于血小板本身无合成环氧化酶的功能，因此阿司匹林对血小板环氧化酶活性的抑制作用是不可逆的。阿司匹林抑制血管内皮中的环氧化酶，使前列环素（PGI_2）合成减少。正常情况下 TXA_2 合成量远远超过 PGI_2 合成量。小剂量阿司匹林对血管内皮细胞环氧化酶的抑制作用较弱，几乎不影响 PGI_2 的合成，却能明显抑制血小板环氧化酶，使 TXA_2 的合成大部分受抑制；大剂量阿司匹林对 PGI_2 和 TXA_2 合成均有很强的抑制作用。另外，阿司匹林还可影响血小板颗粒内容物的释放，如 5- 羟色胺、PF_4 等，并且抑制血小板的释放反应。

本实验采用聚乙烯管连接大鼠一侧颈总动脉和对侧颈外静脉形成旁路血流。在聚乙烯管中段放置一段丝线，当血流通过时，血小板接触丝线或铜圈粗糙面即贴附于丝线上，发生脱颗粒反应，释放内容物 ADP、5-HT 等活性物质，促进血小板聚集于丝线表面，先形成血小板血栓，后有纤维蛋白形成，网罗大量红细胞则形成红色血栓。通过检测血栓干重或湿重、血栓形成抑制率可探讨血栓形成机制和评价抗血栓形成和溶栓药物的药效和作用机制研究。

作用原理如图 5-3-1 所示：

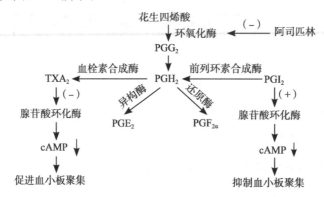

图 5-3-1　阿司匹林拮抗血栓形成作用原理图

【实验器材】

大鼠手术台、手术器械 1 套、动脉夹、聚乙烯管（外径为 1.6 mm 及 1.3 mm 两种）、4 号手术丝线、1 mL 注射器、2 mL 注射器。

【实验对象】

大鼠，250 ~ 300 g，雄性。

【实验药品】

3% 戊巴比妥钠溶液、2% 阿司匹林溶液、肝素生理盐水溶液（50 IU/mL）。

【实验方法与步骤】

（1）每组取大鼠2只，称重，按甲、乙编号。每天清晨灌胃给药，甲鼠给予阿司匹林5 mL/kg，乙鼠给予生理盐水5 mL/kg，一共给药5 d。

（2）末次给药1 h后，将甲、乙两鼠各腹腔注射3%戊巴比妥钠（1.5 mL/kg）麻醉后，仰卧位固定于大鼠手术台上，分离气管，插入一塑料套管（气管分泌物多时可通过此套管吸出），分离右颈总动脉和左颈外静脉。

（3）剪一根长约6 cm的4号手术丝线，称重后放入聚乙烯管中，以肝素生理盐水溶液充满聚乙烯管，当聚乙烯管的一端插入左颈外静脉后，由聚乙烯管精确地注入肝素生理盐水（1 mL/kg）抗凝，然后将聚乙烯管的另一端插入右颈总动脉。

（4）打开动脉夹后，开始计时，血液从右颈总动脉流至聚乙烯管内，返回左颈外静脉。开放血流15 min后中断血流，迅速取出丝线称重，总重量减去丝线重即得血栓湿重。

【实验记录与结果】

计算甲、乙两鼠所测得的血栓湿重，填入表5-3-1中。

表5-3-1 阿司匹林的抗血栓形成作用

组别	药物	剂量（mL）	血栓湿重/g
甲鼠	阿司匹林		
乙鼠	生理盐水		

【注意事项】

（1）对照组和给药组动物体重要严格配对。

（2）聚乙烯管经拉细后才能插入血管，管端径口大小应严格控制。注意聚乙烯管插入血管后勿使血管扭曲。

（3）手术过程要求迅速，技术操作熟练，肝素用量要合适。手术应在15 min内完成。

（4）注意及时吸出气管分泌物，保持呼吸畅通。

【练习题】

1.阿司匹林防止血栓形成的机制是 _____。

A. 直接对抗血小板聚集　　　　　B. 减少 TXA2 生成

C. 降低凝血酶活性　　　　　　　D. 激活抗凝血酶 E，增强维生素 K 的作用

2. 大鼠灌胃容量通常为 _____mL。

A. 0.2 ~ 0.8　　　　B. 1 ~ 4　　　　C. 5 ~ 6　　　　D. 6 ~ 7

3. 阿司匹林用于抗血栓形成时常用 _____。

A. 小剂量　　　　B. 中剂量　　　　C. 大剂量　　　　D. 极量

【思考题】

（1）阿司匹林对大鼠血栓的形成有何影响？

（2）它影响血栓形成的机制是什么？有何临床意义？

【知识拓展】

"柳树中走出的妙药"——阿司匹林

公元前 4 世纪，"医学之父"希波克拉底用柳树叶煮汤治头痛，让孕妇咀嚼柳树皮以缓解生产时的疼痛并减轻后续发热症状。1763 年，人们发现用柳树皮粉可以治疗疟疾引起的发热。直到 1829 年，活性成分水杨苷被成功提取，并被发现其在体外有很强的药理活性，为日后研发阿司匹林奠定基础。由于从柳树中提取水杨酸的过程比较复杂，1859 年科学工作者第一次人工合成了水杨酸，并再次验证该药物具有良好的解热镇痛作用。但是，随着临床上的广泛应用，人们发现水杨酸可导致胃溃疡、呕吐等不良反应。1897 年，德国拜耳公司的科学家霍夫曼因其父亲身患风湿病，而长期服用水杨酸不良反应非常大，故对化合物结构进行改良，合成了乙酰水杨酸。通过动物试验和临床试验，人们发现乙酰水杨酸的解热镇痛作用比水杨酸更好，而且不良反应小。1899 年，德国拜耳公司将乙酰水杨酸注册专利，并命名为阿司匹林。在 20 世纪 40 年代，美国医生克莱文在给扁桃体发炎的患者使用相对大剂量的阿司匹林时，发现患者有流血过多的现象，从而发现了阿司匹林有抗血栓的作用，可于心肌梗死的预防。

勤劳智慧的中华民族在上古时期便有神农尝百草的传说，我国的医药学先贤也在中医四大经典著作之一《神农本草经》、东方药学巨典《本草纲目》中记载了柳树的药用价值，其活性成分即为水杨酸。《神农本草经》载，"柳之根、皮、枝、叶均可入药，有祛痰明目，清热解毒，利尿防风之效，外敷可治牙痛。"李时珍《本草纲目》载，"柳叶煎之，可疗心腹内血、止痛，治疗疮；柳枝和根皮，

煮酒，漱齿痛，煎服制黄疸白浊；柳絮止血、治湿痹，四肢挛急。"

（赵　超）

第四节　缩宫素对豚鼠离体子宫平滑肌的作用

【实验目的】

（1）观察不同剂量缩宫素对离体子宫的作用。

（2）学习离体子宫平滑肌样本的制备方法。

【实验原理】

缩宫素是一种多肽类激素，化学结构见图 5-4-1。不同剂量的缩宫素对子宫的作用不同。小剂量缩宫素使宫底节律性收缩，利于胎儿娩出。大剂量则引起强直性收缩，利于产后止血。雌激素提高子宫对缩宫素的敏感性，孕激素则降低此敏感性。

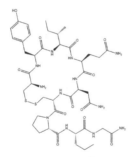 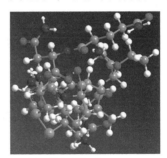

缩宫素分子结构　　　　　　　缩宫素 3D 结构

图 5-4-1　缩宫素化学结构示意图

人体子宫平滑肌胞质膜存在特异性的缩宫素受体，并且在妊娠期的不同阶段，缩宫素受体表达的密度会有所不同。缩宫素发挥宫缩作用的基础是与缩宫素受体结合。缩宫素作用于子宫平滑肌细胞 G 蛋白偶联受体，可激活磷脂酶 C（PLC），使三磷酸肌醇（IP_3）生成增多，随后 Ca^{2+} 向子宫平滑肌细胞内大量转移，从而增强子宫平滑肌的收缩力，并使其收缩频率增加。

【实验器材】

BL422 生物机能实验系统、超级恒温水浴、肌力换能器、浴管、试管、L 形钩、铁支架、双凹夹、螺旋夹、弹簧夹、万能夹、烧杯、氧气、针头、培养皿、缝线、缝针、剪刀、镊子、1 mL注射器。

【实验动物】

雌性未孕豚鼠，体重300 g左右。

【实验药品】

0.005 U/mL缩宫素溶液、0.5 U/mL缩宫素溶液、乐氏液、0.5 mg/mL己烯雌酚。

【实验方法】

1. **实验前用药**　实验前24～36 h，腹腔注射0.5 mg/mL己烯雌酚0.5 mg（促使其进入动情期）。

2. **信号记录系统连接**　打开BL422生物机能实验系统，连接换能装置，调节生物信号，将恒温水浴温度调整在（37.0±0.5）℃，向浴槽中加入乐氏液，以能够浸没标本为宜。

3. **制备标本**　取豚鼠1只，击头致死，迅速剖腹，找出子宫，在子宫两角相连处下端剪断，取出子宫，置于盛有乐氏液的培养皿中，仔细剪除子宫周围的结缔组织和脂肪组织，将子宫两角相连处剪开。

4. **系统调试**　取其中一角，用线结扎其两端，一端固定于L型钩上。放入盛有15 mL乐氏液的浴槽内，另一端与肌力换能器连接，调节静息张力1～2 g，通氧、稳定10 min。描记一段正常曲线。

5. **加药**　① 0.005 U/mL缩宫素溶液0.1 mL，观察子宫平滑肌节律性收缩，作用稳定后冲洗；② 0.5 U/mL缩宫素溶液0.1 mL，观察子宫平滑肌强直性收缩。

6. **观察与记录**　加药后，观察平滑肌的张力变化并记录。

【实验记录与结果】

将实验记录和结果填入表格中，具体见表5-4-1。

表5-4-1　缩宫素对子宫平滑肌的影响

药物	浓度（U/mL）	剂量体积（mL）	给药时间	平滑肌张力（g）	备注
缩宫素	0.005	0.1			
缩宫素	0.5	0.1			

【注意事项】

（1）制作标本时动作要轻，切勿过度牵拉子宫，操作时间越短越好。

（2）浴槽内乐氏液的量要恒定。

（3）浴槽内的工作温度偏低时（32～35℃），标本能保持更长的工作时间；温度偏高时（37～39℃），标本更敏感，但工作时间要缩短。

【练习题】

1. 缩宫素的给药方式不包括 _____。

A. 肌注　　　　　　B. 口服　　　　　　C. 静注　　　　　　D. 喷雾

2. 缩宫素的药理作用不包括 _____。

A. 收缩子宫　　　　B. 排乳　　　　　　C. 收缩血管平滑肌　D. 催产

3. 缩宫素的禁忌证不包含 _____。

A. 产道异常　　　　B. 胎位不正　　　　C. 前置胎盘　　　　D. 初产妇

【思考题】

（1）孕期用药的注意事项有哪些？

（2）孕妇可选用的药物种类有哪些？

【知识扩展】

缩宫素恰到好处的应用

缩宫素可以称得上是产科的"神药"之一，在防治产后出血中发挥重要作用。20世纪90年代，2名英国产妇因注射缩宫素导致死亡，经调查发现与缩宫素注射引起的心血管系统并发症有关。南非也报道了2例缩宫素引起的产妇死亡事件，其中一例是急诊剖宫产中静脉注射缩宫素直接导致心脏骤停。因此，缩宫素虽然为产妇带来福音，但若使用不当仍存在安全隐患。

缩宫素，又名催产素，最初是从猪、牛等垂体后叶提取得来的，然而由于生产工艺限制，提取纯度不高，容易引起过敏性休克等严重不良反应。1953年美国科学家文森特·迪维尼奥（Vincent du Vigneaud）通过人工合成缩宫素，使其生产工艺迎来巨大变革。人工合成缩宫素的出现是医药发展史上划时代的成果，文森特·迪维尼奥也因此获得诺贝尔奖，其制备工艺简单，但杂质含量仍然较高。

1984 年随着多肽药物固相合成法的发明，99% 纯度的缩宫素横空出世，其发明者罗伯特也因此摘得诺贝尔生理学或医学奖。

（王　琳）

第五节　利尿药对动物尿量的影响

【实验目的】

（1）观察呋塞米对麻醉家兔的利尿作用和特点。

（2）了解膀胱插管法和输尿管插管法的急性利尿实验方法。

视频 10

【实验原理】

尿液的生成包括肾小球滤过、肾小管分泌和重吸收三个过程，而影响肾小管重吸收的过程，可引起明显的尿量改变。

呋塞米通过作用于肾小管髓袢升支粗段，竞争性地抑制 Na^+-K^+-$2Cl^-$ 共同转运子的作用，抑制 Na^+、Cl^- 的重吸收，进一步影响肾脏对尿液的稀释和浓缩功能而产生强大的利尿作用。正常状态下，持续大剂量给予呋塞米，可使成年人 24 h 的排尿量达到 50 ~ 60 L。

【实验器材】

BL-422 生物机能实验系统、兔手术台、导尿管、膀胱漏斗（连接橡皮管、小滴管）、静脉输液装置、注射器、计滴器、婴儿秤、手术刀、组织剪、眼科剪、血管钳、量筒、弹簧夹等。

【实验动物】

家兔，2.0 ~ 2.5 kg。

【实验药品】

20% 乌拉坦溶液、生理盐水、1% 呋塞米溶液。

【实验方法】

1. **麻醉**　取家兔 1 只，实验前禁食不禁水 12 ~ 24 h，将家兔称重后，于实验前 0.5 h 用生理盐水 30 mL/kg 灌胃，增加水负荷。自耳缘静脉缓慢注入 20% 乌拉坦溶液（1.0 g/kg），待动物麻醉后仰卧位固定于兔手术台上。

2. **手术**　下腹部剪毛，从耻骨联合向上作长为 3 ~ 5 cm 的正中切口，沿腹白线打开腹腔，暴露膀胱，将膀胱翻出腹外。仔细分离两侧输尿管，在分离出的输尿管下方穿一条线，将膀胱上翻用线结扎膀胱颈部以阻断其流向尿道的通路，然后在膀胱腹侧面靠近膀胱尖避开血管作一长约 1 cm 的切口，放入已充满水的套管（套管连有小滴管，膀胱漏斗应对准输尿管口），结扎固定。将滴管尖端向下并低于膀胱，松开夹在套管橡皮管上的弹簧夹，可见尿液滴出，引出的尿液应滴在记滴器的接触点上，通过记滴装置记录尿滴或直接记录尿量毫升数。最后将膀胱回纳腹腔（切勿扭曲），用盐水纱布覆盖切口，如图 5-5-1 所示。

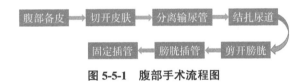

图 5-5-1　腹部手术流程图

3. **安装调节实验装置及记录**　按程序打开计算机及 BL422 生物机能实验系统，单击菜单实验项目栏，在"实验项目"菜单下选择"泌尿系统实验"的"影响尿生成的因素"项，测试尿液记滴、时间描记及刺激符号等记录是否良好。待尿液恒定后收集记录正常每分钟尿液滴数或 5 min 内总尿量（表 5-5-1）。

4. **给药**　耳缘静脉注入 1% 呋塞米 0.5 mL/kg（5 mg/kg），连续收集并记录给药后每分钟尿液滴数或每 5 min 尿量，持续 20 min。

【实验记录与结果】

表 5-5-1　呋塞米对家兔尿量的影响

药物	排尿情况（尿滴／分及尿量 mL/5 min）				
	给药前	给药后			
		0 ~ 5 min	5 ~ 10 min	10 ~ 15 min	15 ~ 20 min
5 mg/kg 呋塞米					

【输尿管插管法】

将兔麻醉后仰卧固定于手术台上,从耻骨联合向上沿中线作长为 3 ~ 5 cm 的切口,沿腹白线打开腹腔,暴露膀胱,在膀胱底两侧找出并仔细地分离两侧输尿管,在其下方各穿两根线,一线结扎近膀胱端,在结扎线上方用眼科剪朝肾脏方向剪一小口插入聚乙烯导管,用另一线结扎固定。将两根导管的游离端一并放入量筒内,收集记录尿量。注意:家兔输尿管纤细脆弱,插管时动作应细致轻巧,切忌将输尿管插穿。

【注意事项】

（1）分离两侧输尿管时要注意避开血管进行钝性分离。

（2）插管前膀胱漏斗及连接的橡皮管应提前注满水。

【练习题】

1. 呋塞米主要的不良反应是 _____。

A. 心律失常　　　　B. 电解质紊乱　　　　C. 血压升高　　　　D. 精神失常

2. 既可治疗高血压又可治疗尿崩症的药物是 _____。

A. 呋塞米　　　　B. 依他尼酸　　　　C. 氢氯噻嗪　　　　D. 螺内酯

3. 对磺胺药过敏的患者可选用的高效能利尿药是 _____。

A. 呋塞米　　　　B. 依他尼酸　　　　C. 布美他尼　　　　D. 氢氯噻嗪

4. 螺内酯可用于治疗 _____。

A. 高钾血症　　　　B. 肝硬化伴水肿　　　　C. 心律失常　　　　D. 心绞痛

5. 伴有高脂血症的高血压患者可选用的利尿药是 _____。

A. 呋塞米　　　　B. 吲达帕胺　　　　C. 维拉帕米　　　　D. 氢氯噻嗪

【思考题】

（1）呋塞米的临床应用及注意事项有哪些?

（2）呋塞米为何被称为高效能利尿药?

【知识拓展】

呋塞米被世界反兴奋剂机构列为违禁药品之一

在体育竞技中如举重、跆拳道、武术、格斗等需要按体重分级别进行比赛的项目中，运动员为了减轻体重，在称量体重前使用利尿剂，通过大量地排尿，快速减轻体重，以参加低级别的比赛；也有运动员服用了其他兴奋剂，在兴奋剂检查前，服用呋塞米来增加尿量，冲淡尿液中的兴奋剂的浓度，来避免被查出尿中的违禁物质。2020 年 12 月 18 日，中国反兴奋剂中心公布一则兴奋剂违规处理结果，知名山地车运动员马皓因在 2019 年 12 月 1 日于赛外被测出禁用物质呋塞米，被处以禁赛两年的处罚。业余马拉松运动员杨庆超在 2024 年鹤壁马拉松赛中以 2 h 31 min 38 s 的成绩获得全马男子季军，赛后检测显示，使用了利尿剂呋塞米，将面临全面调查。诸如此类的案例还有很多，服用兴奋剂虽然可以提高运动成绩，但有悖于比赛公平公正的原则，同时也可对人体造成危害，如呋塞米可造成脱水而降低运动能力，可引起血液缺钾而发生疲劳、痉挛等症状。因此呋塞米被世界反兴奋剂机构（WADA）明确列为违禁药品之一，禁止运动员在赛内和赛外使用。

（王　琳）

第六节　氢化可的松对二甲苯所致小鼠耳郭肿胀的影响

【实验目的】

（1）观察氢化可的松对小鼠耳廓毛细血管通透性的影响，分析其抗炎作用特点。

（2）了解实验性炎症的发生机理。

视频 11

【实验原理】

炎症的基本病理改变是变性、渗出和增生。糖皮质激素具有很强的抗炎作用，能抑制各种炎症的发生。急性炎症初期，能增加血管的紧张性，减轻充血，降低毛细血管的通透性，以此减轻渗出、水肿；同时抑制白细胞浸润及吞噬反应，减少各种炎症因子的释放，从而缓解红、肿、热、痛等症状。糖皮质激素通过基因组和非基因组效应发挥抗炎和免疫抑制作用。经典的基因组效应是由糖皮质激素的细胞质受体介导的，它可以上调细胞核中的抗炎蛋白表达或抑制促炎转录因子从细胞质转入细胞核（图 5-6-1）。非基因组效应可能是由糖皮质激素的膜受体所介导的。将二甲苯涂于鼠耳部，可致局部细胞损伤，促使组胺、缓激肽等致炎物质释放，造成耳部急性炎性水肿，炎症部位明显肿胀，体积增大。本实验通过称重鼠耳重量，可知肿胀程度，从而观察药物的抗炎作用。

糖皮质激素抗炎作用机制（基因组效应）如图 5-6-1 所示：

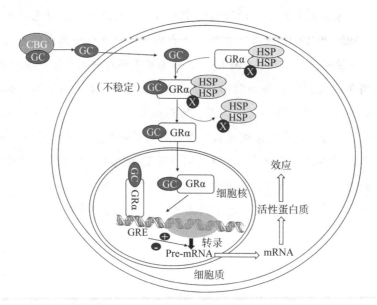

图 5-6-1　糖皮质激素类药物的基因调节机制

注：CBG：皮质类固醇结合球蛋白，GC：糖皮质激素类，GR：糖皮质激素受体，HSPs：热激蛋白，GRE：糖皮质激素受体元件。

【实验器材】

电子天平、1 mL 注射器、鼠笼、移液枪、粗剪刀、8 mm 直径打孔器、精密天平。

【实验药品】

0.5% 氢化可的松注射液、二甲苯、生理盐水、苦味酸。

【实验动物】

雄性小鼠，25 ~ 30 g。

【实验方法】

（1）取小鼠 2 只，称重，苦味酸标记。甲鼠腹腔注射 0.5% 氢化可的松注射液 0.05 ~ 0.1 mL/10 g，乙鼠腹腔注射等容量生理盐水。30 min 后，两鼠左耳前后两面用移液枪均匀涂布二甲苯 0.05 ~ 0.1 mL 致炎，右耳不涂药物作为自身空白对照。

（2）2 h 后将小鼠脱臼处死，沿耳廓线剪下双耳，分别用 8 mm 直径打孔器在左右两耳相同部位打下耳片，用精密天平分别称重。每鼠左右两耳片的重量差即为肿胀程度，并按以下公式计算肿胀度和肿胀率。

$$肿胀度 = 左耳片重 - 右耳片重$$

$$肿胀率（\%）= \frac{左耳片重 - 右耳片重}{右耳片重} \times 100\%$$

【实验记录与结果】

汇总全实验室的实验结果，将对照鼠与给药鼠的肿胀程度进行统计学处理，数据以 $\bar{x} \pm s$ 表示，做组间 t 检验（表 5-6-1）。

表 5-6-1　药物对二甲苯所致小鼠耳部炎症的作用

分组	药物	鼠数	平均肿胀度（mg）	平均肿胀率（%）
甲	氢化可的松			
乙	生理盐水			

【注意事项】

（1）本实验宜在室温进行，温度过低，影响实验结果。

（2）涂擦二甲苯应均匀，剂量准确，涂擦部位应与取下的耳片相吻合。

（3）小鼠耳廓炎症模型还可用含 2% 巴豆油的 70% 乙醇溶液代替。

（4）打孔器应锋利，一次性取下耳片，各组打耳片的部位必须一致。

【练习题】

1. 关于小鼠腹腔注射，不正确的是 _____。

A. 给药时小鼠腹部朝上，头部高位

B. 给药时小鼠腹部朝上，头部下倾

C. 进针部位不宜太高，刺入不能太深，以免伤及内脏

D. 取 30° 角将针头从一侧下腹部向头端刺入腹部

2. 按动力学特点的药物分类，氢化可的松属于 _____。

A. 超长效糖皮质激素　　　　　　　　B. 长效糖皮质激素

C. 中效糖皮质激素　　　　　　　　　D. 短效糖皮质激素

3. 下列不属于糖皮质激素药理作用的是 _____。

A. 抗休克作用　　　　　　　　　　　B. 免疫抑制与抗过敏的作用

C.抗炎作用 D.抗风湿作用

【思考题】

（1）糖皮质激素对抗急性炎症的作用机制是什么？

（2）氢化可的松局部用药和全身用药的效果有何差异？为什么？

【知识拓展】

糖皮质激素是把双刃剑

　　事物矛盾双方既统一又对立，促使事物不断地由低级向高级发展，该理论在糖皮质激素的双重性中得到完美的体现。人体自身分泌的糖皮质激素能在应激反应中有效地抵抗有害刺激的伤害。作为治疗药物，它具有抑制免疫应答、抗炎、抗毒、抗休克作用，在临床上应用广泛。但是同时它有许多的不良反应，比如长期不规范使用糖皮质激素可造成医源性库欣综合征，表现出向心性肥胖，同时还可造成血压高、血糖代谢紊乱、对胃肠黏膜的损害、骨质疏松等。糖皮质激素对下丘脑-垂体有负反馈调节作用，如果长期大量使用糖皮质激素，可抑制腺垂体，使ACTH的分泌长期减少，使患者肾上腺皮质功能减退，甚至萎缩，此时骤然停用，可造成严重后果，危及生命。因此，糖皮质激素必须规范使用，而不是滥用。作为医学院校的学生，应当努力打好基础，具备扎实的理论功底，在未来工作中树立良好的医德医风，始终将患者安危放在第一位，做一名有责任有担当，集医术和医道于一体的医务工作者。

（赵　超）

第七节　硫酸镁、生大黄对小鼠肠管推进作用的影响

【实验目的】

（1）观察硫酸镁、生大黄对小鼠肠管运动的影响。

（2）掌握小鼠的解剖方法及小肠全长的测量方法。

视频12

【实验原理】

硫酸镁属于渗透性泻药，口服后在胃肠道解离成 Mg^{2+} 和 SO_4^{2-}，由于其脂溶性低，在胃肠道难吸收，在肠道内形成高渗压，吸附肠道外的水分进入肠道并阻止肠道内水分吸收，扩张肠道，从而促进肠道蠕动而致泻，兼有促进胆汁分泌的作用（图 5-7-1）。生大黄是一味具有很强的泻下作用的中药，其泻下攻积的作用可用于湿热引起的积滞便秘，其所含的蒽醌类物质能够刺激肠道，引起肠蠕动增加，并抑制肠内水分吸收，促进排便。本实验通过灌胃给药，观察硫酸镁和生大黄对小鼠肠管推进作用的影响。

炭末推进法是一种常用的实验方法，用来评估药物对小鼠胃肠蠕动的影响。此法通过观察炭末在小鼠胃肠道内移动的距离来评价药物效应。

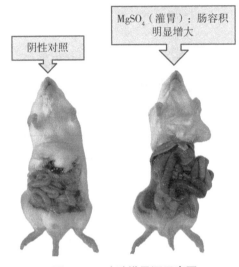

图 5-7-1　硫酸镁导泻示意图

【实验器材】

手术剪、眼科剪、眼科镊、直尺、灌胃针头、注射器（1 mL）、棉球、天平。

【实验动物】

小鼠，体重 23 ~ 25 g，雌雄不拘。

【实验药品】

硫酸镁（15%）、活性炭粉、生大黄水煎液（1 g/mL）、羧甲基纤维素钠。

【实验方法】

1. **实验准备** 取禁食 24 h 小鼠 6 只，称重、苦味酸标记，均分成 3 组，备用。

2. **给药** 分别用混 5% 炭末的硫酸镁溶液、混有 5% 炭末的生大黄溶液和混有 5% 炭末的生理盐水，按 0.2 mL/10 g 体重分别给 3 组小鼠灌胃给药，并记录灌胃完成的时间。

3. **给药后处理** 给药后 20 min 颈椎脱臼处死小鼠，打开腹腔分离肠系膜，剥离胃肠道，剪取上端至幽门，下端至回盲部的肠管，置于托盘中拉成直线，测量肠管长度作为"小肠全长"，测量自幽门至炭末前沿的距离作为"炭末推进距离"。

4. **计算小肠推进率** 小肠推进率（%）＝ 炭末推进距离 / 小肠全长 ×100%。

【实验记录与结果】

记录实验结果，根据公式计算出各组小鼠的小肠推进率，计入表 5-7-1 的表格中，也可收集全实验室统计结果进行统计分析。

表 5-7-1 硫酸镁、生大黄对小鼠肠推进作用的影响

组别	鼠号	体重（g）	药物剂量	小肠全长(cm)	炭末推进距离(cm)	推进率(%)
硫酸镁组						
生大黄组						
生理盐水组						

【注意事项】

（1）给药至处死动物的时间必须准确，以免时间不同造成实验误差。

（2）实验动物体重越相近越好，平均体重在 23 ~ 25 g 的小鼠，肠管比较粗大，易于操作。

（3）肠容积变化观察，可以上、下段结扎，称取重量，以定量化。

（4）肠推进距离观察的着色剂，可用 10% 活性炭溶液或其他颜料（1% 卡红溶液），0.2 mL/10 g 体重灌胃。

（5）打开小鼠腹腔时需用镊子将腹部皮毛提起剪开，避免剪开时破坏肠道。

【练习题】

1. 硫酸镁的临床应用不包括 _____。

　A. 便秘　　　　　B. 食物中毒　　　　　C. 子痫　　　　　D. 高血压的常规用药

2.生大黄的泻下作用与哪一类泻药相似？

A. 容积性泻药　　　　　　　　　　B. 渗透性泻药

C. 刺激性泻药　　　　　　　　　　D. 润滑性泻药

3.关于泻药的描述错误的是 _____。

A. 临床主要用于功能性便秘

B. 老人、妊娠及经期女性不宜应用剧烈的泻药

C. 巴比妥类药物中毒时首选硫酸镁导泻

D. 排出毒物宜选用盐类泻药

【思考题】

（1）临床上使用的泻药有哪几类？作用机制和临床适应证分别是什么？

（2）除了炭末法，还可以用哪些方法观察小鼠的肠推进性作用？

【知识拓展】

泻药也会滥用吗？

　　泻药具有良好的增加胃肠蠕动、促进排便的作用，临床上用于功能性便秘的短期缓解。便秘指的是大便次数每周少于三次，伴排便困难、粪便干燥。但是近年来许多人会长期服用泻药达到排毒和减肥的功效，造成了泻药滥用的趋势。其实有些泻药如果长期服用对我们的健康存在非常大的影响，例如果导片，或者中药中具有泻下作用的大黄、番泻叶、芦荟等，这些刺激性泻药如果长期服用可能会出现非常严重的不良反应。首先，如果经常用此类泻药来加速排便，会导致肠道自主蠕动的功能越来越弱，最后可能会使便秘症状越来越严重，更有甚者，还会出现不服用泻药就不能自主排便的情况；其次，长期服用此类泻药还会由于频繁腹泻导致电解质紊乱；如果是为了减肥而吃此类泻药，会由于肠蠕动过快食物无法吸收，出现营养不良的现象；更为严重的是，长期吃此类泻药可能会导致肠道黑变病，还可能会诱发肠道肿瘤。当然，如果是膳食纤维类的容积性泻药或是含油脂的润滑性泻药，其不良反应就相对较轻。因此，药物滥用不仅仅指精神类药物。作为医学院校的学生，掌握相关的药理学知识对提升我们的临床合理用药能力具有非常重要的意义。我们在临床使用药物时，一定要根据患者的情况合理选用，以科学、严谨、实事求是的态度照护患者，为健康中国战略的推进贡献力量。

（王雅娟）

第八节　药物对小鼠凝血时间的影响

视频 13

【实验目的】

（1）学习测定小鼠凝血时间的简易方法。

（2）观察促凝药和抗凝药对小鼠凝血时间的影响。

【实验原理】

血液凝固指血液从流动的液体状态变成不能流动的胶冻状凝块的过程，可分为内源性凝血途径和外源性凝血途径。内源性凝血途径指参与凝血的因子全部来自血液系统，通常因血液与带负电荷的异物表面（如胶原纤维）接触而启动。外源性凝血途径指由组织因子（tissue factor，TF）启动的凝血过程。血液凝固的关键过程是血浆中的纤维蛋白原转变为不溶的纤维蛋白。凝血时间是血液离开血管体外发生凝固的时间，一般以血液流出血管至出现纤维蛋白细丝所需的时间。

本实验通过给小鼠注射止血敏溶液、肝素溶液和生理盐水，观察促凝药和抗凝药对小鼠凝血时间的影响。酚磺乙胺（止血敏）可增强血小板聚集性和黏附性，并可降低毛细血管通透性，使血管收缩，起到促凝血作用；肝素可促进血液中的抗凝血酶Ⅲ（antithrombin Ⅲ，AT Ⅲ）的作用，发挥体内和体外的强大抗凝作用。

【实验器材】

1 mL 注射器、玻璃毛细管、载玻片、针头、秒表、棉球。

【实验动物】

小鼠，体重 18 ~ 22 g，雌雄不拘。

【实验药品】

2.5% 的止血敏溶液、50 U/ml 肝素溶液、生理盐水、苦味酸溶液。

【实验方法】

1. **实验准备**　取小鼠 3 只，称重、苦味酸标记。

2. **给药**　1 号鼠腹腔注射 2.5% 酚磺乙胺溶液 0.2 mL/10 g（5 mg/10 g），2 号

鼠腹腔注射 50 U/mL 肝素溶液 0.2 mL/10 g（10 U/10 g），3 号鼠腹腔注射生理盐水 0.2 mL/10 g。

3. **取血**　给药 30 min 后，以毛细管给小鼠做眼眶内眦穿刺取血，当血液充满整根毛细管时，立即启动秒表开始计时。眼眶内眦穿刺为刺破小鼠眼底静脉丛取血，具体方法如图 5-8-1 所示。

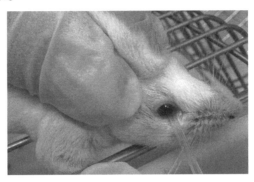

图 5-8-1　小鼠眼眶内眦穿刺取血示意图

4. **测定凝血时间**　每隔 30 s 折断毛细玻璃管一小段（5 ~ 10 mm），观察有无血凝丝出现，直至两段玻管之间有血凝丝连接时，表示血液已经凝固。计算从计时开始到出现血凝丝的时间，即为凝血时间。

5. **玻片法测定凝血时间**　以一小截毛细管做眼眶内眦穿刺后迅速取血，于清洁干燥的玻片的两端各滴血一滴，并立即启动秒表，每隔 15 s 用干燥针头拨动血液一次，到针头能挑起纤维蛋白丝为止。另一滴血供复验，同上法记录凝血时间。

6. **统计分析结果**　汇聚全实验室试验结果，计算酚磺乙胺组、肝素组和生理盐水组小鼠的平均血凝时间，并作均数之间差异的显著性检测，从而得出关于酚磺乙胺和肝素对小鼠凝血时间的影响的结论。

【实验记录与结果】

记录全实验室的实验结果，并进行统计分析。具体见表 5-8-1。

表 5-8-1　药物对小鼠凝血时间的影响

组别	小鼠只数	剂量	血凝时间均值 ± 标准差		P 值	
			毛细管法	玻片法	毛细管法	玻片法
酚磺乙胺组						
肝素组						
生理盐水组						

【注意事项】

（1）凝血时间可受温度影响，本实验室温最好在 15℃左右。

（2）毛细管的内径最好为 1 mm，并均匀一致。

（3）折断毛细管的动作宜轻，折断后向两边慢慢拉开两端的毛细管，检查中间有无纤维蛋白细丝（血凝丝）出现。

【练习题】

1. 肝素的临床应用不包括 _____。

A. DIC 早期　　　　　B. 心肌梗死　　　　　C. 体外抗凝　　　　　D. 早产儿出血

2. 香豆素类药物的抗凝机制是 _____。

A. 抑制血小板聚集

B. 竞争性抑制肝脏合成凝血因子 Ⅱ、Ⅶ、Ⅸ、Ⅹ

C. 拮抗血液中的凝血因子

D. 激活纤溶酶 _____。

3. 直接输血时，每 100 mL 血中加入 2.5% 的枸橼酸钠溶液 _____。

A. 5 mL　　　　　B. 10 mL　　　　　C. 15 mL　　　　　D. 20 mL

【思考题】

（1）影响凝血时间的主要因素有哪些？

（2）目前临床上常用的促凝药和抗凝药主要作用于血液凝固的哪些环节，在临床上都有哪些常见的用途？

【知识拓展】

凝血酶和血凝酶

凝血酶和血凝酶看起来差不多，实际上完全不一样，给药途径千万别搞错。凝血酶与血凝酶二者均能起到止血作用，临床应用广泛。然而，虽然二者名称相似，但用法完全不同。凝血酶是局部止血药，可以生理盐水配制成溶液喷雾或以干粉喷洒于创面，或口服、灌注用于消化道止血，严禁血管内、肌内或皮下注射，否则可能导致广泛性血栓形成而危及生命。血凝酶（又名立止血、巴曲酶）是一种速效、长效、安全的止血药。可静脉注射、肌内注射、皮下注射，也可局部用药。凝血酶为机体本来就存在的凝血因子之一，而血凝酶为非凝血因子，有类凝血酶作用，易在体内降解而不致引起弥散性血管内凝血（DIC），两者作用相似，给药途径不同。差之毫厘，谬以千里。作为医护工作者，我们直接为人的生命和健康服务，每个环节、每个细节都要严谨细致，容不得有半点的马虎和侥幸，因为我们 1% 的疏忽却有可能会给患者带来 100% 的危害。

（王雅娟）

第九节　喷托维林的镇咳作用观察

【实验目的】

（1）学习小鼠氨水引咳法。

（2）观察镇咳药喷托维林的镇咳作用。

【实验原理】

镇咳药可分为中枢性镇咳药和外周性镇咳药。喷托维林为胺基酯类衍生物，具有中枢和外周性镇咳作用，吸收后可轻度抑制支气管内感受器及传入神经末梢，减弱咳嗽反射，并可使痉挛的支气管平滑肌松弛，减低气道阻力，具有镇咳作用，可缓解各种原因引起的干咳。

咳嗽为机体的保护性反射之一，当呼吸道受到异物刺激时会诱发咳嗽反射。动物实验中常用的引咳法包括氨水引咳法、枸橼酸引咳法和辣椒素引咳法。浓氨水是一种较强的化学刺激物，可刺激呼吸道感受器引发咳嗽。本实验采用氨水引咳法，通过小鼠吸入氨水气雾后，刺激呼吸道感受器诱发咳嗽反射，并在此基础上观察喷托维林对小鼠的镇咳作用（图 5-9-1）。

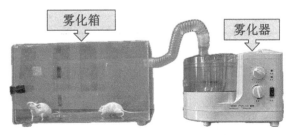

图 5-9-1　氨水引咳法实验装置示意图

【实验器材】

小鼠灌胃针头、雾化器、雾化箱、秒表、1 mL 注射器。

【实验动物】

小鼠，体重 18 ~ 22 g，雌雄不拘。

【实验药品】

浓氨水（分析纯）、生理盐水、枸橼酸喷托维林片、桔梗水煎剂、苦味酸溶液。

【实验方法】

1. **实验准备**　取健康合格小鼠 6 只，称重、标记，随机均分成 3 组，即生理盐水组、喷托维林组和桔梗组。

2. **给药**　各组小鼠分别灌胃给药 0.2 mL/10 g 体重，并记录给药时间。

3. **镇咳作用观察**　灌胃后 30 min 将小鼠放入密闭的雾化箱中，将 10 mL 的浓氨水放入雾化器的储液杯中密封，开启雾化器 15 s，观察各组小鼠出现典型咳嗽动作（腹肌收缩，同时张大嘴，有时可有咳嗽声）的次数，记录小鼠自氨水雾化吸入到出现咳嗽的时间（咳嗽潜伏期）。

【实验记录与结果】

记录各组小鼠的咳嗽潜伏期和咳嗽次数，计入表 5-9-1 中。

表 5-9-1　镇咳药的镇咳作用观察

组别	鼠号	体重（g）	剂量（mg/kg）	咳嗽潜伏期（s）	咳嗽次数
喷托维林组					
桔梗组					
生理盐水组					

【注意事项】

（1）观察小鼠的咳嗽动作必须仔细。

（2）雾化器中每次放入 10 mL 的浓氨水，需将前一次的残液倒尽后再重新加入。

（3）喷雾时最好将实验组和对照组动物交叉进行。

【练习题】

1. 以下镇咳药不属于中枢性镇咳药的是 _____。

A. 可待因　　　　　B. 那可丁　　　　　C. 右美沙芬　　　　　D. 喷托维林

2. 中枢性镇咳药适用于 _____。

A. 感冒咳嗽　　　　B. 痰多咳嗽　　　　C. 无痰干咳　　　　D. COPD 咳嗽

3. 下列镇咳药作用强度的比较，正确的是 _____。

A. 喷托维林＞苯丙哌林＞可待因　　　　B. 可待因＞苯丙哌林＞喷托维林

C. 苯丙哌林＞喷托维林＞可待因　　　　D. 苯丙哌林＞可待因＞喷托维林

【思考题】

（1）镇咳药物可通过哪些环节起到镇咳作用？

（2）中枢性镇咳药的优缺点有哪些？临床上如何合理应用？

【知识拓展】

"止咳药"右美沙芬被"列管"！

2024 年 5 月 7 日，国家药监局、公安部、国家卫生健康委发布关于调整精神药品目录的公告，将右美沙芬、含地芬诺酯复方制剂、纳呋拉啡、氯卡色林列入第二类精神药品目录，7 月 1 日起正式实施。右美沙芬，一般指氢溴酸右美沙芬类止咳药物，其镇咳作用与可待因相仿，但无镇痛作用，适用于感冒、急慢性支气管炎、咽喉炎、支气管哮喘及其他上呼吸道感染引起的少痰咳嗽。尽管右美沙芬在临床治疗上具有显著的优点，但随着该药物的广泛使用，滥用与依赖的现象也逐渐在人群中显现。右美沙芬超剂量服用时，可引起欣快、幻觉等症状，而且随时间增加，极易成瘾，长期滥用会对大脑造成损伤、出现精神错乱。因此，右美沙芬存在被滥用的风险。

近年来，右美沙芬的管理一直在不断强化。2021 年 12 月，国家药监局发布公告，将右美沙芬口服单方制剂由非处方药转为处方药。公告还对药品说明书进行了修订，增加了过量服用右美沙芬可能产生的症状如精神错乱、兴奋、紧张等，删除了长期服用无成瘾性和耐受性的表述。2022 年 12 月 1 日，国家药监局制定的《药品网络销售禁止清单（第一版）》开始施行，右美沙芬被网络禁售。2023 年，国家药监局、公安部、国家邮政局发布关于进一步加强复方地芬诺酯片、右美沙芬口服单方制剂等药品管理的通知，要求通知相关部门严格控制药品生产量、加强药品生产环节监管、加强寄送渠道查验、严厉打击违法违规行为等事宜。对于右美沙芬管理上的一系列变化体现了我国对人民健康的重视，作为医药专业的学生，我们应认识到医药工作的重要性和特殊性，在培养自身医疗水平的同时还要增强法律意识，避免药物滥用，为未来的医疗工作做好充分准备。

（王雅娟）

第六章　化疗药物药理

第一节　链霉素的毒性反应及解救

【实验目的】

观察硫酸链霉素阻断神经肌肉接头的毒性反应及氯化钙的解救作用。

视频 14

【实验原理】

链霉素大剂量肌内注射给药或给药速度过快有神经肌肉接头阻断作用，引起心肌抑制、血压下降、四肢无力以及呼吸抑制。主要机制为：链霉素与突触前膜钙结合部位结合，抑制钙离子中和突触前膜负电荷的作用，阻止钙离子参与的乙酰胆碱的释放，使乙酰胆碱释放减少，出现四肢无力和呼吸抑制等症状。使用新斯的明或者钙剂可对抗链霉素引起的肌松作用。

【实验器材】

1 mL、2 mL 注射器，婴儿秤。

【实验动物】

豚鼠（300 g 左右）。

【实验药品】

25% 硫酸链霉素、5% 氯化钙溶液，苦味酸溶液。

【实验方法】

1. **称重、标记**

取豚鼠 2 只，用苦味酸标记、编号，称重。观察动物的呼吸体位、步态、四肢肌张力等。

2. 给药与观察

甲鼠：25% 硫酸链霉素肌内注射，给药剂量为 0.24 mL/100 g，注射 15 min 后观察动物反应（呼吸快慢、体位、四肢肌张力）。如果出现呼吸抑制，腹腔注射 5% 氯化钙溶液进行抢救，给药剂量为 1 mL/100 g，观察其能否恢复。

乙鼠：25% 硫酸链霉素肌内注射，给药剂量为 0.24 mL/100 g，注射 15 min 后观察动物反应（呼吸快慢、体位、四肢肌张力），观察其能否恢复，如图 6-1-1 所示。

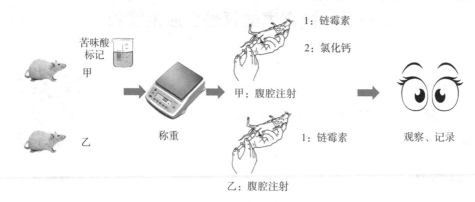

图 6-1-1 实验操作步骤示意图

【实验记录与结果】

实验记录与结果见表 6-1-1。

表 6-1-1 链霉素的毒性反应及氯化钙的解救作用观察

动物	药物处理	呼吸情况	体位	四肢肌张力
甲	用链霉素前			
	用链霉素后			
	用氯化钙后			
乙	用链霉素前			
	用链霉素后			

【注意事项】

（1）链霉素肌内注射后毒性反应较慢，一般给药后 10 min 出现反应，并逐渐加重。

（2）$CaCl_2$ 溶液预先抽取好待用，用过的注射器冲洗干净。

（3）第一次 $CaCl_2$ 解救效果不好，可再次给予半量。

【练习题】

1.链霉素属于哪一类抗生素?

A.喹诺酮类　　　　B.大环内酯类　　　　C.氨基糖苷类　　　　D.四环素类

2.下列属于链霉素药物不良反应的是 _____。

A.二重感染　　　　B.神经肌肉麻痹　　　C.肝损伤　　　　　　D.骨髓抑制

3.下列用于链霉素毒性解救的是 _____。

A.新斯的明　　　　B.盐酸阿托品　　　　C.硫酸镁　　　　　　D.生理盐水

【思考题】

通过本实验观察到链霉素的哪些毒性反应? 为什么?

【知识拓展】

链霉素的故事

青霉素的发现极具神奇和戏剧性, 开启了抗生素的新时代。链霉素发现的意义, 一点也不亚于青霉素, 但它的发现是经过精心设计、长期努力的结果。"结核病"与黑死病齐名, 因患者咳嗽咯血、面色苍白, 称为白色瘟疫, 也被称为"会传染的癌症"。结核病是由一种结核分枝杆菌复合群引起的慢性传染性疾病。美国罗格斯大学土壤学教授塞尔曼·瓦克斯曼, 注意到肺结核菌在土壤中会被迅速杀死, 并在土壤中寻找能杀死结核菌的微生物, 分离出一种对结核分枝杆菌有致命作用的物质——链霉素, 结核病的大肆泛滥才得以中止。瓦克斯曼首先将链霉素用于治疗肺结核患者, 因此获得 1952 年诺贝尔生理学或医学奖。

（张朋飞）

第二节　头孢拉定血药浓度的检测

【实验目的】

（1）利用高效液相色谱仪检测血药浓度, 观察头孢拉定血药浓度的变化。

（2）掌握药代动力学参数的计算方法和临床意义。

【实验原理】

视频 15

血浆半衰期（half-life，$t_{1/2}$）指血药浓度下降一半所需要的时间，反映了药物在体内消除速度的快慢，以 $t_{1/2}$ 表示。临床常用药物中多数药物在体内按一级动力学消除，消除速率与瞬时药物浓度成正比，即单位时间内药物浓度按照恒定比例消除，其血药浓度（对数值）- 时间曲线为直线。按照零级动力学消除的药物，其血药浓度（对数值）- 时间曲线为抛物线，属于非线性动力学消除。零级消除动力学是由于体内消除药物的能力达到饱和所致，血药浓度 - 时间曲线为直线，通过药物血药浓度的测定可计算出血浆半衰期等重要的药动学参数。

头孢拉定（cefradine）是 1972 年研究成功的第一代半合成头孢类抗菌药物，其适应证为用于敏感菌导致的各种呼吸道、泌尿生殖道及皮肤软组织感染等。除注射剂外，头孢拉定可制成多种口服制剂，包括头孢拉定干混悬剂、头孢拉定片、头孢拉定胶囊和头孢拉定颗粒。

【实验器材】

离心机、离心管、胶头滴管、注射器、手术器材一套、高效液相色谱仪。

【实验动物】

大鼠，体重 250 ~ 300 g，雌雄不拘。

【实验药品】

注射用头孢拉定、头孢拉定对照品、甲醇、乙腈、磷酸、磷酸氢二钠和磷酸二氢钾、0.9% 氯化钠注射液、超纯水。

【实验方法】

1. **动物处理**　取体重 250 ~ 300 g 大鼠，禁食不禁水 12 h 后，受试期间用统一标准餐。眼眦取血 1 mL，5 min 后静脉注射头孢拉定（0.2 g/kg），分别于给药后 5 min、35 min 等各眼眦取血 1 mL，所有血样放置于采血管，静置 15 min 以上，6000 r/min，离心 10 min，分离血清。

2. **样品制备**　分别取 300 μL 血清并加入 450 μL 的甲醇和 450 μL 乙腈，将样品涡旋离心 5 min 后，在 4000 rpm、4 ℃ 条件下离心 10 min，取上清过滤即得。

3. 色谱条件设置 采用 OSAKASODA CAPCELL PAK C_{18}（4.6 mm × 250 mm，5 μm）色谱柱；流动相 A 为磷酸盐缓冲液（0.02 mol/L 磷酸二氢钾溶液并用磷酸溶液调节 pH 值至 3.0），流动相 B 为甲醇；梯度洗脱：0 ～ 2.5 min（3% ～ 3%B）→ 2.5 ～ 11 min（3% ～ 25%B）→ 11 ～ 13 min（25% ～ 40%B）→ 13 ～ 16 min（40%B）→ 16 ～ 19 min（40% ～ 80%B）→ 19 ～ 20 min（80% ～ 3%B）→ 20 ～ 30 min（3%B）；流速为 1.0 mL/min，检测波长为 220 nm，进样量 10 μL，柱温 30℃（图 6-2-1）。

4. 对照品制备 精密称定头孢拉定对照品适量，加流动相 A 溶解，制成含 60 μg/mL 的溶液，作为对照品溶液。

5. 数据处理及分析 以外标法进行定量计算，测得血药浓度 - 时间数据，用 3p87 药动学程序，在微机上进行房室拟合，得药动学参数。

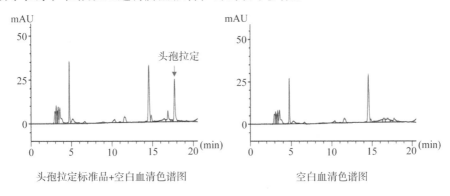

图 6-2-1　色谱图

【实验记录与结果】

记录实验结果，根据公式计算出用药后 5 min 和用药后 35 min 时头孢拉定的血药浓度、$t_{1/2}$。具体见表 6-2-1。

表 6-2-1　头孢拉定血药浓度和血浆半衰期测定

取样时间	血样（mL）		血清（mL）	甲醇（mL）	乙腈（mL）		上清液（mL）	峰面积	浓度（mg/mL）
给药前	1	离心	0.3	0.45	0.45	离心	0.9		
给药后 5 min	1		0.3	0.45	0.45		0.9		
给药后 35 min	1		0.3	0.45	0.45		0.9		

【注意事项】

（1）采血时，需剪去大鼠胡须，避免溶血。

（2）采血管注意不能剧烈晃动，避免溶血。

（3）离心时，离心管的放置注意配平。

（4）流动相 A 和 B 配置后需要过滤，清除不溶性杂质，防止阻塞色谱柱。

（5）流动相 A 和 B 过滤后需要超声去除气泡，以防影响结果。

【练习题】

1. 属于第一代头孢菌素是 _____。

A. 头孢他啶　　　　　B. 头孢拉定　　　　　C. 头孢曲松　　　　　D. 头孢呋辛

2. 使用时需进行治疗药物监测的抗菌药物是 _____。

A. 头孢克洛　　　　　B. 阿莫西林　　　　　C. 万古霉素　　　　　D. 克拉霉素

3. 服用磺胺类药物时加服 $NaHCO_3$ 的目的是 _____。

A. 增强抗菌效果　　　　　B. 促进药物吸收

C. 抑制药物排泄　　　　　D. 碱化尿液，增加磺胺类药物在肾小管的溶解度

【思考题】

（1）抗菌药物的血药浓度监测有何意义？临床上哪些抗菌药物在使用时需要监测血药浓度？

（2）不同患者，给药剂量相同而血药浓度不同，可能的原因有哪些？

【知识拓展】

庆大霉素——我国自主研发的抗生素

庆大霉素作为第一个中国自主研发的抗生素，是中国人的骄傲，也因其造成耳聋等严重不良反应而饱受诟病。我国中国科学院福建维生素研究所的王岳教授在 1965 年从福州湖泥中分离出一株小单孢菌，发现它产生的抗生素正是 Gentamicin，并在 1969 年生产用于临床，当时正值新中国成立 20 周年大庆、"中共九大"召开之际，故取名为"庆大霉素"。庆大霉素弥补了青霉素、链霉素的不足，而且过敏反应发生率低，在 20 世纪七八十年代应用十分广泛。但随着庆大霉素的广泛使用，人们发现庆大霉素存在明显的耳毒性，能够导致永久性耳聋。2005 年春晚的经典节目"千手观音"的演员中就有许多是因为使用此类药物（包括庆大霉素、链霉素、卡那霉素）导致的药物性耳聋。庆大霉素虽然曾经辉煌也饱受诟病，但它至今仍然在临床上用于痢疾、肠炎等疾病以及败血症等严重感染

的治疗。抗生素是科技创新的结晶，它的发现和应用源于卓越的科学家们的积极探索和大胆尝试。

（王　蕾）

第三节　注射剂的溶血实验

【实验目的】

视频 16

（1）认识溶血现象，掌握溶血实验体外试管法的基本操作。

（2）掌握家兔心脏采血的方法及红细胞悬液的制备方法。

【实验原理】

溶血性指药物制剂经血管给药时，对全身产生的毒性，为临床前安全性评价的组成部分。药物的原形及其代谢物、辅料、有关物质及理化性质（如 pH 值、渗透压等）均有可能引起溶血性的发生，因此注射剂在临床应用前应研究其使用后引起的局部和（或）全身毒性，以提示临床应用时可能出现的毒性反应、毒性靶器官、安全范围。溶血反应指红细胞膜被破坏或出现多数小孔，或由于极度伸展致使血红蛋白从红细胞流出的反应；凝集是一种血清学反应，指颗粒性抗原与相应抗体结合，在有电介质存在的条件下，出现肉眼可见的凝集小块。

本实验取一定量的枸橼酸咖啡因注射液加到 2% 兔血生理盐水中，在一定时间范围内，观察溶血和凝集反应情况，验证注射剂的安全性。

【实验器材】

兔固定器、磅秤、离心机、水浴锅、试管、试管刷、烧杯、试管架、离心管、移液枪、吸头、10 mL 注射器。

【实验动物】

家兔，体重 1.5 ~ 3.0 kg，雌雄不拘。

【实验药品】

蒸馏水、生理盐水、枸橼酸咖啡因注射液。

【实验方法】

1. **实验准备**　取家兔 1 只，称重备用。

2. **家兔心脏采血**　家兔背位固定（或助于用左右手分别捉住兔的后肢和前肢，将兔右侧卧位于桌角），在左胸第 2 ~ 4 肋间剪毛一块，用碘酒和酒精消毒。然后用配有 7 号针头的 10 mL 注射器，在心跳最明显处作穿刺。针头刺入心腔，即有血液流入注射器（或边穿刺边抽）。采血完毕，迅速将针头拔出，使心肌上穿孔容易愈合。

3. **红细胞悬液的制备**　取家兔 1 只，自心脏采血 10 mL，立即置于用生理盐水预先荡洗过的烧杯中；用生理盐水清洗过的试管刷，轻微搅拌去除纤维蛋白；将血移入含有 5 ~ 10 mL 生理盐水的离心管中，混匀后以 2500 r/min 转速离心 5 min，弃去上清液，如此方法用生理盐水反复洗 3 ~ 4 次至上清液呈无色透明为止。将洗涤好的红细胞用生理盐水配制成 2% 的细胞悬液，备用。

4. **药物体外溶血测定**

5. **结果判定**

（1）全溶血：溶液澄明红色，管底无红细胞残留（图 6-3-1 中 7 号管）。

（2）部分溶血：溶液澄明或棕色，管底有少量红细胞残留。

（3）无溶血：红细胞全部下沉，上层液体无色澄明（图 6-3-1 中 1 ~ 6 号管）。

（4）凝集：不溶血，红细胞在试管底部凝集，振摇后细胞不能分散。

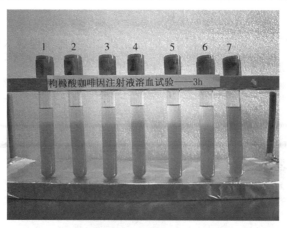

图 6-3-1　枸橼酸咖啡因注射液溶血试验结果示意图

6. **结论**

（1）在 0.5 h 出现部分溶血、全溶血，或出现凝集反应的制剂，不能静脉内用药。

（2）在 3 h 不出现溶血和凝集反应的制剂，判断为溶血试验符合规定。

【实验记录与结果】

观察 0 h、0.25 h、0.5 h、0.75 h、1 h、2 h、3 h 时的溶血试验结果，计入表 6-3-1 的表格中。

表 6-3-1 溶血试验设计

项目	试管号						
	1	2	3	4	5	6	7
供试药液（mL）	0.1	0.2	0.3	0.4	0.5		
生理盐水（mL）	2.4	2.3	2.2	2.1	2.0	2.5	
蒸馏水（mL）							2.5
2% 红细胞悬液（mL）	2.5	2.5	2.5	2.5	2.5	2.5	2.5
结果							

注：6 号管为空白对照组，7 号管为阳性对照组；结果以"+"表示溶血、"−"表示不溶血。

【注意事项】

（1）家兔的心脏一般在第 2 ~ 4 肋间，要在心室的位置进针，针尖进入心室，会有血液喷射到针管内，此时需仔细观察，一旦有血液进入针管，就停止进针，然后慢慢抽血。

（2）受试药物为出厂浓度，不要稀释。

（3）试管要洁净干燥。

（4）接触血液的烧杯和试管一定要用生理盐水润洗。

【练习题】

1. 患者发生溶血反应时，排出的尿液呈浓茶色或酱油色，主要因为尿中含 _____。

A. 胆红素　　　　　B. 红细胞　　　　　C. 血红蛋白　　　　　D. 淋巴液

2. 溶血反应时指红细胞在遇到某些因素时发生 _____。

A. 红细胞凝集　　B. 红细胞破裂　　C. 红细胞变形　　D. 红细胞增生

3. 家兔心脏采血的位置是 _____。

A. 1 ~ 2 肋间　　B. 3 ~ 4 肋间　　C. 5 ~ 6 肋间　　D. 2 ~ 6 肋间

【思考题】

（1）药物制剂的哪些因素会引起溶血？

（2）临床上发生溶血反应时应采取哪些措施？

【知识拓展】

药源性免疫性溶血性贫血

　　药源性免疫性溶血性贫血（drug-induced immune hemolytic anemia，DIIHA）是药物临床应用过程中合并的一种罕见并发症（发病率约为 1/1000000/ 年），常常漏诊[1]。DIIHA 通常会导致严重不良后果，包括多脏器功能衰竭甚至死亡。头孢曲松是一种广谱的第三代头孢类抗生素，在临床上广泛应用于治疗各种细菌感染，临床上曾出现头孢曲松引起的 DIIHA 及多例溶血反应[1, 2]。有文献报道，对于儿童、老年和有基础疾病及免疫功能较差的患者，头孢曲松有致严重的免疫性溶血的可能[3]。头孢曲松引起溶血的机制是形成免疫复合物：静脉给药后红细胞中可出现头孢曲松 IgM 抗体，该抗体进而与头孢曲松或其代谢产物形成免疫复合物，此复合物与红细胞膜上的特异性靶蛋白结合，激活补体系统，破坏红细胞，导致红细胞破裂，最终引起严重的溶血反应。由这种抗体激活补体系统引发的溶血通常是血管内溶血。因此，对儿童、老人和有基础疾病的患者建议临床谨慎使用头孢曲松，且密切观察患者临床症状。

（邹莹莹）

第四节　注射剂的热原检查

【实验目的】

（1）学习用家兔检查注射剂内热原的方法和判断标准。

（2）掌握家兔肛温检测的方法。

【实验原理】

　　热原又称为致热原，主要来自细菌的代谢产物。中草药含有有利于细菌生长繁殖的淀粉、糖、蛋白质等成分，如果在提取过程中在空气中暴露的时间过长，则容易被细菌污染而产生热原。含热原的输液注入人体约 0.5 h 后，患者会出现寒战、高热、出汗和恶心呕吐的症状，严重者出现昏迷、休克，甚至危及生命的现象。家兔法是一种体内热原试验法，其原理是依据家兔对热原的反应与人类相似，该方法通过将供试品注入家兔耳缘静脉，在规定时间内多次测量动物体温，以观察体温变化，从而评价供试品是否存在诱发机体发热反应的潜在可能性，此法也是我国药典规定的热原检查法。

本实验以临床常用的 25% 或 50% 葡萄糖注射液（其他注射液也可）为供试药品，观察其静脉注射后是否会对家兔的体温产生影响。

【实验器材】

兔固定盒、磅秤、肛门温度计、10 mL 注射器及针头、镊子、酒精棉球和干棉球。

【实验动物】

家兔，体重 1.7 ~ 3.0 kg，雌雄不拘（雌兔应排除妊娠）。

【实验药品】

供试品（25% 或 50% 葡萄糖注射液或其他注射液）、液体石蜡。

【实验方法】

实验操作步骤如下，见图 6-4-1。

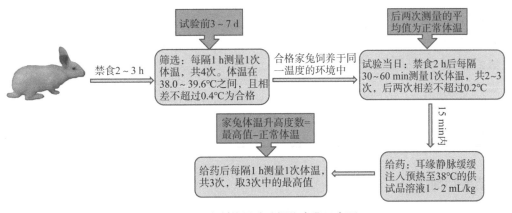

图 6-4-1 家兔热原试验操作步骤示意图

1. 试验前准备 在做热原检查前 1 ~ 2 d，供试家兔应尽可能处于同一温度的环境中。凡未经使用于热原检查的家兔，应在试验前 7 d 内预测体温，进行挑选。于禁食 2 ~ 3 h 后，用肛温表每隔 1 h 测量体温 1 次（测温时应尽可能避免对家兔刺激，温度计插入的深度应相同，一般约 5 cm），共 4 次。若 4 次体温都在 38.0 ~ 39.6℃ 范围内，且最高最低体温差数不超过 0.4℃的家兔方可供试验用。

2. **检查法**　试验当日家兔禁食 2 h 后，用肛门温度计每隔 30 ~ 60 min 测家兔体温 1 次，共 2 ~ 3 次，末两次体温之差不得超过 0.2 ℃，即以这两次体温的平均值作为该兔的正常体温。正常体温应在 38.0 ~ 39.6 ℃ 内，各兔间的温差不得超过 1 ℃。取适用的家兔 3 只，在测定其正常温度后 15 min 内，自耳缘静脉缓缓注入预热到 38 ℃规定剂量的供试品溶液 1 ~ 2 mL/kg，然后每隔 1 h 按前法测体温 1 次，共 3 次。以 3 次体温中最高的一次减去正常体温，即为该兔体温的升高度数。

【实验记录与结果】

记录家兔的肛温测量结果，填入表 6-4-1 中。

表 6-4-1　注射剂的热原检查

检查日期		室温		检查者	
检查名称		理化性状和含量		批号	
兔号	1	2	3	4	5
体重					
第 1 次测量					
第 2 次测量					
平均体温					
注射供试品时间					
第 1 次测量					
第 2 次测量					
第 3 次测量					
注射前后温差					
检查结论					

【结果判断】

（1）在 3 只家兔中，如果体温升高均在 0.6 ℃以下，并且 3 只家兔的体温升高总数在 1.4 ℃以下，应认为供试品符合规定。

续表

（2）如 3 只家兔中仅有 1 只体温升高 0.6 ℃或以上；或 3 只家兔体温升高均在 0.6 ℃以下，但总数达到 1.4℃或以上，应另取 5 只家兔复试。复试时，在 5 只家兔中，体温升高 0.6 ℃或以上的兔数不超过 1 只，并且初、复试合并 8 只家兔的体温升高度数不超过 3.5 ℃时，均应认为供试品符合规定。

（3）在初试 3 只家兔中，体温升高 0.6℃或以上的家兔数超过 1 只时；或在复试的 5 只家兔中，体温升高 0.6℃或以上兔数超过 1 只；或在初、复试合并 8 只家兔的体温升高总数超过 3.5 ℃时，均应认为供试品不符合规定。

【注意事项】

（1）热原检查法是一种绝对方法，没有标准品同时进行试验比较，是以规定动物发热反应的程度来判断的。影响动物体温变化的因素较多，因此必须严格按照要求的条件进行试验。

（2）试验用的注射器、针头及一切与供试品接触的器皿，应置 250 ℃的烘箱中加热 30 min 或在 180 ℃的烘箱中加热 2 h，除去热原。

（3）给家兔测温或注射时动作应轻柔，以免引起动物挣扎而使体温波动。测温时，在肛门温度计的水银头上涂以液体石蜡，轻轻插入肛门 5 cm 深，测温时间至少 1.5 min，每兔各次测温最好用同一温度计，且测温时间相同，以减少误差。

（4）本实验记述的方法主要供教学试验之用，其他事项可参阅药典。

（5）可以在供试品中加入适量伤寒 - 副伤寒菌苗，或自制的非灭菌葡萄糖液，使学生观察到阳性结果。

【练习题】

1. 注射剂的热原检查采用 _____。

A. 鲎试剂法 　　　B. 家兔法 　　　C. 凝胶吸附法 　　　D. 超滤法

2. 下述关于注射剂质量要求的表述错误的是 _____。

A. 无菌 　　　　　　　　　　　B. 无色

C. 无热原 　　　　　　　　　　D. pH 值要与血液的 pH 值相等或接近

3. 热原的主要成分是 _____。

A. 异性蛋白 　　　B. 脂多糖 　　　C. 胆固醇 　　　D. 磷脂

【思考题】

（1）热原检查对家兔有何要求？试验中须注意什么？

（2）注射剂中的热原由哪些途径产生？如何去除？

【知识拓展】

警惕注射剂热原反应！

　　注射剂中热原的产生是多方面的，如从原料中带入、从配制注射剂的用具或容器中带入、从注射剂的溶媒中带入、在制备过程中污染等，需要从包装材料、注射用水、原辅料、生产设备、制备过程等多个环节进行严格控制和管理，以减少热源的产生和污染。临床上在进行静脉滴注大量输液时，如果药液中含有热原，患者会在 0.5～1 h 内出现冷战、高热、出汗、昏晕、呕吐等症状，高热时体温可达 40 ℃，严重者甚至可休克，这种现象称为热原反应。据不完全统计，目前在中国上市的中药注射液约有百余种，这些注射液当中，也有部分不良反应案例，监管部门也对相关中药注射液的使用进行收紧与限制，如 2022 年 1 月 11 日，国家药监局宣布，自即日起停止莲必治注射液在我国的生产、销售、使用，注销药品注册证书。已上市销售的产品，由药品上市许可持有人负责召回。因此，药品生产企业需要严格控制药品质量，确保药品安全有效；监管部门也应加强对药品的监管，及时发现并处理存在质量问题的药品，保障公众用药安全。作为医药学专业的学生，无论今后从事的是药品生产还是临床使用的相关工作，都需要警惕注射剂的热原反应，保障人民群众的用药安全。

（邹莹莹）

第五节　多柔比星体外抑制肿瘤细胞生长的作用

【实验目的】

（1）利用 MTT 法观察多柔比星对体外肿瘤细胞生长的抑制作用。

（2）掌握应用 MTT 法进行细胞生长检测的实验方法。

【实验原理】

多柔比星又名阿霉素（结构式如图 6-5-1 所示），是一种抗肿瘤药，其作用机理是嵌入肿瘤细胞 DNA，干扰转录和复制过程，导致 DNA 损伤和细胞周期停滞，最终诱导细胞死亡。抗瘤谱较广，对多种肿瘤均有作用，对各种生长周期的肿瘤细胞都有杀灭作用，属周期非特异性药物。临床上用于治疗急性白血病、淋巴瘤、乳腺癌、肺癌、膀胱癌等恶性肿瘤。

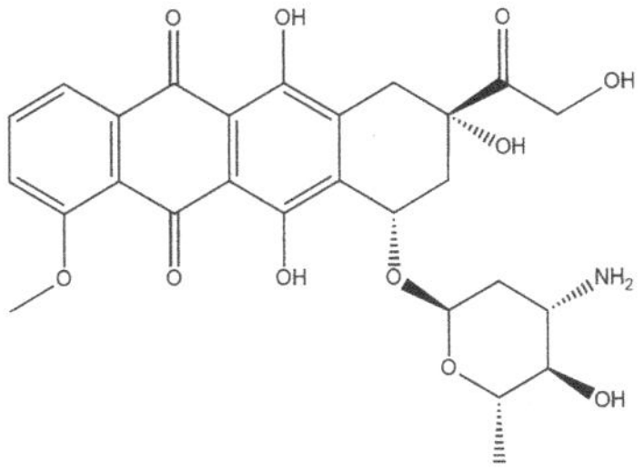

图 6-5-1　多柔比星的化学结构

MTT〔3-(4,5-二甲基噻唑-2-基)-2,5-二苯基四氮唑溴盐〕是一种黄色四唑盐，可以被活细胞中的线粒体脱氢酶还原为紫色的甲酰胺。MTT 的还原程度可以反映细胞的活性，从而用于评估药物对细胞生长的抑制效果。

【实验器材】

医用净化工作台、座式离心机、酶联分析仪、CO_2 细胞培养箱，实验用移液管、吸管、离心管等玻璃器材均经高压消毒处理，无菌 96 孔培养板等。

【实验细胞株】

人非小细胞肺癌 A549 细胞株。

【实验药品】

多柔比星（贮存浓度为 5 mg/mL）、RPMI-1640 细胞培养液、胎牛血清、MTT（贮存浓度为 5 mg/mL）、DMSO、0.25% 胰酶溶液、锥虫蓝（台盼蓝）染料。

【实验方法】

1. 细胞培养与传代　将复苏后的细胞使用含有 10% 胎牛血清、100 U/mL 青霉素和链霉素的 RPMI-1640 培养液进行培养。培养条件为 37℃、5% CO_2 的饱和湿度环境。

当细胞覆盖率达到 70% ～ 80% 时，进行传代。首先，轻轻倒出培养液，用中性 PBS 洗涤细胞 1 ～ 2 次。然后，添加预热至 37℃的适量胰酶，轻轻旋转培养瓶以确保胰酶与细胞层充分接触。室温下消化 2 ～ 5 min 或在 37℃培养箱中孵育 1 min，直至细胞质浓缩。吸出胰酶后，加入含血清的新鲜培养液以终止消化过程，通过轻轻吹打使细胞形成单细胞悬液。以 800 L/min 离心 5 ～ 10 min，收集细胞，并按 1∶2 或 1∶4 的比例进行传代。

2. 药物处理　选取处于对数生长期的细胞，使用锥虫蓝进行染色并计数，调整细胞浓度至 2.5×10^4 个 /mL。将细胞接种于 96 孔培养板，每孔 200 μL。细胞贴壁过夜后，向各组分别加入不同终浓度的多柔比星（0.5、1、2、4、8、16 μg/mL），而阴性对照组则加入完全培养基，继续培养 48 h，每组设立 4 个复孔。显色步骤：培养 48 h 后，向每孔加入 20 μL 的 5 mg/mL MTT 溶液，继续孵育 4 h。

3. 终止培养与吸光度测定　吸去孔内上清液后，向每孔加入 150 μL DMSO，并低速震荡 10 min 以溶解形成的结晶物。使用酶联免疫分析仪，在 570 nm 波长下测定各孔的吸光度，并记录数据。

【实验记录与结果】

记录测定的各实验组吸光度值，并分析结果。

结果分析方法

生长抑制率（GI）=1-（药物组 OD 值 / 阴性对照组 OD 值）×100%。采用 NDST 软件，根据 Bliss 法计算药物作用 48 h 后的 IC_{50} 值。

【注意事项】

（1）细胞接种浓度适当，以每孔 10^3 ～ 10^4 个细胞为宜，测得 OD 值在 0.4 ～ 0.8 范围为线性关系最佳。

（2）96 孔培养板最外周孔的数值在读数时有偏差，一般不使用；设置不加细胞只加培养液的空白对照。其他试验步骤保持一致，最后比色以空白调零。

【练习题】

1. 多柔比星产生抗肿瘤活性的作用机制是 _____。

A. 抑制 DNA 复制　　　　　　　　B. 与 DNA 发生甲基化

C. 抑制二氢叶酸还原酶　　　　　　D. 干扰细胞有丝分裂

2. MTT 法测细胞活性时，用酶联免疫检测仪在 _____nm 波长处测定其光吸收度。

　　A. 570　　　　　　　B. 480　　　　　　　C. 400　　　　　　　D. 440

【思考题】

　　（1）MTT 法检测药物对肿瘤细胞生长的抑制作用基本原理。

　　（2）多柔比星抑制肿瘤细胞生长的分子机制。

　　（3）除了 MTT 法外，还有哪些可以评估细胞增殖能力的实验方法？

【知识拓展】

多柔比星的发现

　　多柔比星最初是在 20 世纪 60 年代中期从放线菌属中提取和分离的，这类细菌以其在土壤中的天然存在而闻名。其在临床上广泛应用于乳腺癌、肺癌、淋巴癌、卵巢癌等多种癌症的治疗，效果显著，已成为癌症治疗科研领域的"明星"药物。柔红霉素被认为是蒽环类抗生素的原型，研究工作人员已发现多种蒽环类抗生素或类似物，据统计目前已有超过 2000 种多柔比星类似物。我国自主研发的抗肿瘤药物盐酸多柔比星脂质体注射液于 2012 年成功上市，为医生和患者提供了强有力的"武器"。

（史立宏）

第六节　青霉素 G 的体外抗菌作用

【实验目的】

　　（1）熟练掌握体外测定抗生素抗菌活性的实验方法，包括数据记录和分析。

　　（2）理解并掌握试管法和纸片法测定抗生素最低抑菌浓度（MIC）的实验技术和科学原理。

【实验原理】

　　青霉素 G 是一种在细菌快速繁殖期发挥作用的杀菌剂，对革兰阳性细菌和革兰阴性球菌具有显著的抗菌效果，然而，其对革兰阴性杆菌的杀菌作用相对较弱。青霉素 G 的杀菌机制主要在于其能够干扰细菌细胞壁肽聚糖的合成过程，导致细胞壁结构受损。这种损伤使细菌失去其天然的保护屏障，进而导致菌体膨胀并最终裂解死亡。

在评估药物的体外抗菌活性时，我们通常使用最低抑菌浓度（minimum inhibitory concentration，MIC）和最低杀菌浓度（minimum bactericidal concentration，MBC）这两个关键指标。MIC 指的是在体外培养条件下，能够抑制病原菌生长的最低药物浓度，通常在给药 18 ~ 24 h 后进行测定；而 MBC 则指能够完全杀灭培养基内细菌的最低药物浓度。如果一种药物能在较低浓度下有效抑制或杀灭致病菌，我们称该致病菌对药物表现为"敏感"。相反，如果药物在较高浓度下仍无法抑制或杀灭细菌，则称之为"不敏感"或"耐药"。

为了检测细菌对不同药物的敏感性或耐药性，我们通常会进行药敏试验。在体外培养条件下，常用的方法有试管法和纸片法。

试管法，也称为稀释法，将药物在一系列容器中进行倍比稀释，然后加入试验菌，经过一定时间的培养后，观察细菌对药物的反应。由于不同药物浓度下试验菌的生长速度和数量存在差异，这将导致培养基的混浊程度不同，从而反映出药物的抗菌效果。

纸片法则是扩散法的一种形式，通过将含有药物的纸片放置在接种有待测菌的固体培养基上，观察药物在培养基中的扩散情况以及是否形成抑菌环。抑菌环的出现与否及其大小，可以推断出药物对细菌生长的抑制效果。药物扩散的距离越远，表明其抑菌能力越强。根据抑菌环的大小，我们可以对药物的抗菌效果进行评估：抑菌圈小于 10 mm 表示不敏感；10 mm 表示轻度敏感；11 ~ 15 mm 表示中度敏感；16 ~ 20 mm 表示高度敏感。

金黄色葡萄球菌是一种革兰阳性球菌，而大肠埃希菌则是一种革兰阴性杆菌。通过应用试管法和纸片法，我们可以观察青霉素 G 对这两种临床常见致病菌的抗菌活性差异，从而初步了解青霉素 G 的抗菌作用特点。

【实验器材】

灭菌小试管、试管架、吸管（0.5 mL，2 mL）、灭菌小棉签、小镊子、圆形滤纸（直径 6 mm）、培养皿、肉汤琼脂平板。

【实验菌株】

金黄色葡萄球菌标准株（ATCC 29213）、大肠杆菌标准株（ATCC 35218）。

【实验药品】

灭菌牛肉膏汤、MH 培养基、青霉素 G。

【实验方法】

（一）试管法（稀释法）操作步骤：

1. **试管准备** 选择 10 支干净、透明、无裂纹的无菌试管，编号 1～10。

2. **培养基添加** 向每个试管中精确加入 0.5 mL 预先配制好的牛肉膏汤培养基。

3. **药物稀释准备** 准备 40 U/mL 的青霉素 G 母液，并放置于室温下回温。

4. **倍比稀释过程** 将 0.5 mL 母液加入 1 号试管中，作为起始浓度；使用移液枪或移液管，将 1 号试管中的药液混合均匀后，吸取 0.5 mL 加入 2 号试管；重复此过程至 9 号试管，每次转移前需充分混匀；9 号试管中的 0.5 mL 药液弃去，以减少误差。

5. **对照组设置** 10 号试管作为对照组，不加药物，仅加入培养基和菌液。

6. **细菌接种** 准备金黄色葡萄球菌和大肠埃希菌的菌液，调整至大约 10^8 CFU/mL 的浓度；向每个试管中加入 0.5 mL 的菌液，并轻轻摇动试管使菌液与培养基混合均匀。

7. **孵育条件** 将所有试管放入 37℃的孵箱中，孵育 18～24 h。

8. **观察与记录** 孵育结束后，观察每个试管中是否有细菌生长的迹象，如混浊或沉淀；记录下细菌不生长的最高药物浓度，这将是青霉素 G 的最低抑菌浓度。

（二）纸片法（扩散法）操作步骤：

1. **培养基准备** 将 MH 培养基熔化并调整至 45～50℃，倒入无菌平板中，待其凝固。

2. **菌液调整与接种** 使用麦氏比浊管调整菌液至 0.5 麦氏单位，确保菌液浓度均匀；使用无菌棉签蘸取菌液，均匀涂布在培养基表面，注意不要用力过猛，避免损伤琼脂表面。

3. **药物浓度准备** 根据所需浓度，将青霉素 G 稀释至 62.5～2000 U/mL 的不同浓度。

4. **滤纸片处理** 选择适当大小的无菌圆形滤纸片，每两张浸入同一浓度的药液中，确保纸片完全浸湿；取出纸片，用无菌镊子轻轻甩去多余药液，避免药液积聚在纸片边缘。

5. **贴附滤纸片** 将浸有药液的纸片放置在接种好的培养基表面，注意保持纸片间的间距和位置准确；纸片一旦放置，不得移动或调整，以避免影响药物扩散。

6. **孵育条件** 将平板翻转，避免纸片干燥或移动，然后放入 37℃孵箱中孵育

18 ~ 24 h。

7. 观察与测量 孵育结束后，从平板背面观察每个纸片周围是否形成清晰的抑菌圈；使用游标卡尺测量抑菌圈的直径，并记录数据。

8. 数据分析 根据抑菌圈的大小，评估青霉素 G 对金黄色葡萄球菌和大肠埃希菌的抗菌效果，并进行比较。

【实验记录与结果】

记录实验结果，如表 6-6-1 和表 6-6-2 所示。

表 6-6-1 试管法检测青霉素 G 对金黄色葡萄球菌的作用结果记录

管号	1	2	3	4	5	6	7	8	9	10
稀释倍数	1	2	4	8	16	32	64	128	256	0
终浓度 (U/mL)	10	5	2.5	1.25	0.625	0.313	0.16	0.08	0.04	—
有无混浊										

表 6-6-2 青霉素 G 对金黄色葡萄球菌和大肠埃希菌抑菌圈直径 (mm)

细菌类别	青霉素 G 浓度 (U/mL)					
	2000	1000	500	250	125	62.5
金黄色葡萄球菌						
大肠埃希菌						

【注意事项】

（1）金黄色葡萄球菌和大肠埃希菌均为潜在的致病菌，因此在实验过程中，应严格遵循个人防护措施，同时注意防止细菌污染其他物品或环境。

（2）在操作过程中，确保液体的量取精确无误。在使用试管法时，观察应细致入微，而在进行纸片法实验时，应事先精心规划纸片的放置位置。

（3）无菌操作，实验前应彻底清洁实验台，并使用紫外灯或消毒剂进行消毒。

（4）培养基的制备和灭菌，确保培养基成分准确无误，并且在灭菌过程中避免过度加热，以免破坏培养基中的营养成分。

（5）实验器材的准备，在实验前应检查所有器材是否完好，避免在实验过程中因器材问题影响结果。

（6）实验结果的记录和整理，实验过程中应详细记录每个步骤的条件和观察到的现象，实验结束后应及时整理数据。

（7）实验后的清洁和消毒，实验结束后，应对所有使用过的器材进行彻底的清洁和消毒，以防止交叉污染。

（8）实验安全，在处理潜在的致病菌时，应穿戴适当的个人防护装备，如实验服、手套和口罩。

【思考题】

（1）关于青霉素 G 对金黄色葡萄球菌和大肠埃希菌抗菌活性存在差异的原因？

（2）纸片法实验中，观察到某个青霉素 G 浓度下的抑菌圈直径明显小于其他浓度，应如何解释这一现象？

【知识拓展】

青霉素发现的故事

青霉素的发现是一个充满偶然性和科学洞察力的故事。1928 年，英国细菌学家亚历山大·弗莱明在伦敦大学圣玛丽医学院的实验室中，意外地发现了这种具有革命性意义的抗生素。当时，他正准备去度假，却留下了一些未清洗的培养皿。当他返回时，发现其中一个培养皿被一种青绿色的霉菌污染了。这种霉菌周围形成了一个没有细菌生长的空白区域，这一现象引起了弗莱明的极大兴趣。

弗莱明发现，这种霉菌——后来被确认为青霉菌，能够杀死多种细菌，包括金黄色葡萄球菌，这是一种常见的致病菌。他意识到这可能是一种具有强大杀菌作用的物质，于是开始研究并最终分离出了青霉素。然而，弗莱明在提取和纯化青霉素方面遇到了困难，他的研究在一段时间内并未得到广泛的认可或应用。

直到 1939 年，牛津大学的霍华德·W. 弗洛里和恩斯特·B. 钱恩重复了弗莱明的工作，并成功地提纯了青霉素，使其能够用于临床治疗。在第二次世界大战期间，青霉素的大规模生产和应用拯救了无数生命，标志着抗生素时代的开始。弗莱明、弗洛里和钱恩因其在青霉素发现和应用上的贡献，共同荣获了 1945 年的诺贝尔生理学或医学奖。

青霉素的发现不仅开启了抗生素治疗的新纪元，也促进了对其他抗菌物质的寻找和研究，极大地改善了人类的健康状况和预期寿命。尽管随后出现了对青霉素的耐药性问题和过敏反应，但青霉素的发现无疑是医学史上的一个里程碑。

（史立宏）

第七章　实验设计

第一节　实验设计的目的和意义

实验设计指一种有计划的研究，是科学研究工作的核心环节，实验设计的科学性、合理性和可行性直接决定实验结论的可靠性。广义的实验设计是科学研究的一般程序，包括问题提出、假说形成、变量选择、实验方法等过程到结果分析、论文写作等科学研究的全过程。狭义的实验设计特指设计出一个可靠的实验方案，并按照方案实施实验及其相关的统计分析过程，着重解决从建立假说到作出结论这一过程。本章有关的药理学实验设计属后者。

实验设计的目的是通过合理的变量、条件设置和数据分析，以获取对研究对象的深刻认识和理解，从而对事物的本质特征、规律性、功能等方面进行探究，为研究者提供真实可靠的数据基础，推动科学知识不断更新和发展。对药理学实验而言，由于实验误差及实验对象（如实验动物、离体器官等）之间的差异性，必须严格控制实验条件，排除可能对结果产生干扰的因素，以期获得精确可靠的实验结论，从而进一步认识药物与机体相互作用的规律。

实验设计的意义在于通过有目的、有计划、有步骤地设计各种实验因素，严格控制实验误差，从而用较少的人力、物力和时间，最大限度地获得丰富而可靠的资料。一个周密而完善的实验设计能够正确地反映事物发展的内在规律性，为科学研究和技术应用提供有益的指导和参考，推动科学领域的发展和技术创新。

总之，实验设计是实验过程的依据，是实验数据处理的前提，也是提高科研成果的重要保证。在医学科研工作中，无论实验室研究、临床疗效观察或现场调研，在制订研究计划时，均应根据实验的目的和条件，结合统计学的要求，针对实验的全过程，认真做好实验设计。

（王姿颖）

第二节　实验设计的基本要素与原则

一、实验设计的基本要素

实验设计包括实验对象、处理因素和观察指标三个基本要素。

1. 实验对象

实验对象又叫受试对象，指被实验的客体，可以是正常的，也可以是病理性的。药理学实验的实验对象主要是人和动物，包括其整体及离体组织和器官等。

人是临床药理学研究的实验对象，包括健康志愿者和患者。人体实验必须遵循《赫尔辛基宣言》，即在人体实验过程中，对受试者健康的考虑必须优先于对科学和社会的兴趣，必须坚持符合医学目的的科学研究，必须维护受试者权益，必须尊重受试者人格和知情同意权。

一般来讲，不同实验动物对同一药物的反应相似，但有时也会因为种属和品系的差异，不同实验动物对药物的反应会出现量和质的不同。因此应根据实验目的、方法及动物自身的特点选择不同的实验动物。

药理学实验常用的实验动物包括大鼠、小鼠、豚鼠、蛙类、家兔、猫、狗、羊等，特殊情况下可选用非人灵长类动物。

2. 处理因素

处理因素指对实验对象施加的外部干预，包括物理因素（如声、光、热、射线等）、化学因素（如毒素、营养液等）、生物因素（如细菌、病毒等）、药物因素以及外伤、手术等因素。应用处理因素的目的包括 2 个方面：一是复制人类疾病模型，观察疾病的表现，分析疾病的病因和发病机制；二是观察药物或其他治疗手段的干预效果。

在实验设计过程中，处理因素可以单一也可以多种。单因素设计指只涉及一种处理因素，观察其对实验对象产生的效应；多因素设计指给予多种处理因素，观察对实验对象引起的效应。多因素分析又称多变量分析或多元分析，是研究多个相关因素之间的关系及具有这些因素的样品之间关系的一类分析方法，该方法的主要目标是使复杂问题简单化，抓住事物的主要矛盾，同时减少工作量。正交试验、回归分析、聚类分析等均属于多因素分析的方法。

3. 观察指标

观察指标是反映实验对象在经过处理因素处理后生理或病理状态变化的标志。观察指标的选择应在科学性、重复性和可行性的前提下，尽可能选用先进的仪器，采用稳定的技术和定量指标，减少主观性对实验结果判定的影响。

二、实验设计的基本原则

实验设计是建立在逻辑推理和统计分析基础上的一门科学，应遵循重复、对照、随机三个基本原则。

（一）重复原则

重复原则亦称重现性。由于个体差异或实验误差，仅根据一次实验或一个样本所得的结果往往很难获得可靠的结论。在一定范围内重复越多，则结果越可靠。除增加正确性和可靠性外，增加样本量还可使我们了解变异情况。但样本量过大，会增加人力、物力和时间的消耗，不符合经济原则。所以在进行药理学实验设计时，首先应该考虑如何用适量的样本进行实验，才能保证结果的可确性。

样本大小的估算主要考虑以下因素：①变异系数（CV）越大，样本应大；反之，变异系数小，需较小样本就可得到显著的差别。②可信限要求小，样本需增大；反之，可信限设定的范围大，样本就可较小。③概率（p 值）要求小，样本必须加大，反之亦然。

在动物实验时，小动物（大小鼠、蛙等）计量资料每组不少于 10 例，计数资料不少于 30 例；中等动物（家兔、豚鼠等）计量资料每组不少于 6 例，计数资料不少于 20 例；大型动物（犬、猫、羊等）计量资料每组不少于 5 例，计数资料不少于 15 例。在临床研究时，难治病（癌症、狂犬病等）为 5 ~ 10 例；急重病（休克、心衰、流脑等）为 30 ~ 50 例；一般病或慢性病为 100 ~ 500 例。

（二）对照原则

对照是比较的基础，在实验过程中，为了观察处理因素对实验对象产生的影响，要进行处理前后或不同组间的比较，所以实验设计必须设计对照组，并遵照"齐同对比"的原则，即除了所研究的因素外，其他条件应一律齐同，从而消除非处理因素对实验结果的干扰。从处理因素上，对照可分为阴性对照和阳性对照，从实验对象上，对照可分为自身对照和组间对照。

1. 阴性对照

阴性对照包括：①空白对照，即以不给予任何处理因素的正常动物作对照，又称正常对照；②假处理对照，即除不用被研究的处理因素（如药物）外，对照组的动物要经受同样的处理如麻醉、手术、注射不含药物的溶媒等，该对照方法较为常用；

③安慰剂对照，安慰剂是一种本身无特殊药理活性的物质制成的外形似药的制剂，是临床试验常用的阴性对照。

2. 阳性对照

阳性对照又称标准对照，即实验结果与标准值进行对比，包括①标准品对照，即以典型药物或标准品作为对照，以便评定药物的作用强度；②阳性对照，指以有国家批准文号的有效药品作为对照，如果新药优于老药，并有显著意义，则可肯定新药的价值。

3. 自身对照

自身对照指对同一实验对象处理前后进行自身对比。

4. 组间对照

组间对照指在实验中设计若干平行组进行组间比较。

（三）随机原则

由于实验对象对处理因素的反应存在个体差异，分组应按随机原则，使每一个体在实验中都有同等的机会接受处理，以避免或减少有意或无意造成的偏差。常用的随机分组法包括完全随机分组法、随机区组法、拉丁方阵随机法和配对随机法等，其中较常用的是随机区组法，分组过程为①排队：将所有动物按某一条件排序；②区组：将所有动物划分成几个区域，使每一区域的动物数与所分组数相等；③取随机数字：参考附表 X 随机数字表，注意表中数字必须连续使用，但使用方向较灵活（横向、纵向均可）；④确定除数：即为每个区组中每只动物分到各组的可能性；⑤计算余数：以随机数字除以对应的除数，得到余数。注意可能会出现整除或被除数小于除数的两种特殊情况，均以除数代替余数；⑥确定组别：根据余数的数字将每个区组的动物进行分配。以 14 只小鼠分成 4 组为例，分组步骤见表 7-2-1、表 7-2-2。

表 7-2-1　随机区组分组举例

编号	1	2	3	4	5	6	7	8	9	10	11	12	13	14
体重（g）	18	18	18	19	19	19	19	19	19	20	20	21	21	21
随机数字	68	65	84	68	95	23	92	35	87	02	22	57	51	61
除数	4	3	2	1	4	3	2	1	4	3	2	1	4	3
余数	4	2	2	1	3	2	2	1	3	3	2	1	3	1
组别	4	2	3	1	3	2	4	1	3	4	2	1	3	1

表 7-2-2　分组结果表

组别	动物号（体重）			
一组	4（19）	8（19）	12（21）	14（21）
二组	2（18）	6（19）	11（20）	
三组	3（18）	5（19）	9（19）	13（21）
四组	1（18）	7（19）	10（20）	

（王姿颖）

第三节　实验设计的基本内容与方法

实验设计的基本内容包括以下几点：

（一）明确实验目的和任务

进行实验设计前，首先要明确实验的目的，即本实验要探讨的核心问题，确保实验的方向和目标清晰，再围绕这一目标设计实验。实验目标必须突出，不可贪多。

（二）确定实验设计的基本要素

1. 选择合适的实验对象

在实验设计中，要根据实验观察的目的与内容，结合实验对象的生理特点及对处理因素反应的敏感性和实际情况（如样本来源、实验条件和经费等），明确规定采用什么样的实验对象，实验对象中的每个实验单位必须具备的条件与要求，以保证实验对象的一致性和代表性，详见本章第二节。

2. 确定稳定可靠的处理因素

处理因素指的是在实验研究中计划施加给实验对象的某些因素，如营养实验的营养液、饲料等，治疗某种疾病的几种疗法或药物，药理研究中某药的不同剂量等。实验设计时应选用公认、可靠的处理方法。如研究调血脂药的作用，常用以一定配比的高脂饲料喂养实验动物造成实验性高脂血症模型的方法。如需改进或创新实验方法，除了要有科学依据外，尚需对该方法的稳定性和灵敏性进行检验，并与标准方法对比，确系可靠方可应用。在实验的全过程中，处理因素要始终保持恒定。如果实验的处理因素是药物，药物的成分、含量、出厂批号等必须保持不变。如果实验的处理因素是手术，则应该在实验之前手术者的熟练程度要保证稳定一致。

3. 选择可靠的观察指标

观察指标是实验因素作用在实验对象上所产生的反应的标志。观察指标应满足以下要求：①能反映被研究问题的本质，具有专一可靠性；②尽可能客观，避免或减少主观因素的干扰；③尽可能为量反应，可定量测定以取得准确的数据。

（三）体现实验设计的三大原则

实验设计中要通过确定样本大小来体现重复原则；通过设立适当的对照组，体现对照原则；通过对实验对象进行随机分组，体现随机原则。具体采用的方案详见本章第二节。

（四）实验的组织与实施

包括实验步骤、技术手段、控制途径与实施办法，以确保实验的顺利进行。

（五）拟定实验记录格式

原始记录是实验的重要档案，是实验结果判断的根据。在进行实验设计时，应拟好实验记录的格式，以保证实验有条不紊地进行。实验记录一般应包括①实验对象的条件：如实验动物的种类、性别、体重等；②处理因素的设定：如药物的来源、批号、剂型、浓度、给药剂量、给药途径等；③实验的环境条件：如实验室的温度、湿度等；④实验日程安排、方法、步骤；⑤观察指标变化的数据或图形；⑥实验者信息等。

（六）实验结果的统计处理方法

实验资料分为计量资料和计量资料，对应药理效应中的量反应与质反应。前者指有连续量变的资料，可用具体的工具测量，如体重、血压、血糖等；后者指效果出现与否（全或无，阳性或阴性），如死亡与存活、有效与无效等。在实验设计时应拟定好实验结果的统计处理方法。一般来讲，计量资料可用 t 检验或方差分析，计数资料可用卡方检验或 Fisher 直接概率法等。

总之，实验设计应理清设计思路，即根据实验目的提出假设，围绕假设确定被试和变量，按照实验变量采取相应的方法、手段、依从变量控制安排实验步骤、选择合适器材和反应条件等。在实施过程中要特别重视对比和控制，确保实验的科学性和有效性。

（王姿颖）

第四节　实验设计的类型

实验设计涵盖了从基础科学研究到实际应用领域的多种类型。研究者可根据不同的研究目的和条件选择适合的实验设计类型。常用的实验设计包括以下类型：

1. 因素设计

根据实验中自变量的数量进行设计，可以分为单因素设计和多因素设计。单因素设计简单易行，适用于情况较为简单的情况；多因素设计则考虑多个影响因素，适用于复杂情况。

2. 准实验设计

考虑到某些无关变量可能影响实验结果，但又难以在实际中妥善控制时，可采用准实验设计，其特点是没有采用随机化程序，即被试的选择和编组、处理分配等都不是随机安排的。

3. 非实验设计

用于确定自然存在的临界变量及其相互关系。包括自然观察法、相关法、访谈法等多种研究方法。

4. 预实验设计

在进行正式实验前，先进行小规模的实验以测试实验的可行性和效果。

5. 真实验设计

在严格控制条件下进行的实验，通常涉及随机分配和对照组的设置。

6. 市场测试

特定于市场研究领域的实验设计类型，用于评估产品或服务的市场反应和效果。

7. 平行组设计

平行组设计又称成组设计，将符合条件的受试对象随机分配到试验组和对照组，分别接受不同的处理，并收集其有效性及安全性信息，通过比较说明干预效果。这种设计的优点在于能有效避免选择偏倚，增加处理组的均衡可比性。

8. 析因设计

将两个或多个处理因素的各水平进行组合，对各种可能的组合进行评价，适用于分析多个因素的主效应及交互作用。

9. 配对设计

将研究对象按一定条件配成对子，再将每对中的两个研究对象随机分配到不同的处理组进行试验研究。

10. 随机区组设计

先将条件相近的研究对象配成组，然后按随机化方法分配到不同的处理组中，增强各处理组间的均衡性。

11. 重复测量设计

在多个时间点上对同一个受试对象的效应指标进行重复观察，探讨同一研究对象在不同时间点的变化情况。

12. 单盲设计和双盲设计

涉及实验参与者的知情状态，单盲设计中参与者不知道自己属于实验组或对照组，而双盲设计中参与者和研究人员对分组信息均不知情。

选择适当的实验设计类型对于确保研究的科学性和有效性至关重要。研究者应根据研究的具体需求和资源条件，选择最合适的实验设计方案。

（王姿颖）

第五节　实验设计的步骤与要求

（一）实验设计的步骤

实验设计的步骤指在具体的实践中，实验者按照一定的程序和方法进行实验设计。具体为：

1. 立题

在进行实验设计之前，需要明确研究问题，此为实验的出发点和基础。通过查阅与实验有关的文献，了解国内外发展动态及先进的方法，明确研究问题的科学性、创新性与可行性。

2. 制定实验目标

根据研究问题，明确实验的目标和预期成果。实验目标应该与研究问题密切相关，且具有具体的可测量标准。

3. 确定实验变量

实验变量是对实验过程中可能影响实验结果的因素进行控制与调整的对象。实验设计时应明确独立变量和因变量，并进行操作性定义。

4. 设计实验步骤

根据研究问题和实验目标，确定实验的具体步骤和操作流程。实验步骤应该有一定的系统性和逻辑性，确保实验的可靠性和有效性。

5. 确定实验对象和样本量

根据研究问题和实验目标，确定实验所需的有代表性的研究对象类型和样本量。

6. 制定实验数据采集和处理方法

根据研究问题和实验目标，确定实验数据的采集方法和数据处理方法。数据采集方法应该具有一定的准确性和可重复性，数据处理方法应该与研究问题和实验目标相匹配。

7. 进行预实验

在进行正式实验之前，开展预实验有助于检验实验步骤和操作方法的可行性，并及时发现和解决潜在问题。

8. 进行正式实验

按照实验设计和实验方案的要求，进行正式实验。在实验过程中，需认真记录实验原始数据和实验操作过程，确保实验的可靠性和可复制性。

9. 数据分析和结果解释

根据实验数据，进行数据分析和结果解释。数据分析应该遵循科学的统计方法和数据处理原则，结果解释应该与实验目标和研究问题相一致。

10. 获得实验结论

通过对实验数据、结果进行客观分析和评价，提出对研究问题的回答和进一步研究的建议。

（二）学生实验设计的要求

学生实验设计是在本学科学习的基础上，由学生自立题目、自行设计并实施实验的一种自主性学习活动。通过实验设计，可培养学生查阅文献、独立思考和分析解决问题等能力，为其具备初步的科学研究能力打下基础。学生实验设计书的基本要求包括：①实验题目；②立题依据（含主要参考文献）；③实验目的；④实验材料；⑤实验方法；⑥预期结果；⑦预期结论。

（王姿颖）

第八章　案例分析

案例 1

【病例】

患者张某，女，42岁。因腹部剧烈疼痛入院。入院前患者曾间歇性上腹绞痛发作数年，并伴有恶心、呕吐、腹泻等症状。经医院诊断为胆石症、慢性胆囊炎。本次入院前，患者因疼痛注射过吗啡，用药后出现剧烈呕吐，呼吸变慢，腹泻却得到控制。入院后，给予头孢拉定静脉滴注，并肌注哌替啶 50 mg，阿托品 0.5 mg，每隔 3～4 h 一次，同时进行手术治疗。术后患者伤口疼痛，仍继续使用哌替啶。患者要求注射哌替啶，若一天不用则四肢怕冷、情绪不安、手脚发麻、气急、说话含糊，甚至情绪暴躁。现患者每天要注射哌替啶 4 次，每天 300～400 mg，晚上还需加镇静催眠药方能安静入睡。根据以上情况随后将患者转入精神病院。

【讨论】

（1）试分析该患者在入院前后对吗啡和哌替啶的使用是否合适？

（2）患者出院后继续使用哌替啶的可能原因是什么？

（3）哌替啶配伍阿托品使用的依据是什么？

（4）患者在入院前使用吗啡后出现呼吸变慢，腹泻却得到控制的原因何在？

（高　伟）

案例 2

【病例】

患者杨某，男，66岁。因气胸入院。患者患有风湿性关节炎病史10年，并且患有慢性咳嗽 30 多年，长期不规则口服泼尼松。本次入院以慢性支气管炎、肺结核伴气胸入院。患者入院后抽气、胸腔闭式引流，给予抗感染及抗结核治疗。住院期间患者反复发热、咳嗽、吐痰及其气胸发作，并出现精神症状，考虑为肺性脑病。静脉滴注肺脑合剂（含地塞米松）及强的松，4 天后出现明显上腹痛及黑便，血压下降，于出血后第 4 天死亡。

【讨论】

（1）试分析该患者在使用激素后出现了哪些并发症？发生机理是什么？

（2）请谈一下如何正确使用糖皮质激素，从本案例中获得哪些体会。

（高　伟）

案例 3

【病例】

患者吴某，女，55 岁。高血压和冠心病病史 10 年，医生建议每天口服阿司匹林 100 mg，患者严格按照医嘱服药。最初一切正常，但其在服用阿司匹林 3 个月后，开始出现上腹部隐痛、恶心等消化不良症状。起初，患者以为是饮食问题未予重视，但症状持续加重，并且开始出现黑便。患者意识到情况严重，立即到医院就诊。经检查，医生诊断为阿司匹林引起的胃溃疡出血。患者被紧急安排住院治疗，接受止血和胃黏膜保护的药物治疗，并停用阿司匹林。医生在与患者及其家属沟通后，建议改用替代药物如氯吡格雷，并给予质子泵抑制剂保护胃黏膜。在随后的复查中，患者的症状逐渐好转，胃溃疡愈合良好。

【讨论】

（1）本案例中阿司匹林使用的依据是什么？

（2）试分析本案例中阿司匹林使用后出现的不良反应的机理。除此之外，还可能会出现哪些不良反应？

（高　伟）

案例 4

【病例】

　　患者王某，男，45 岁。因急性呼吸道感染服用头孢克肟 3 天。经治疗，患者病情迅速好转，第 4 天与朋友聚会时饮用 4 瓶啤酒。几小时后，患者开始出现面部潮红、头痛、恶心、心悸等症状，并感觉身体不适。他被立即送往医院，经诊断怀疑其出现了"戒断反应"，即双硫仑样反应（类似于双硫仑戒酒反应）。给予对症处理，包括补液、止吐和监测生命体征。病情好转，身体逐渐恢复，在此过程中，患者被告知发生双硫仑反应的严重风险。

【讨论】

　　（1）请分析双硫仑反应发生的机理？

　　（2）服用头孢类药物同时饮酒危险在哪里？

（高　伟）

第九章　常用实验仪器设备

第一节　信息化集成化信号采集与处理系统

【实验目的】

（1）学习信息化集成化信号采集与处理系统的使用方法。

（2）掌握信息化集成化信号采集系统与处理系统的操作方法。

【实验原理】

随着科技和社会的不断进步，电子计算机已被广泛应用于管理、金融、信息网络、科研等多个领域。在药理学实验中，通过将生物信号采集系统与计算机结合，可以实现多数实验操作。尽管不同的制造商生产的信号采集设备和分析软件可能存在差异，但其核心组件和基本原理大体相似。生物体发出的信号形式多样，其中只有电信号可以直接输入放大器，而非电信号（如血压和张力）则需要通过相应的传感器转换为电信号后才能输入放大器。电信号经过放大和滤波处理（以去除生物信号中的干扰信号，例如 50 Hz 的交流电源干扰，这些干扰信号的强度往往大于生物电信号本身，若不滤除会掩盖实际信号），随后转换为数字信号供计算机处理，从而获得清晰的生物信号图像。

生物信号采集与处理系统就是一款集成信号采集、处理与显示功能的系统。它能够替代传统实验设备，如放大器、记录仪、刺激器、示波器和心电图机，并具备数据处理能力，在国内各大高校得到了广泛应用。这一系统的应用显著改进了实验教学方式，实现了教育手段的网络化、数字化和集成化。该系统由计算机、系统主机、传感器、相关软件和打印机组成，主要用于观测和检测生物体或离体组织中的生物电信号以及非电信号，如张力、压力和温度等，并能记录并分析生物体在不同实验条件下的变化。本章节着重介绍生物信号采集与处理系统的使用方法和注意事项。

【实验器材】

BL-422I 信息化集成化信号采集与处理系统。

【实验动物】

可进行家兔、蟾蜍、大小鼠等实验动物机能信号的检测与记录。

【实验药品】

根据药理学实验项目而定。

【实验方法】

该部分主要介绍 BL-422I 生物机能实验系统组成和基本使用方法。

1. 系统组成

BL-422I 生物机能实验系统采用一体化设计原则，同时集成了可移动实验平台、生物信息采集系统、呼吸系统、测温系统、照明系统以及同步演示系统。实验数据、报告处理无纸化，协助教师进行实验信息化管理。帮助科研工作者获取更客观、全面的实验数据，可运用于各项生理学、药理学、病理生理学等实验。

BL-422I 生物机能实验系统是配置在微机上的多通道生物信号采集、放大、显示、记录与处理系统，主要由计算机、系统硬件、生物信号显示与处理软件和控制单元等四部分构成。该系统从生物体内或离体器官中探测生物电信号或张力、压力等非电信号，并可对实验数据进行储存、分析及处理。

2. 开关机操作

1）开机操作

（1）请按机器右侧背后的总电源按钮，如图 9-1-1 所示。

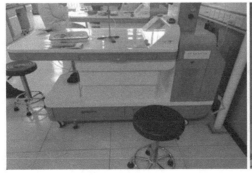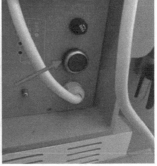

图 9-1-1 BL-422I 生物机能实验系统开机示意图

（2）按下总电源后，等待 Windows 系统进入桌面。

（3）使用平板连接 BL-422I 生物机能实验系统后即可正常实验。

2）关机操作

（1）务必使用平板关闭 Windows 系统（请按照图 9-1-2 操作）。

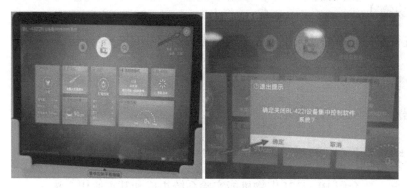

图 9-1-2　BL-422I 生物机能实验系统关机示意图

（2）务必等待 1 min 左右（待集成化系统全部停止运行后）再关闭机器总电源。

3. 主界面操作简要步骤

软件面板界面：BL-422I 配套软件是该系统主要硬件 420N 生物采集设备共用的软件，以 Windows 系统为软件平台，应用中英文双语和图形化操作界面，预置十大类 55 个实验模块。根据实验项目决定具体操作步骤。软件主界面见图 9-1-3。启用软件后，按照操作提示插入相应的换能器或配件，然后按照操作提示操作即可（见图 9-1-4）。

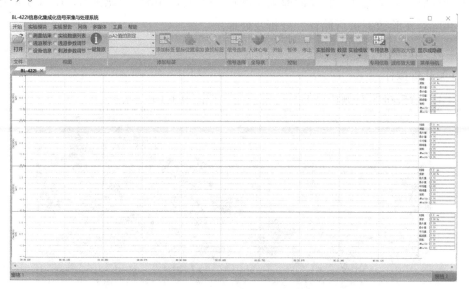

图 9-1-3　BL-422I 生物机能实验系统主界面

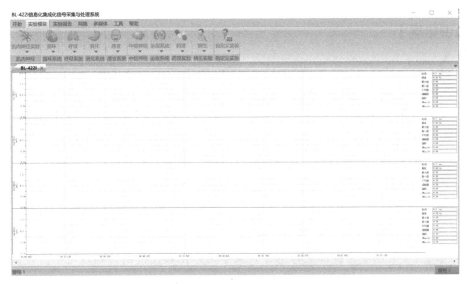

图 9-1-4　BL-422I 生物机能实验系统可选择的实验项目

【注意事项】

（1）务必按照开关机操作说明进行，尤其是不要使用 Windows 界面关机。

（2）爱护设备，杜绝暴力插入换能器和拆解设备。

【练习题】

1. BL-422I 信息化集成化信号采集与处理系统最主要优势是 _____。

A. 突出智能化　　　　　　　　　　B. 集成生物信息采集功能

C. 突出信息化　　　　　　　　　　D. 以上都不对

2. BL-422I 信息化集成化信号采集与处理系统工作原理是 _____。

A. 智能 AI　　　　　　　　　　　　B. 生物信号转化为电信号和数字信号

C. 人工输入数字信号　　　　　　　D. 根据实验动物而异

【思考题】

（1）生物信息采集系统的工作原理是什么？

（2）如何使用信息化集成化信号采集与处理系统设计一个关于磺胺嘧啶药物对家兔肾功能的影响作用的实验？

【知识拓展】

我国在医疗科技领域的不断创新

在民生科技领域，我国取得了显著的进展。医用重离子加速器、磁共振、彩超、CT 等高端医疗装备的国产化替代取得了重大突破。习近平总书记在两院院士大会和中国科协第十次全国代表大会上对这些国产高端医疗装备给予了高度评价。

CT、彩超、磁共振等高端医疗设备作为现代医疗诊断的重要工具，为健康中国战略提供了强有力的支持。特别是在抗击突发公共卫生事件的过程中，CT 作为关键的诊疗设备发挥了至关重要的作用。根据《2020 年中国医疗影像产业链研究报告》，CT 已成为我国医疗影像产业中国产化程度较高的领域之一，许多国产高端 CT 设备已经达到了国际先进水平。然而，二十年前，无论是三甲医院还是县级医疗机构，CT 设备不仅数量有限，而且全部依赖进口，高昂的价格让基层医疗机构难以承受，普通民众也难以负担得起检查费用。

面对这一挑战，一批本土医疗影像设备企业坚持自主研发，逐步打破了外国品牌的垄断局面。如今，多家中国企业已经成功研发并生产出了高端 CT 设备，实现了从依赖进口到自主生产的转变。这一转变不仅降低了医疗成本，提高了医疗服务的可及性，也提升了我国医疗科技领域的自主创新能力和国际竞争力。

（崔晓栋）

第二节　分光光度计

【实验目的】

（1）学习分光光度计的使用方法。

（2）掌握分光光度计的操作方法。

【工作原理】

分光光度计的基本工作原理是基于物质对光（光的波长）的吸收具有选择性。不同的物质都有其各自的吸收波长，所以当光色散后的单色光通过溶液时，某些波长的光线就会被溶液吸收（光能量减弱）。因此，在一定波长下，溶液中物质的浓度与光能量减弱的程度有一定比例关系，也符合比耳定律（Beer's Law）。

721 型分光光度计是一种简洁易用的分光光度法通用仪器（图 9-2-1），能够在 360 ~ 800 mm 的允许测定范围内，进行透射比、吸光度和浓度的测定。由于其构造比较简单，测定的灵敏度和精密度较高，被广泛用于医学卫生、临床检验、生物化学、石油化工、环保检测质量监控等部门做定性定量分析使用。

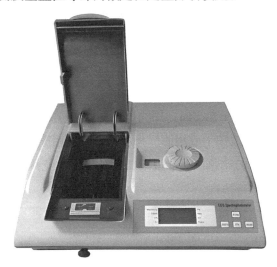

图 9-2-1　721 型分光光度计

【使用方法】

分光光度计可通过系列分光装置，将成分复杂的光，分解为特定波长的单色光。单色光照射测试的样品时,部分光线被吸收,通过测定透过样品前后的入射光和透射光能量，可检测被测物质在特定波长处或一定波长范围内对光的吸收度，进而对该物质进行定性和定量分析。常用的波长范围为 200 ~ 400 nm 的紫外光区、400 ~ 760 nm 的可见光区、2.5 ~ 25 μm 的红外光区。所用仪器相应可分为紫外分光光度计、可见光分光光度计、红外分光光度计或原子吸收分光光度计。

1. **仪器的使用前准备**　①首先接通电源，打开电源开关，指示灯亮，打开比色皿暗箱,预热 20 min。②转动波长选择按钮，选择所需要的单色光波长。③按动 MODE 键，选择到透射比（T），打开比色皿暗箱盖，放入比色皿，按动零调节按钮（即 0%T），使屏幕显示 0.00；将比色皿暗箱盖合上，推进比色皿拉杆，使比色皿处于空白矫正位置，按动 OA 按钮调节（即 100%T），使屏幕显示 100，稳定后按动 MODE 键选择到吸光度（A），即可进行测定工作。

2. **样品检测**　将装有溶液的比色皿置于比色皿架中，盖上比色皿暗箱盖，拉动比色皿拉杆，使样品溶液置于光路上，读出吸光度值，读数后应立即打开比色皿暗箱盖。测定三次，取平均值。测量完毕，取出比色皿，洗净后倒置于滤纸上晾干，电源开关置于"关"，拔下电源插头。

【注意事项】

（1）使用仪器时要认真、谨慎、严格按照操作要求进行。

（2）仪器要放置于固定且不受震动的仪器上，严防振动、潮湿、磁场和强光直射。

（3）被测样品要使溶剂和溶质充分溶解稳定，无悬浮物和挥发性，以免造成仪器检测不稳定。

（4）严禁用手拿比色杯光学面，用完比色杯后应立即用自来水冲洗，再用蒸馏水洗净，洗净后比色杯倒置晾干或用滤纸将水吸去，再用擦镜纸轻轻揩干。

（5）不同测试项目的比色皿不能混用，紫外光区比色用石英比色皿，可见光区比色用玻璃比色皿。

【练习题】

1. 721 型分光光度计是基于物质对 _____ 具有选择性。

A. 电　　　　　　　B. 光　　　　　　　C. 水　　　　　　　D. 原子

2. 721 型用手拿比色杯的 _____。

A. 光学面　　　　　B. 毛玻璃面　　　　C. 顶面　　　　　　D. 侧面

【思考题】

（1）721 型分光光度计的工作原理是什么？

（2）721 型分光光度计操作时应注意什么？

第三节　生理、药理电子刺激仪

【实验目的】

学习生理和药理电子刺激仪的工作原理和使用方法。

【工作原理】

YLS-9A 生理、药理电子刺激仪为多用途方波刺激仪，见图 9-3-1。输出的电压范围宽，最高可达200 V，具有限流保护功能，限制电流可调；最大输出电流为2 mA，刺激输出与控制电路完全隔离；可通过参数设定，定制多种类型的输出方波；输出可通过开关触发，也可通过外接输入信号触发，在外接输入信号触发时可设为延时输出，延时时间可调。输出的方波包括：正脉冲、正脉冲＋间隙＋负脉冲、正脉冲＋负脉冲三种波形，输出的脉冲数可调，输出过程电压电流可调整，能适合生理、药理等各类实验的需要。仪器采用液晶面板中文显示当前输出参数，非常直观，可存储8个设定的波形参数，方便实验人员的操作。

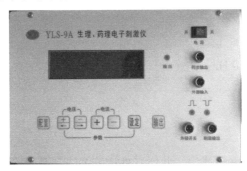

图9-3-1　YLS-9A生理、药理电子刺激仪

仪器特点：

（1）双向脉冲：双向脉冲解决了长时间用一种极向刺激使电极周围产生极电解反应的问题，从而保护了与电极接触的神经、肌肉、血管等组织，避免了组织极化效应。

（2）高电压：高电压可用于对动物的强刺激，如惊厥、激怒、刺痛和对大动物的刺激如猪、狗、猴、兔等，解决了一些生物信号采集处理系统刺激电压较低的问题。

（3）限电流：一方面保护刺激对象不受大电流伤害，另一方面保护仪器不过流损坏，当输出电流超过限流值时仪器自动降低脉冲幅度，使电流不超过设定值。

（4）梯度增压：当设定为连续波变压输出模式时，输出将按原设定值和递增间隔以及增量自动增压输出（也可减压输出），用于刺痛和激怒实验非常方便。

（5）外触发输出：外触发输出是在给外部输入一个脉冲信号或一组脉冲信号后在输出端输出一个或一组同极性的信号，因其输出电压和电流是可调的，从而起到了信号放大和波形整形的作用。

（6）便携式结构方便移动和堆放。

【主要技术指标】

方波输出类型：单波输出、单波断续输出、连续波输出、连续波断续输出、连续波变压输出、外方波输入、变压变流输出。

方波参数：

电压：1 ~ 200 V 增量为 1 V。

电流：0.01 ~ 2.00 mA 可调限流（配置 8 为 4.00 mA）调整步长为 0.01 mA。

波宽：50 μs ~ 4.99999 s。

间隙：50 μs ~ 4.99999 s。

触发延时：0 或 20 μs ~ 4.9999 s。

触发信号电压：±2 ~ 12 V。

间断：1 ms ~ 999.999 s。

脉冲前沿上升时间≤ 1 μs。

电源电压：220 V 50 Hz。

输入功率：10 VA。

【使用方法】

用电源线将仪器与电源连接，并插好外接开关线和刺激输出线，打开电源开关。

（1）参数设置：设定方法首先按动设定键，液晶显示屏上的参数项由阳文显示变为阴文显示，变为阴文显示的项目是可设定项目，不断按动设定键可循环变项（注意电压和电流限流可随时调整，可不预设）。

（2）配置键的使用：仪器设有 8 个存储设定模式，使用者可提前将常用的刺激参数分别设置在 8 个配置中，使用时只需按动配置键就可方便地调出某组实验参数。

（3）外接开关使用：仪器配有手控开关，能在观察受试动物的情况下同时控制刺激输出，方便了实验人员，提高了实验的准确性。

（4）指示灯显示：按动输出键或按动手控开关后输出指示灯亮，刺激输出端按设定好的方波参数输出方波，同时方波相位指示灯也按输出情况在闪动。

（5）输出设定与配置：仪器在输出状态下除电压、电流可调整外，其他参数不能改动，仪器在设定状态下无法输出，仪器在非输出非设定状态下才可选择配置。

【注意事项】

（1）使用后请切断电源，存放在通风干燥处。

（2）内有高压请不要自行拆卸，避免发生危险。

【练习题】

1. YLS-9A 生理、药理电子刺激仪使用的脉冲类型是 _____。

A. 单向脉冲　　　　B. 双向脉冲　　　　C. 负向脉冲　　　　D. 正向脉冲

2.YLS-9A 生理、药理电子刺激仪可输出的方波不包括 _____。

A. 正脉冲　　　　　　　　　　　B. 正脉冲 + 间隙 + 负脉冲

C. 正脉冲 + 负脉冲　　　　　　　D. 负脉冲 + 间隙

【思考题】

生理、药理电子刺激仪主要完成哪些实验指标检测？

（李文涛）

附　录

附录1　药理实验中药物的浓度及剂量换算

（一）药物剂量单位

药物剂量的法定单位包括重量单位和容量单位。

重量单位主要有克（g）、毫克（mg）、微克（μg）、纳克（ng）及匹克（pg）。换算关系是：$1\ g=10^3\ mg=10^6\ μg=10^9\ ng=10^{12}\ pg$。

容量单位主要有升（L）、毫升（mL）、微升（μL）。

换算关系是：$1\ L=10^3\ mL=10^6\ μL$。

此外，国际单位（IU）和单位（U）也是法定计量单位的一部分。对于中药饮片，其剂量通常以克（g）为单位。在处方中，药品剂量与数量需要用阿拉伯数字书写，以确保准确性与一致性。

（二）给药容量

注射用药前应首先考虑该种动物在特定注射途径所能允许的最大容量（一般为mL），只有确定容量之后才能决定溶液配成多大浓度合适。通常动物血容量约占体重的1/3，静脉注射药液容量过大，可影响到循环系统正常功能，故静脉注射容量最好在体重的1/100以下，静脉外注射（皮下、肌内及腹腔）容量最好在体重的1/40以下。如体重20 g的小鼠，尾静脉注射不宜超过0.2 mL；肌内、皮下、腹腔等部位注射不宜超过0.5 mL。

（三）药物浓度

药物浓度指定量液体或固体制剂中所含药物的分量，常用的液体制剂有下列几种表示方法：

1. 百分浓度

以每一百份溶液中所含药物的份数来表示，简写成%。

（1）重量/容量（W/V）法：表示每 100 mL 溶液中含有药物的克数。如 5% 葡萄糖指 100 mL 溶液中含有 5 g 葡萄糖，不加特别说明时的药物 % 浓度即指这种方法。

（2）容量/容量（V/V 法）：适用于液体药物的配制，表示 100 mL 溶液中含有药物的 mL 数。如 75% 乙醇即 100 mL 中含无水乙醇 75 mL；换言之，用 75 mL 无水乙醇加蒸馏水至 100 mL 即可制得 75% 乙醇。

2. 比例浓度

用来表示稀溶液的浓度，如 1：10000 肾上腺素溶液即指 0.01% 肾上腺素（1 mL 中含 0.1 mg 肾上腺素）。

3. 摩尔浓度

摩尔/升（M 或 mol/L）指 1 L 溶液中所含溶质的摩尔量，称为该溶液的摩尔浓度，如 0.1 M NaCl 表示 1 升溶液中含有 0.1 摩尔量，即 5.844 g NaCl（NaCl 分子量为 58.44）。

4. 剂量换算

动物实验所用的药物剂量，一般是按 mg/kg（有时也用 g/kg）计算，给药时需从已知药物浓度换算成相当于每 kg 体重（为方便起见，大鼠、豚鼠也可按每 100 g 体重，小鼠、蟾蜍可按每 10 g 体重）应该注射的药液量（mL）。有时则需根据药物剂量和给药容量计算出合适的药物浓度；有时还须进行浓度之间换算（如百分浓度和比例浓度间）以便进行分析和计算。

（1）由药物剂量 mg/kg 以及药液百分浓度换算成每 kg 体重注射药量（mL），进而计算出每只动物应该注射多少 mL。

例：小白鼠体重 22 g，腹腔注射盐酸吗啡 10 mg/kg，药物浓度 0.1%，应该注射多少 mL？

计算方法：0.1% 的盐酸吗啡溶液每 mL 含药物 1 mg，10 mg/kg 相当于 10 mL/kg，动物 22 g 体重换算成 0.022 kg，10 mg/kg × 0.022 kg =0.22 mL。为计算方便，也可将上述 10 mL/kg 首先换算成 0.1 mL/10 g，小白鼠体重改写成 2.2×10 g，则计算 0.1 mL/10g × 2.2 × 10 g=0.22 mL。

（2）由药物剂量 mg/kg 和设定的药液容量 mL/kg，计算应该配制的药物浓度。

例：家兔静脉注射盐酸吗啡 10 mg/kg，注射容量 1 mL/kg，应该配制的药液浓度是多少？

计算方法：10 mg/kg 相当于 1 mL/kg，即 1 mL 药液应该含 10 mg 盐酸吗啡，1：10=100：X，X=1000（mg）=1 g，故配成的浓度 100 mL 含 1 g，即 1% 的盐酸吗啡。

（李成檀）

附录 2　常用生理溶液的成分和配置

试剂类型和主要用途	生理盐水		任氏液			乐氏液	任-乐氏液	台式液	克氏液	无钙原液
试剂成分	冷血动物	温血动物	离体蛙心	冷血动物	温血动物	温血动物心脏	温血动物肌等	温血动物小肠等	细胞培养取材时组织块漂洗	离体主动脉
NaCl	6.5	9.0	6.76	6.5	9.5	9.0	9.0	8.0	6.6	69.544
$CaCl_2$			0.117	0.12	0.20	0.24	0.2	0.2	0.28	
KCl			0.09	0.14	0.12	0.42	0.2	0.2	0.35	3.578
$NaHCO_3$			0.225	0.2	0.15	0.1 ~ 0.3	0.3	1.0	2.1	
NaH_2PO_4				0.1				0.05		
KH_2PO_4									0.162	1.633
$MgCl_2$								0.1		
$MgSO_4 \cdot 7H_2O$									0.294	3.451
CO_2						充气 10 min				
Glucose				或 1.0	或 1.0	1 ~ 2.5	1	1	2.0	
Na_2EDTA										0.05
O_2						含氧	含氧	含氧	含氧	含氧
ddH_2O	1000	1000	1000	1000	1000	1000	1000	1000	1000	1000

单位：固体为克，液体为毫升。

（张朋飞）

附录 3　药物的剂型及处方

一、药物剂型

药物剂型指任何药物在供给临床使用前，均须按照药典或处方制成适合医疗和预防应用的形式。常用剂型按形态分为液体剂型、固体剂型、半固体剂型和气雾剂等。

1. 液体剂型

（1）溶液剂

一般为化学药物的澄清水溶液，供内服或外用。

（2）注射剂

第一种是溶液型注射剂，亦称安瓿剂，是药物的灭菌溶液或混悬液，供注射用。

第二种是粉末型的注射液，通常称为粉针剂，有的药物在溶液中不稳定，则以其灭菌的干燥粉末封装于安瓿中，临用时配成溶液。

第三种是乳剂型注射剂，多为静脉滴注用，通常是不溶于水的溶质。

第四种是混悬液注射剂，通常是难以溶于水或者需要延长作用时间的药物。

（3）煎剂是用水煎煮的生药（单味药或复方）煎出液。中草药常用这种剂型，须新鲜制备。

（4）合剂是多种药物配制成透明或混悬的水性液体制剂，供内服。

（5）酊剂一般指生药用乙醇萃取或溶解制成的澄清液体制剂。

（6）流浸膏剂指生药的浸出液经除去部分溶媒而成为浓度较高的液体剂型。

（7）乳剂指互不相溶的两种液体经过乳化剂的处理制成的均匀而较稳定的乳状液体。

（8）洗剂主要指饮片经适宜的方法提取制成的供皮肤或者腔道涂抹或清洗用的不溶性药物混悬液。

（9）糖浆剂指含有药物、药材提取物或芳香物质的近饱和浓蔗糖水溶液。

（10）醑剂指一般是挥发性药物的浓乙醇溶液。

2. 固体剂型

（1）片剂：将药物加入赋形剂经压制而成的小圆片。可分为多层片、植入片、肠溶片、外用片等类型。

（2）丸剂：将药物细粉或药物提取物加适宜的辅料制成的球形或类球片形固体制剂。

（3）胶囊剂：将药物盛装入空硬胶囊或软胶囊中制成的制剂。

（4）散剂：一种或数种药物均匀混合而制成的干燥粉末状制剂。

（5）膜剂：将药物溶解于或混悬于多聚物的溶液中，经涂膜、干燥而制成。

（6）颗粒剂：将化学药物制成干燥颗粒状的内服制剂。

3. 半固体剂型

（1）硬膏剂：由药物和适当的基质混合而成，具有黏性而供贴敷的外用制剂。

（2）软膏剂：指药物加入适宜基质制成的半固体外用制剂。

（3）栓剂：药物与适宜基质混合制成的专供人体不同腔道给药的一种软性制剂。

（4）浸膏：药材浸出液浓缩后的粉状或膏状固体剂型。

4. 气雾剂

气雾剂指药物与抛射剂（液化气体或压缩气体）一起封装于密闭的、带有阀门的耐压容器内的液体制剂。分为吸入气雾剂、非吸入气雾剂和外用气雾剂三种类型。

二、药物处方

1. 处方的意义

处方是医师根据患者病情所开具的用药剂量、用法等，以便药剂师按照处方配药和发药的一项重要的书面文件。处方意义在于确保患者正确、安全地使用药物，达到治疗疾病的目的。

2. 处方的基本结构

完整的处方可分作六部分，依次排列如下。

（1）处方前项：包括医院全名、患者的姓名、性别、年龄、门诊号或住院号以及处方的日期等。

（2）处方头：写处方都以 Rp（或 R）起头，Rp 是拉丁文 Recipe 的缩写，是"请取"的意思。

（3）处方正文：包括药物的名称、剂型、规格和用量。如果一张处方中有几种药，则每一药物均应另起一行书写，药品数量一律用阿拉伯数字表示，药量应写在药品的后面。

（4）配置：对于完整的处方，医师开完药物后，还要写明调配方法。简单处方没有这一项。

（5）用药方法：用药方法通常以 sig. 或 S.（拉丁文 signa 的缩写）表示。具体用时既可用中文书写，也可用拉丁文缩写表示。内容包括处方药物用量、用法、每日次数等。

（6）医师签名：医师写完处方，仔细核对确保无误后签名交给患者。药师必须认真审核、评估、核对处方，如发现错误，有权退还医师改正，确认无误后再进行配制和发药，最后在处方笺上签名。

3. 书写处方的注意事项

（1）药物用量单位一律按药典规定书写。固体或半固体药物以克（g）为单位，液体药物以毫升（mL）为单位，如果用 mg、kg 或 IU 为单位时则必须写明。

（2）一般药物开 2 ~ 3 d 的量（慢性病除外），慢性病、老年病或特殊情况可酌情延长，但医师应注明。

4. 处方类型

主要有完整处方和简化处方两大类型，常用的处方类型为简化处方（附表 3-1）。

附表 3-1　处方中常用简写拉丁文字及其意义

简写字	拉丁文	意义	简写字	拉丁文	意义
aa	ana	各	M.f.	Misce,fiat	混合制成
a.c	ante cidul	饭前	N 或 N.	numero	数目
ad	ad	加至	p.o	post oibum	饭后
add	adde addatur	加，须加入	p.r.n.	pro re nata	必要时用
b.i.d	bis in die	1 日 2 次	q4h	quaque4h ora	每 4 小时
D.t.d	dentur tales doles	给予同量	q.i.d	quter in die	每日四次
gtt	gutta	滴	q.s.	quantum sufficiat	适量
h.s.	hora somni	临睡前	Sig. 或 S.	signa	标记，用法
i.h.	injectio hypodermica	皮下注射	S.O.S.	Si opus sit	必要时
i.m.	injectio intrausculosa	肌肉注射	S.S.	semisse	一半
i.v.	injectio intravenosa	静脉注射	St 或 stat	statim	立即
M	misce	混合	t.i.d.	ter in die	1 日 3 次

（1）完整处方：医师根据病情需要，自己设计开出的比较复杂处方，包括主药、佐药、赋形药、矫味药等。

（2）简化处方：书写已经制成各种剂型的药物。在处方正文中写明一个药物的名称、剂型、规格、取量，以及每次用量、每日次数、给药时间、给药途径。

处方练习：

（1）田某，男，46 岁。开罗红霉素分散片，150 mg/ 片，每日 2 次，每次 1 片，3 日用量。

（2）张某，女，32岁。开艾司唑仑片，1 mg／片，1 mg睡前口服，三日量。

（3）李某，男，50岁。开地塞米松注射液1支，规格1 mL：2 mg，皮下注射1 mg。

（4）工某，男，68岁。开磺胺嘧啶片（0.5 g／片）与碳酸氢钠片（0.5 g／片），二药同时口服，每次各服1 g，每日2次，首剂加倍，三日量。

（李　鑫）

附录4　实验报告的撰写

【实验报告撰写要求】

实验报告是学生完成实验后，对某项实验的目的、实验方法、实验结果如实记录并进行整理写出的书面总结。实验报告要充分体现实验内容的科学性、创造性和实用性。实验报告的书写要求如下：

1. 实验名称

实验名称要力求明确、能准确反映实验的内容。如观察苯巴比妥的抗惊厥效果，可写成"巴比妥类药物的抗惊厥作用"。

2. 实验人员信息

姓名、班级、学号，实验时间（×年×月×日）。

3. 实验目的

简要说明进行实验的主要目的，实验需要解决的问题及实验要达到的预期效果。

4. 实验材料

列出实验所用的仪器设备名称（型号）、实验耗材、实验动物（体重、性别）、和实验药品（浓度）等。

5. 实验方法

简要描述本实验所采用的实验方法、实验技术路线、给药顺序、观察指标和实验数据的收集方法等。

6. 实验结果

根据实验目的的不同，详细记录原始数据。对原始记录进行整理、归类，以供统计分析。同时应记录实验时间、条件、环境或出现的特殊情况。

注：对原始资料不允许更改、编造，不可主观选择、任意取舍。

7. 实验结果分析与讨论

对实验中所收集的数据，首先进行统计学处理，然而结合所学专业理论知识对实验进行分析和解释，讨论实验中出现的一般性规律和特殊规律之间的关系。

8. 结论

根据对实验结果的分析、判断，得出结论。结论是对实验结果归纳出的概括性总结。结论应回答实验提出的问题，要简明扼要、符合逻辑，具有理论意义。

【实验报告示例】

实验 X 药物的量效关系实验实验报告

专业班级：_____　　指导教师：_____

实验时间：_____

小组成员：姓名：_____　学号：_____

　　　　　姓名：_____　学号：_____

　　　　　姓名：_____　学号：_____

　　　　　姓名：_____　学号：_____

一、实验目的

了解药物的量效关系及测定量效关系的实验方法和量效曲线的绘制。

二、实验器材
三、实验步骤
四、实验过程记录表

实验时间点	操作内容	实验现象	备注

五、主要实验结果记录及分析

量效曲线：请画出实验中出现的量效关系的示意图（说明，根据具体实验安排以老师要求为准）。

检测指标：各浓度对应的效应值记录（说明）。

实验现象分析。

六、结论

七、实验体会（非必选）

请写明本实验中获得的体会。

（赵春贞）

附录5　练习题参考答案

第一章　药理学总论

第一节　1. A　2. D　3. B
第二节　1. A　2. D　3. B
第三节　1. A　2. B　3. B
第四节　1. B　2. C　3. B
第五节　1. C　2. C　3. B
第六节　1. B　2. C　3. B
第七节　1. B　2. C　3. B
第八节　1. A　2. C　3. D
第九节　1. A　2. A

第二章　传出神经系统药理

第一节　1. C　2. B　3. D
第二节　1. A　2. C　3. C
第三节　1. B　2. A　3. B
第四节　1. A　2. A　3. B
第五节　1. B　2. C　3. D

第三章　中枢神经系统药理

第一节　1. A　2. B　3. C　4. C

第二节　1. D　2. D　3. B

第三节　1. B　2. D　3. D

第四节　1. C　2. A　3. A

第五节　1. B　2. C　3. B

第六节　1. C　2. C　3. B

第七节　1. D　2. A　3. C

第八节　1. B　2. B　3. B

第九节　1. A　2. C　3. B

第四章　心血管系统药理

第一节　1. A　2. C　3. D

第二节　1. D　2. D　3. D　4. C

第三节　1. A　2. A　3. B

第四节　1. A　2. B　3. A

第五节　1. D　2. A　3. B

第五章　激素内脏药理

第一节　1. B　2. D　3. C

第二节　1. A　2. D　3. B

第三节　1. B　2. B　3. A

第四节　1. B　2. C　3. D

第五节　1. B　2. C　3. B　4. B　5. B

第六节　1. A　2. D　3. D

第七节　1. D　2. C　3. C

第八节　1. D　2. B　3. B

第九节　1. B　2. C　3. B

第六章　化疗药物药理

第一节　1. C　2. B　3. A

第二节　1. B　2. C　3. D

第三节　1. C　2. B　3. B

第四节　1. B　2. C　3. B

第五节　1. A　2. A

第九章　常用实验仪器设备

第一节　1. B　2. D
第二节　1. B　2. B
第三节　1. B　2. D

英文部分练习题参考答案同上。

（赵春贞）

Chapter 1　General pharmacology

Section 1　Basic knowledge of experimental animals

[Definition of experimental animals]

Experimental animals refer to animals that have been artificially feeded, controlled for carrying microorganisms, have clear genetic backgrounds or sources, and are used for scientific research, teaching, production, verification, and other scientific experiments.

Experimental animals refer to animals used in experiments. It only indicates the purpose of using such animals for experiments, not the quality attributes or the standardization of their use. Experimental animals have the following characteristics: ① Have clear genetic background. ② Monitor the carrying microorganisms and parasites. ③ Artificial reproduction under specific environmental conditions. ④ Have clear application scope. ⑤ There is a licensing system and quality supervision system established by the government to regulate laws and regulations.

[Types of experimental animals]

Experimental animals are an important part of modern life science research, served as the foundation and important supporting conditions for life science, especially biomedical research. Functional validation and safety evaluation are inseparable from experimental animals which play an irreplaceable role as compared to other research techniques and methods. According to national standards, experimental animals are divided into four levels such as ordinary level, clean level, specific pathogen free level, and sterile level.

Conventional animals refer to experimental animals that do not carry specified zoonotic pathogens and animal infectious disease pathogens.

Clean animals refer to experimental animals that do not carry pathogens that are harmful to animals or interfere with scientific research, in addition to pathogens that should be excluded for conventional animals.

Specific pathogen free animals (SPF) refer to experimental animals that do not carry major potential infections, conditional pathogens, or pathogens that interfere greatly with scientific experiments, in addition to pathogens that should be excluded for clean animals.

Experimental animals are controlled by the microorganisms they carry. The quality of experimental animals must be ensured mainly through regular laboratory testing, controlling the contamination of the environment and animals by biological and chemical factors.

[Characteristics of experimental animals]

Animal experimental methods are indispensable and important tools in pharmacological research. In pharmacological experiments, the vast majority of experiments need to be conducted on animals. Common experimental animals include toads, mice, rats, guinea pigs, rabbits, cats, dogs, etc.

1. Toads

Amphibian class, anura and bufonidae. The detached heart of toads can contract rhythmically and persistently, which was often used to observe the physiological functions of the heart and the effects of drugs on the heart. Gastrocnemius and sciatic nerve samples of the toads were used to observe the effects of drugs on peripheral nerves, skeletal muscles, and neuromuscular junctions. The rectus abdominis muscle sample of the toads can also be used to observe the effects of cholinergic drugs.

2. Mice

Chordata, mammalia, rodentia, muridae, mus musculus. Among various pharmacological experiments, mice are the most common ones. At present, there are over 500 distant and inbreeding groups, making it the most extensively studied and widely used mammalian experimental animal in the world. The genetic similarity between mice and humans can reach between 90% and 99%. They are easy to be reproduced in large quantities, inexpensive, and convenient to be reproduced. They are suitable for experiments such as drug screening, various toxicity tests (acute toxicity experiments, subacute and chronic experiments, determination of median lethal dose, etc.). Mice are nocturnal animals, whose eating, drinking, and other activities increase at night. Males are aggressive and have a significant social advantage. They are sensitive to external environmental reactions.

3. Rats

Chordata, mammalia, rodentia, muridae, ratte, and rattus norvegicus family. Similar in appearance to mice, but larger in size. Commonly used rats include Wistar rats, Sprague Dawley (SD) rats, etc. , which are widely used in medical, biological, toxicological, and nutritional research. Wistar rats are the earliest introduced rat species in China, with gentle temperament, strong reproductive ability, strong resistance to infectious diseases, low incidence of spontaneous tumors, and strong resistance to infectious diseases. SD rats grow and develop faster than Wistar rats, with stronger resistance to respiratory diseases, lower spontaneous tumor rates, and better sensitivity to sex hormones.

4. Guinea

Also known as guinea pig or hamster. Belonged to mammalia, rodentia, caviidae, cavia. Guinea pigs originate from the Andes Mountains in South America. The experimental guinea pig is domesticated from wild guinea pigs, with diverse fur colors such as white, black, and sandy white. Guinea pigs have a gentle temperament, precocious puberty, strong anti hypoxia ability, sensitive allergic reactions, poor temperature regulation ability, and are sensitive to changes in environmental temperature. Due to its particular sensitivity to histamine and susceptibility to antigenic substances, it is commonly used to observe the screening of antiasthmatic drugs, antihistamines, and antiallergic drugs, as well as to conduct experimental studies on anaphylactic shock.

5. Rabbits

Mammalia, rodentia, leporidae, oryctolagus. Have high reproductive capacity, good adaptability, and strong disease resistance. Rabbits have a gentle temperament and are easy to perform experimental procedures such as gastric lavage, intravenous injection, and blood collection. They can be used for direct recording of respiration, blood pressure, electrocardiogram, body temperature, and other experimental research. They are commonly used to observe the effects of drugs on the heart and respiration, as well as experiments on organophosphate pesticide poisoning and rescue. They can also be used for the effects of drugs on the central nervous system, body temperature, pyrogen testing, and contraceptive experiments.

6. Cats

Mammalia, carnivora, felidae. Cats are naturally timid and cautious, suspicious and uneasy towards strangers and environments. Cats have strong tolerance to surgical procedures and relatively stable blood pressure, but they are expensive and highly aggressive. They are commonly used in experimental studies on brain rigidity, hypothalamus, and blood pressure.

7. Dogs

Mammalia, carnivora, canidae. Dogs have a keen sense of smell, vision, and hearing, and are highly adaptable to external environments. The blood circulation, nervous system, and digestive system are relatively developed, similar to humans. Commonly used to observe the effects of drugs on cardiac pumping function and hemodynamics, as well as research on antihypertensive and anti-shock drugs. Dogs can also be trained for chronic experimental research, such as conditioned reflex, gastrointestinal motility and secretion experiments, central nervous system experiments, etc.

[Selection of experimental animals]

In pharmacological experiments, the appropriate selection of experimental animals is directly related to the quality of the project and the correctness of the experimental results, which is the first issue to be considered in animal experiments. In order to obtain ideal experimental results, suitable observation objects must be selected according to the experimental purpose. The selection of experimental animals should comply with the following basic principles.

(1) Choose experimental animals that are sensitive to stimuli and similar to humans, including structure, metabolism, health status, and disease characteristics, etc.

(2) Select standardized animals that are suitable for the experimental purpose, content, etc.

(3) Select animals with anatomical and physiological characteristics that meet the experimental requirements, fully utilize the different breeds and strains of animals that have certain anatomical and physiological characteristics, and special reactions that exist.

(4) Select experimental animals that are easy to obtain, raise, and manage, provided that they meet the experimental objectives and do not affect the experimental results.

The expression level and response of experimental animals to human diseases and applied factors are not only related to the physiological characteristics of the animals themselves, but also influenced by their state, such as hunger, sufficient sleep, and the presence of other diseases. In addition, environmental factors also have a strong interference effect on experimental animals. During the experiment, the experimental environment should be chosen to be as consistent as possible with the natural life of the test animals or artificially controlled to meet the conditions.

The selection and application of experimental animals should also follow the international "3R" principles for animal treatment including reduction, refinement, replacement. It also should comply with the corresponding international laboratory practice (GLP) and standard operating procedures (SOP).

[Practice questions]

1. The preferred animal for allergic reaction testing is _____.

A. guinea pig   B. mouse   C. rat   D. rabbit

2. According to national standards, experimental animals are classified into _____ levels.

A. one   B. two   C. three   D. four

3. Which one is the incorrect description about mice?

A. Easy to reproduce and affordable.

B. Strong tolerance to surgical procedures, stable blood pressure, commonly used in blood pressure experiments.

C. High homology with human genes.

D. Used for drug screening, toxicity experiments, etc.

[Thinking questions]

(1) What is the difference between experimental animals and animals used for research?

(2) How should we conduct animal experiments to ensure that we can achieve the experimental objectives while minimizing animal suffering to the greatest extent?

[Knowledye expansion]

Experimental mice

When it comes to experimental animals, what comes to your mind first? It's often said that "don't be a mouse for experiments." But do you really know a mouse? With so many experimental animals to choose, why do scientists focus on mice? There are a huge number of mice, about 1,700 kinds of mice distributed all over the world, which is more than that of the total human population. As early as the 16th century, some scientists had used mice for scientific research. At the beginning of the 20th century, because the research on Mendel's laws of inheritance required verification in different species, mice became an important research object. The world's first pure inbred mouse (DBA mouse) was born. In 1912, Hash Bugg in the United States obtained the BALB/c mouse strain after multiple generations of inbreeding. Since then, mice have officially entered the historical stage of experimental research.

（赵春贞）

Section 2 Common techniques for experimental animals

[Number of experimental animals]

In animal experiments, it is common to conduct experiments with multiple animals simultaneously and group them appropriately. In order to facilitate observation, identification, and recording of changes in the animals, they need to be numbered and labeled before the experiment. There are many methods for marking, and a good marking method should meet the requirements of clear, easy to distinguish, simple, and durable labeling. The commonly used marking methods include staining, imprinting, and ear margin cutting.

1. Dyeing method

Use colored dyes to apply on the hair of animals in obvious positions, and uses different dyes to distinguish between groups of animals. This labeling method is the most commonly used and convenient in the laboratory. The commonly used dyes include 3% ~ 5% picric acid solution (yellow), 0.5% neutral fuchsin (red), and 2% silver nitrate solution (coffee). When marking, dip a cotton swab or brush into the above solution and apply spots on different parts of the animal body to indicate different numbers. The principle of numbering: from left to right, from top to bottom. As shown in Figure 1-2-1, the coating on the left front leg is labeled as number 1, the left waist as number 2, the left hind leg as number 3, the top of the head as number 4, the center of the back as number 5, the base of the tail as number 6, the right front leg as number 7, the right waist as number 8, and the right hind leg as number 9. If the animal number exceeds 10 or a larger number, two different colored solutions can be used, with one color as the single digit and the other color as the ten digit. This interactive use can be coded up to number 99. This labeling method is more suitable for animal experiments with short experimental cycles. Over time, the dye is prone to fading, so it should be relabeled in a timely manner.

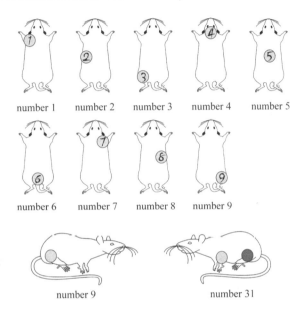

| number 1 | number 2 | number 3 | number 4 | number 5 |

| number 6 | number 7 | number 8 | number 9 |

| number 9 | number 31 |

Figure 1-2-1   Mouse numbering method

2. Imprinting method

Use ear number pliers (also known as ear number pliers) to pierce numbers on animal ears.Then dip a cotton swab in black ink dissolved in vinegar and apply it. It is best to disinfect the imprinting area with alcohol before imprinting, and the imprinting operation should be light and agile. This method is applicable to animals such as rabbits and dogs with relatively large ears.

The number can also be branded on a square or circular metal plate, or the number can be branded on the animal's belt according to the experimental grouping number, and the belt can be fixed on the animal's neck. This method, also known as the number card method, is suitable for larger animals such as rabbits, cats, and dogs.

3. Ear margin cutting method

Use a hole puncher to punch holes at a certain position on the animal's ear, and distinguishe experimental animals based on the location and number of holes punched (also known as punching method). Scissors can also be used to cut the gap, and attention should be paid to twisting it with talcum powder after cutting to prevent the cut from closing after healing (also known as the cutting gap method).

4. Acupuncture method

Remove the animal's fur, dip a small amount of carbon ink with a needle, and puncture the subcutaneous tissue of the animal's ear, front and rear limbs, or tail, leaving a black mark on the affected area.

5. Hair cutting method

Use a shearing knife to cut off the shape of the marked number on one side or back of the animal's body, suitable for large and medium-sized experimental animals such as rabbits, dogs, etc. This method is clearly and reliably labeled and is only for short-term observation use.

[Capture and fixation of experimental animals]

1. Toad

Usually hold in their left hand, with their index and middle fingers gripping their forelimbs, straightening their lower limbs, and using their ring and little fingers to grip them. Press the back with your thumb.

2. Mouse

Lift its tail with its right hand and place it on a cage cover or other rough surface, gently pulling it back and up. Quickly pinch the skin on the back of the mouse's neck with the thumb and index finger of the left hand, and use the little finger and palm ruler to clamp its tail root and fix it in the hand. It can also be operated with only one hand. First, grab the tail of the mouse with the thumb and index finger, then clamp the base of the tail with the palm ruler and little finger, and then pinch the skin on its neck with the thumb and index finger.

3. Rat

Rats are prone to be anger and bite, so when holding them, protective gloves should be worn on the left hand or a thick cloth. The thumb and middle finger of the left hand wrap around the back and armpit of the rat to grab it. If using the right hand at this time, place the index finger in front of the right forelimb and clamp it with the middle finger to make it easier to grasp. For $1 \sim 2$ week old or small-sized rats, gently pinch the skin on their back, grab their entire body, and secure their head to prevent biting.

4. Rabbit

When capturing a rabbit, one hand should grab its neck and back skin, gently lift the rabbit up, and the other hand should support its buttocks, making the rabbit sit in a seated position.

5. Guinea pig

Guinea pigs have a gentle temperament and can be held directly from the back with their left hand on the front trunk. For those who are underweight, they can be held with one hand, while for those who are overweight, they should be held with both hands and supported with their right hand on the buttocks. Guinea pigs can also be fixed with fixators or their limbs can be fixed on wooden boards.

6. Cat

Cats are relatively gentle, Grab their neck skin with one hand and lift them up with the other hand. For more aggressive cats, slowly insert your hand into the cage and gently stroke the cat's back, head, and neck. Use one hand to grab the cat's neck, and use the other hand to grab the skin from the back to the waist after leaving the cage. If cats are not allowed to touch their skin with hands, they can be caught with leather gloves.

7. Dog

For untamed dogs, use a dog catching fork to clamp the dog's neck and press it down, then tie the dog's mouth with a rope. When tying the mouth, first tie a knot with the rope from the corner of the mouth to above the nose, then tie a knot with the rope below the mouth, and then pull the rope to the neck behind the ear and tie it in place before administering the medicine. For domesticated dogs, it is not advisable to to clamp them with iron pliers. You can first caress them, gradually approach them, secure the dog with a mouth cover, and tie the dog's limbs with straps.

[Anesthesia of experimental animals]

In some animal experiments, especially animal surgery experiments, necessary measures are often taken on the animals for ease of operation. Animal anesthesia can choose both general anesthesia and local anesthesia. And different anesthesia methods require different drugs to be used.

1. Commonly used anesthetics

1) Local anesthetics

Such as procaine and lidocaine, have quick effects and commonly be used for local infiltration anesthesia.

2) General anesthetics

(1)Ether Ether inhalation anesthesia is suitable for various animals. And there is a large difference between the anesthetic dose and lethal dose, so the safety level is also high. The depth of animal anesthesia is easy to grasp, and it is easy to wake up after anesthesia. The disadvantage is that it has a strong local stimulating effect and can cause an increase in mucus secretion in the upper respiratory tract. Through neural reflexes, it can affect breathing, blood pressure, and heart rate activity, and is prone to suffocation.

(2) Sodium pentobarbital Commonly used 1% ~ 3% pentobarbital sodium physiological saline solution. And the effective anesthesia time can last for 3 to 5 hours after a single administration. Anesthesia is convenient to use, and a single administration can maintain a long anesthesia time. The anesthesia process is relatively stable, and there is no obvious struggle in the animals. The disadvantage is that the awakening is slow.

(3) Sodium thiopental The commonly used concentration of thiopental sodium is 1% to 5%. After injection, this drug can quickly enter the brain tissue, so anesthesia induction is fast, but recovery is also fast. The anesthesia duration of one administration is only maintained for 0.5 ~ 1 hour.

2. Anesthesia method

1) General anesthesia

(1) Inhalation anesthesia method: Anesthetics are produced by inhaling them through the respiratory tract in a vapor or gas state, and ether is commonly used as the anesthetic. Specific method: when using ether anesthesia for rabbits, rats, and mice, the animals can be placed in a glass anesthesia box, and a small beaker containing a cotton ball soaked in ether can be placed in the anesthesia box.

(2) Abdominal injection and intravenous anesthesia methods: Commonly used anesthetics include pentobarbital sodium, thiopental sodium, etc. Using intraperitoneal injection and intravenous injection anesthesia, with simple operation, is one of the most commonly used methods in the laboratory. Abdominal injection anesthesia is commonly used in rats, mice, and guinea pigs, while larger animals such as rabbits and dogs are often anesthetized by intravenous administration.

2) Local anesthesia

Use local anesthetics to block the impulse conduction of peripheral nerve endings, nerve trunks, ganglia, and nerve plexuses, producing a local anesthetic effect. Its characteristics are that animals remain awake, with minimal interference with important organ function and few anesthesia complications. Local anesthesia for cats is usually administered by injecting 0.5% to 1.0% procaine hydrochloride solution. For rabbits undergoing eye surgery, 0.02% cocaine hydrochloride solution can be dripped into the conjunctival sac, and anesthesia can occur within seconds.

[Administration of experimental animals]

1. Intraperitoneal injection

When conducting experiments with mice and rats, the animal is fixed with the left hand with the abdomen facing upwards and the head in a low position to move the internal organs to the upper abdomen. The injection is directed towards the right (left) lower abdomen and inserted into the skin with the right hand, passing through the abdominal muscles at 45°C. The needle tip is kept still at this point, and the needle plug is withdrawn. If there is no blood or urine return, the medication is slowly injected. If the experimental animal is a rabbit, it is advisable to insert the needle at a position 1 cm away from the white line in the lower abdomen.

2. Intragastric administration

Suitable for animals such as mice, rats, guinea pigs, rabbits, etc. Taking mice as an example, the left hand grasps the skin on the neck and back to fix the animal, the right hand holds a gastric lavage needle and inserts it into the animal's mouth, slowly inserting it into the esophagus along the posterior pharyngeal wall. Animals should be fixed in a vertical position, and there should be no resistance when inserting the needle. If resistance is felt or the animal struggles, the needle should be immediately stopped or pulled out to avoid damaging or puncturing the esophagus and accidentally entering the trachea. The commonly used gastric lavage volume for mice is 0.2 ~ 1 mL, for rats it is 1 ~ 4 mL, and for guinea pigs it is 1 ~ 5 mL.

3. Intravenous injection

1) Tail vein injection

Mice and rats are generally administered via tail vein injection. Fix the animal in the tail vein injector or in the mouse tube during injection, expose the tail. Soak the tail in warm water at 45 ~ 50°C for half a minute or wipe it with a 75% ethanol solution to dilate blood vessels and soften epidermal keratin. Pinch the sides of the tail of the mouse with the left thumb and index finger to fill the veins. Use the middle finger to lift the tail from below, and use the ring finger and little finger to clamp the tip of the tail. Hold the needle with the right hand so that the needle is parallel to the tail vein (less than 30°C), and insert the needle from 1/4 below the tail (about $2 \sim 3$ cm from the tip of the tail). Slowly inject a small amount of medication first, and if there is no resistance, continue to complete the injection.

2) Ear margin injection

Rabbits usually receive ear vein injection. Place the rabbit in a fixed box, first remove the fur from the injection site of the ear vein, and use your fingers to flick or gently rub the ear to fill the vein. Pinch the proximal end of the vein with the index and middle fingers of the left hand, tighten the distal end of the vein with the thumb, and place the ring and little fingers underneath. Use the right hand to hold a syringe and insert it into the blood vessel from the distal end, moving the fingers along the parallel direction of the blood vessel to fix the needle. Release the index and middle fingers, inject the medicine, then remove the needle and use the compressed needle eye for a moment.

4. Intramuscular injection

Choose areas with well-developed muscles and no major blood vessels or nerves passing through, and generally choose the buttocks. Insert the needle vertically into the muscle during injection, and if there is no blood return after withdrawing the needle plug, the injection can be performed. Intramuscular injection can be administered to small animals such as rats and mice, by injecting the medication into the upper lateral muscles of the hind legs.

5. Subcutaneous injection

When injecting, lift the skin with your left thumb and index finger, insert the syringe into the subcutaneous tissue, slowly inject the medication, remove the needle, and gently press the injection site with your fingers to prevent the medication from leaking out. Different experimental animals have different injection sites, with mice usually on the back and dogs and cats mostly on the outer thigh.

6. Intracranial injection

Used to observe the effects of drugs acting on brain lesions. For small animals, precise needle insertion is required. Placement and depth can be assisted by using a brain stereotaxic device for injection. When administering intracranial injections to mice, rats, guinea pigs, rabbits, etc., it is necessary to firstly use a transcranial steel needle to penetrate the skull, and then use a syringe needle to pierce the brain.

[Collection of experimental specimens]

1. Blood collection from tail vein

Mainly used for experiments in rats or mice that require very little blood. Fix the animal and expose the tail of the mouse. Soak the rat tail in warm water at 45 ~ 50 °C or wipe it with xylene to dilate and congestion the blood vessels. Cut open the tail vein with a surgical blade, and the blood will flow out on its own. Also take blood by cutting off the tail tip (cutting off 3 ~ 5 mm of the tail tip) to take blood.

2. Blood collection from the retrobulbar venous plexus

When taking blood, hold the neck between the ears of the mouse with your left hand and gently press down on the scalp on both sides of the back, so as to block the venous return of the head and make the eyeball protrude outward. Hold the capillary blood collection tube (0.5 ~ 1 mm) in your right hand and insert it from the eyelid and eyeball. Push the capillary parallel to the orbital wall towards the larynx for 4 ~ 5 mm, reaching the retrobulbar venous plexus where blood will flow into the tube on its own. Mice can collect 0.2 ~ 0.3 mL of blood each time, and rats can collect 0.4 ~ 0.6 mL of blood each time. This method can be used to collect blood multiple times in a row.

3. Blood collection from orbital arteries and veins

Hold the mouse upside down and compress its eyeball, causing it to become congested and protrude. Quickly remove the eyeball with hemostatic forceps. And then blood will quickly flow out of the box, just drop the blood into a test tube with anticoagulant.

4. Blood collection from the heart

Mainly used for larger animals such as rabbits and dogs. Fix the animal supine on the operating table. Cut off the hair in the precordial area, disinfect the skin with 75% ethanol solution. Touch the 3rd and 4th intercostal spaces on the left edge of the sternum with the left hand, and select the area with the most obvious heartbeat as the puncture point. Hold the syringe in the right hand, insert the needle into the heart. And the blood will automatically enter the syringe with the beating of the heart.

5. Blood collection from the ear margin vein

Commonly used for collecting blood from rabbits. Gently tap the ear shell or apply xylene to the blood collection site to dilate blood vessels. Then wipe clean with alcohol, and use a thick needle to puncture the ear vein to collect blood.

6. Blood collection by cutting off the head

Mainly used for large-scale blood collection in rats and mice. Fix the animal with your loft hand and tilt your head slightly downwards. Use scissors to quickly cut off the animal's head with your right hand, allowing blood to quickly drip into the test tube (containing anticoagulant).

[Execution of experimental animals]

1. Toad

Insert a frog needle into the foramen magnum, destroy the brain and spinal cord, or cut the head with coarse scissors and execute.

2. Rats and mice

1) Spinal cord dislocation method

Grasp the tail of the mouse with your right hand and pull it back with force, while pressing down on the mouse head with your left thumb and index finger to disconnect the brain and spinal cord. The mouse immediately dies. This is the most commonly used method of euthanizing mice.

2) Decapitation method

Cut off the mouse head with scissors at the neck of the mouse.

3) Striking manipulation

Grasp the tail of the mouse with your right hand, lift it up, and forcefully strike its head. The mouse spasms and immediately dies. Or hitting the mouse's head with a small wooden mallet can also be fatal.

4) Acute bleeding method

The method of acute massive blood loss in the orbital arteries and veins of mice can be used to induce immediate death.

3. Dogs, cats, rabbits, guinea pigs

① Air embolism method: Inject a certain amount of air into the animal's vein to cause embolism and death. ② Acute blood loss method: First anesthetize the animal, expose the femoral triangle or abdominal cavity, then cut off the femoral artery or abdominal aorta, immediately spray out blood, rinse with tap water continuously for bleeding, and die within 3 ~ 5 minutes. ③ Striking manipulation: Use a wooden mallet to forcefully strike the posterior brain of a rabbit, causing damage to medulla oblongata and resulting in death. ④ Open pneumothorax method: Open the chest of an animal to create an open pneumothorax, causing the animal to suffocate and die.

[Practice questions]

1. The most commonly used method for numbering experimental animals is _____.

A. dyeing method   B. license plate method

C. imprinting method   D. hair coating method

2. Common methods for euthanizing rats do not include _____.

A. acute bleeding method   B. striking method

C. decapitation method   D. destruction of spinal cord

3. Which method can be chosen for taking small amounts of blood from mice?

A. Cut off the head to collect blood.   B. Collect blood from the tail vein.

C. Heart blood collection.   D. Femoral artery blood collection.

[Thinking questions]

What preparations are needed before animal experiments?

[Knowledye expansion]

Clone mouse "Xiaoxiao"

In 2009, Chinese scientists successfully cloned the live mouse "Xiao Xiao" using iPS cells for the first time. The birth of this mouse announced the wisdom of the Chinese people to the world and continued the legend of cloning the sheep "Dolly". This achievement was published in the journal *Nature*. iPS cells, also known as induced pluripotent stem cells, are stem cells induced from somatic cells and have developmental pluripotency similar to embryonic stem cells. This is a cloned mouse cultivated by Chinese scientists without using embryonic stem cells, which has received high attention from the international stem cell research community. The website of *Nature* magazine praised Chinese scientists for "opening up a new path for cloning adult mammals".

（赵春贞）

Section 3　Ethics of experimental animals

[Welfare and protection of experimental animals]

The ethics of experimental animals is to examine from a moral perspective whether and how experimental animals receive moral treatment and care, and to constrain and regulate human behavior towards the use of experimental animals. Experimental animals are also a part of animals, so in a broad sense, the welfare of experimental animals also belongs to animal protection. Animal protectionism firstly emerged in the West in the 1960s, and research on animal ethics also flourished. The views on animal protectionism are gradually emerging, some of which are too extreme or radical. We need to have a correct view of the ethics of experimental animals, combined with the actual situation in China, which is related to the development of life sciences and medicine in our country.

Animal welfare refers to various measures taken by humans to avoid unnecessary harm to animals, preventing animal abuse, and ensuring that animals survive in a healthy and comfortable state. According to international consensus, the main content of animal welfare includes five freedoms (5F): freedom from hunger and thirst, freedom from discomfort, freedom from pain, injury, and disease, freedom from fear and sadness, and freedom to express normal behavior.

The welfare of experimental animals does not necessarily mean absolute protection from any harm, but rather a balance between exploring scientific issues and meeting the needs of experimental animals to maintain their lives, health, and comfort to the maximum extent possible. Research on the living environment conditions, "inner feelings" of experimental animals, and humane experimental techniques are the main research contents of scientific experimental animal welfare. When conducting activities related to experimental animals, we should aim to serve science and minimize the harm caused to experimental animals as much as possible.

At present, the welfare of experimental animals has caused widespread concern among countries and international organizations around the world.

Nowadays, all scientific research papers related to animal experiments are published or applied for scientific research topics must present a certificate provided by the "Animal

Ethics Committee" to ensure that the animal experimental research complies with animal welfare guidelines.

[Basic requirements of animal experimental ethics]

To resolve the conflict between bioethics and animal experiments, we need to adhere to the 3R principles and 5R concepts.

The "3R" principle refers to: ① "Reduction": minimize the number of animals used in the experiment as much as possible, improving the utilization rate of experimental animals and the accuracy of the experiment. ② Refinement: improve experimental conditions to reduce animal mental stress and pain. ③ Replacement: use single-cell organisms, microorganisms, cells, or other non-animal models instead of live animals for experimentation.

The five concepts of animal welfare are: ① Freedom from hunger and thirst (physiological welfare). ② Freedom from discomfort (environmental welfare). ③ Freedom from pain, injury, and illness, injury and disease (health and welfare). ④ Freedom from fear and distress (behavioral welfare). ⑤ Freedom to express normal behavior (psychological welfare).

Animal welfare not only ensures the survival status of animals, but also protects the existence of animal rights. Animal welfare theory advocates adhering to the "3R" and "5F" principles in the use of animals, explicitly prohibiting the indiscriminate killing and abuse of animals, and constraining human behavior to fully protect animals from suffering.

[Practice questions]

1. The "3R" principle of experimental animal ethics does not include _____.

A. protection   B. reduction   C. refinement   D. replacement

2. The "5F" principle of experimental animal ethics does not include _____.

A. freedom from hunger and thirst

B. freedom from slaughter

C. freedom to live comfortably

D. freedom to express one's nature

3. Which statement about animal welfare is incorrect?

A. Meeting the needs of animals to sustain their lives.

B. Absolutely protecting animals from harm

C. Animal welfare receives attention from various countries

D. Respecting the "inner feelings" of animals

[Thinking questions]

(1) How to understand "euthanasia"?

(2) What kind of animals do you think should be protected?

[Knowledye expansion]

Salute to the "Unknown Hero"

April 24th every year is designated as "World Experimental Animal Day", which was initiated by the UK Association Against Vivisection (NAVS) in 1979 and recognized by the United Nations as an international commemorative day. The week before and after it is called "Experimental Animal Week". The establishment of World Experimental Animal Day aims to promote the scientific and humane conduct of animal experiments, remember the enormous contributions and sacrifices made by experimental animals to human health, and standardize to use experimental animals reasonably.

（成　敏）

Section 4　Determination of plasma half life of sulfadiazine

[Experimental purpose]

(1) To study the methods for measuring and calculating the blood concentration and plasma half-life of sulfadiazine.

(2) To Master the calculation methods and clinical significance of pharmacokinetics.

[Experimental principle]

The plasma half-life ($t_{1/2}$) refers to the time required for blood concentration of a drug to decrease by half in the body, expressed as $t_{1/2}$. Most commonly used drugs in clinics are eliminated in the body according to first-order kinetics, and the blood drug concentration is proportional to the instantaneous drug concentration. It is that the drug concentration is eliminated in a constant proportion per unit time. The blood drug concentration (logarithmic value) - time curve is a straight line. The blood drug concentration (logarithm) - time curve of drugs eliminated according to zero-order kinetics is parabolic, which belongs to nonlinear kinetic elimination. Zero-order elimination kinetics is due to the saturation of the ability to eliminate drugs in the body, and the blood drug concentration-time curve is a straight line.

Sulfadiazine (SD) is a para aminobenzene compound that can ionize the amino group ($-NH_2$) on the benzene ring to form ammonium compounds ($-NH_3^+$) in acidic environments. It can react with sodium nitrite to generate diazonium salts ($-N{=}{=}N^+-$). This diazonium salt undergoes coupling reaction with phenolic compounds (such as thymol) in alkaline solution, producing orange red azo compounds (Figure 1-4-1). The color depth of azo compounds is related to the concentration of sulfadiazine. Measure the optical density using a spectrophotometer, and the drug concentration of sulfamethoxazole can be quantitatively analyzed by comparing it with the optical density of standard samples. According to the changes in plasma drug concentration at different times after medication, pharmacokinetic parameters such as plasma half-life can be calculated.

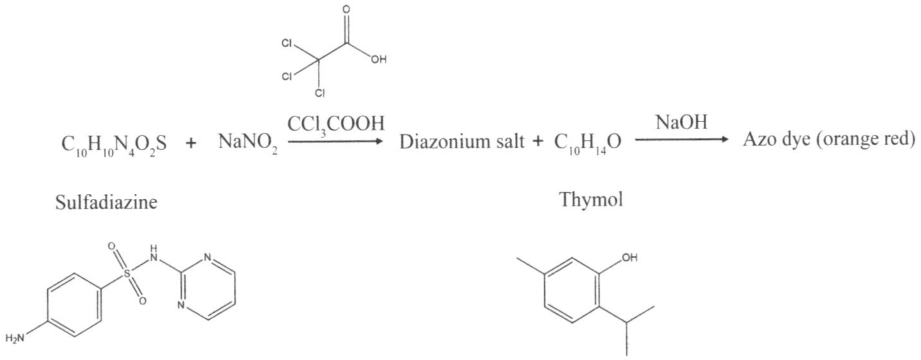

$$C_{10}H_{10}N_4O_2S \; + \; NaNO_2 \xrightarrow{\text{CCl}_3\text{COOH}} \text{Diazonium salt} + C_{10}H_{14}O \xrightarrow{\text{NaOH}} \text{Azo dye (orange red)}$$

Sulfadiazine   Thymol

Figure 1-4-1   Schematic diagram of the color development principle of sulfadiazine

[Experimental materials]

721 spectrophotometer, centrifuge, rabbit fixator, set of surgical instruments, test tube, centrifuge tube, beaker, scale, syringe (1 mL, 5 mL, 10 mL), pipette, pipette tip, test tube holder, toilet paper, cotton ball, plastic basin.

[Experimental animals]

Rabbits, weight 2.0 ~ 3.0 kg, regardless of gender.

[Experimental reagents]

20% sulfadiazine solution, 0.5% heparin saline solution, 0.5% sodium nitrite solution, 0.02% sulfadiazine sodium standard solution, 7.5% trichloroacetic acid solution, 0.5% thymol solution (prepared with 20% NaOH solution).

[Experimental methods]

The experimental operation steps are as follows, as shown in Figure 1-4-2.

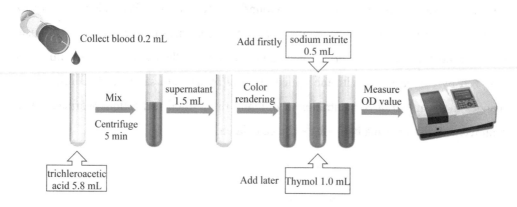

Figure 1-4-2　Schematic diagram of operation steps

1. Experimental preparation

Take 3 test tubes, labeled A, B, and C, and add 5.8 mL of 7.5% trichloroacetic acid solution to each tube. Take another 3 test tubes, also labeled A, B, and C, for spare use.

2. Collect blood before administration

Take one rabbit, weigh and record the weight, calculate the dosage based on the weight, and take the medicine for later use. Take one 1 mL syringe, rinse with 0.5% heparin saline solution, and collect 0.2 mL of blood from one ear vein of the rabbit. Keep the needle, remove the syringe, inject the blood into tube A, shake well and set aside.

3. Medication administration

After the first blood collection of the rabbit, immediately switch to another syringe (5 mL) and inject 2 mL/kg of 20% sulfadiazine solution from the original needle (calculate the corresponding administration volume based on the dosage). Record the time of injection completion.

4. Collect blood after administration

At 5 and 35 minutes after administration, the same method was used to collect blood from the other ear edge. Take 0.2 mL of blood from each vein and inject it into tube B and C. Accurately record the time of obtaining blood samples and calculate the time difference between two blood samples.

5. Color rendering

Shake the three test tubes A, B, and C well, centrifuge at a speed of 1500 r/min for 5 minutes, take 1.5 mL of the supernatant after centrifugation with a pipette, add it to the corresponding labeled test tube, and add 0.5 mL of 0.5% sodium nitrite solution and 1.0 mL of 0.5% thymol solution in sequence, mix well.

6. Color comparison

Adjust the sample tube A to zero and calibrate it before administration. Place the solution in each tube after the reaction into a 1.0 mL colorimetric cup of a 721 spectrophotometer. Measure the optical density values of each sample tube and standard tube at a wavelength of 525 nm.

7. Calculate drug concentration

According to the principle that the concentration of the same solution is proportional to the optical density, a standard tube without blood can be used to calculate the concentration of sulfadiazine in the blood at a certain time point based on its optical density value. The formula is as follows.

Concentration of sample tube /concentration of standard tube = optical density of sample tube / optical density of standard tube

$$C_{measurement} = OD_{measurement}/OD_{standard} \times C_{standard}$$

8. Calculate the plasma half-life ($t_{1/2}$)

The formula for calculating the half-life of one room model is: $t_{1/2}/T = \log(1/2)/\log R_T$

In the formula, T represents the interval time. R_T is the retention rate of drugs in the body after metabolism during the T time period (the ratio of drug concentrations taken twice after administration). In this experiment, it is the ratio of the blood drug concentration corresponding to 35 minutes to the blood drug concentration corresponding to 5 minutes, which can be replaced by OD_C/OD_B.

[Experimental records and results]

Record the experimental results and calculate the blood concentration and $t_{1/2}$ of sulfadiazine at 5 minutes and 35 minutes after medication according to the formula. Please refer to Table 1-4-1 for details.

Table 1-4-1　Blood concentration and plasma half-life determination of sulfadiazine

sampling time	blood sample (mL)	trichloroacetic acid (mL)		supern- atant (mL)	NaNO₂ (mL)	thymol (mL)	OD value (A)	concentration (mg/mL)
before administration	0.2	5.8	centrifuge	1.5	0.5	1.0		
5 min after administration	0.2	5.8		1.5	0.5	1.0		
35 min after administration	0.2	5.8		1.5	0.5	1.0		
Standard product	(standard solution) 0.2	5.8		1.5	0.5	1.0		

[Precautions]

(1) The syringe must be rinsed with heparin saline solution before taking a blood sample.

(2) When taking a blood sample, the syringe must be replaced and cannot be mixed.

(3) Each tube must be thoroughly mixed after adding a reagent, and the order of sample addition cannot be reversed.

(4) Each suction tube should be used separately, the colorimetric cup should be cleaned thoroughly, and the liquid should be accurately aspirated.

(5) Pay attention to the balance of the centrifuge tube during centrifugation.

(6) Blood collection can also be done using the cardiac method.

[Practice questions]

1. The blood collection from the ear vein should start from _____.

A. proximal end

B. distal end

C. any position

D. inner edge of the back of the ear

2. What is the correct description of first-order elimination kinetics?

A. The half-life of a drug is not a constant value.

B. Its elimination rate represents the actual percentage of elimination per unit time.

C. The elimination rate is directly proportional to the amount of drugs in the body.

D. It is the elimination method for a small portion of drugs.

3. What is the incorrect description regarding the operation of the centrifuge?

A. Preheat for 5 ~ 10 minutes before use.

B. The centrifuge tubes must be placed adjacent to each other and should not be too far apart.

C. Centrifugal tubes should not be filled too full.

D. Overloading is prohibited.

[Thinking questions]

(1) Is the plasma half-life of a drug fixed and unchanging? What is the guiding significance for clinical medication?

(2) The half-life of sulfadiazine varics among individuals. Apart from individual differences, what other factors affect it?

[Knowledye expansion]

The legendary discovery of Sulfonamids

Sulfadiazine, is a sulfonamide dye. It was discovered by German biochemist Gerhard Johannes Paul Domagk in 1932 and was the world's first commercially available antibacterial chemotherapy agent. Originally called "Prontosil", it is an industrial dye that was found to contain some disinfectant ingredients and was used to treat erysipelas and other diseases. However, it was found in experiments that it did not have a significant bactericidal effect in test tubes, and therefore did not receive much attention from the medical community. The earliest patient of Domagk was his 6-year-old daughter, who contracted an infection due to improper use of unsterilized needles. Her condition was worsened and doctors have begun to consider amputation. Desperate Domagk gave his daughter Prontosil, a medication that has not yet completed clinical trials. Fortunately, his daughter recovered and was discharged from the hospital after 2 days. Domagk was awarded the Nobel Prize in Physiology or Medicine for his discovery of the antibacterial properties of Prontosil .It was found that Prontosil can only kill streptococcus in the body, but not *in vitro*. It can be broken down into sulfamethoxazole, and animal experiments have found that "sulfonamide" is the same as Prontosil. The name sulfonamide quickly spread widely in the medical community.

（赵春贞）

Section 5　Determination of LD_{50} of procaine

[Experimental purpose]

To determine LD_{50} of procaine using sequential method.

[Experimental principle]

The dosage of a drug that can cause a positive reaction in 50% of experimental animals, and if the effect is death, is called the median lethal dose (LD_{50}). LD_{50} is one of the indicators for measuring the toxicity of drugs and is one of pharmacological data that must be provided during new drugs application. Median effective dose (ED_{50}) refers to the amount of medication that can cause 50% of the maximum reaction intensity in a quantitative reaction. The ratio of LD_{50} to ED_{50} is called the therapeutic index (TI), which is used to evaluate the safety of drugs. Generally speaking, drugs with higher TI value are relatively safer than those with lower TI value, but they are not entirely reliable.

Procaine is a local anesthetic with a molecular structure shown in Figure 1-5-1. It can temporarily block the conduction of nerve fibers and has anesthetic effects. When absorbed in large amount, it will produce systemic toxic reactions, mainly manifested as central nervous system excitation followed by inhibition, initially manifested as dizziness, restlessness, muscle tremors, and then developed into neurological disorders, convulsions, coma, respiratory depression, etc. Patients may die due to respiratory failure.

There are many methods for determining LD_{50}, such as the weighted probit method (Bliss method), Karber's method, sequential method, etc. The Bliss method is currently recommended as it does not have strict requirements for dose grouping and does not require a 0% or 100% mortality rate for dose groups. It is widely recognized as the most accurate measurement method. But this method is cumbersome to calculate, so computer programs are now commonly used for calculation. According to the regulations of the Ministry of Health of our country, the Bliss method is a necessary method for determining the LD_{50} of new drugs.

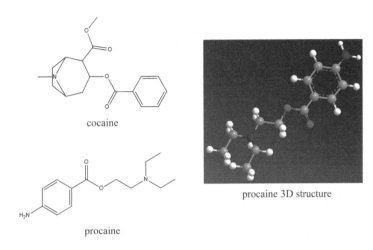

cocaine

procaine 3D structure

procaine

Figure 1-5-1   Molecular structure of procaine and cocaine

Sequential method, also known as sequential design method or sequential testing method, is an experimental measurement method that involves conducting experiments and analyzing them one by one. The advantage of this method is that it saves test animals and is easy to observe experimental results, making it suitable for drug experiments with relatively fast reactions after medication.

[Experimental materials]

Syringe, electronic balance, squirrel cage, functional calculator.

[Experimental animals]

Mice (18 ~ 22 g), sex in half.

[Experimental reagents]

2% procaine solution, 2% picric acid solution.

[Experimental methods]

(1) Determine the dosage for administration Pre-determine the drug dosage before the experiment, and arrange adjacent doses in equal proportions (with equal logarithmic differences), as shown in Figure 1-5-2.

Dose (mg/kg)	LogD	Animal status (Dead "+" or Not Dead "−")										R	R · logD
		1	2	3	4	5	6	7	8	9	10		
125	2.097	+										1	2.097
87.5	1.942		+		+							2	3.884
61.3	1.787			−		+		+		E		4	7.148
42.9	1.632						−		−			2	3.264
Total												9	13.363

Figure 1-5-2   Example of experimental results of intraperitoneal injection of pentylenetetrazol in mice

(2) Ten mice were selected in each experimental group, with sex in half. After weigh the mice, label them with picric acid.

(3) Administration and result recording First, take one mouse and inject the first dose of 2% procaine 0.1 mL/10 g intraperitoneally. If death occurs, the next animal will receive the lower dose. If no death occurs, the next animal will receive the higher dose. Record the results in a table, with "+" indicating animal death and "−" indicating survival. If there are two consecutive occurrence of "−" in the same dose, the next experiment will end and the last animal will not be tested, but it needs to be marked with "E" in the table.

(4) Calculation of experimental results

$$LD_{50}=\log{-1}(C/N) \text{ mg/kg}$$

In the formula： $C=\sum(R \cdot \log D)$;

R= Number of animals in the dosage group;

LogD= The logarithmic value of dose D;

N= Total number of experimental animals = $\sum R$.

[Experimental records and results]

The table of experimental result record is as follows (Table 1-5-1).

Table 1-5-1 Experimental results of intraperitoneal injection of procaine in mice

Dose (mg/kg)	LogD	Animal status (Dead "+" or Not Dead "–")										R	R · logD
---	---	1	2	3	4	5	6	7	8	9	10		
222	2.347												
200	2.301												
180	2.255												
162	2.209												
145.8	2.163												
Total													

[Precautions]

(1) This experiment is a quantitative experiment, and the injection dose must be accurate.

(2) After administration, the animal's reaction should be carefully observed and the mice should not be moved too much to avoid affecting the experimental results.

(3) Because weight has a significant impact on the mortality rate of this drug, the weight distribution of each group of animals should be consistent.

[Practice questions]

1. Which of the following statements about intraperitoneal injection in mice is incorrect?

A. When injecting into the abdominal cavity, it is not advisable to stab the internal organs with the animal's head down.

B. Before administering medication via intraperitoneal injection, the air bubbles in the syringe should be emptied firstly.

C. The injection needle should be tightly attached to the skin and inserted parallel as much as possible.

D. When the needle tip passes through the abdominal muscles and enters the peritoneal cavity, the resistance disappears.

2. The relationship between LD_{50} and toxicity evaluation is that_____.

A. LD_{50} is directly proportional to the toxicity level

B. LD_{50} is directly proportional to the toxic dose

C. LD_{50} is inversely proportional to toxicity level

D. LD_{50} is inversely proportional to acute threshold dose

3. The most accurate method for determining LD_{50} is _____.

A. karber's method

B. bliss method

C. sequential method

D. cumulative method

[Thinking questions]

(1) What is the significance of LD_{50} measurement?

(2) What other toxicity indicators should be considered in the safety evaluation of drugs besides LD_{50}?

[Knowledye expansion]

The classic "transformation" process of procaine from a "drug" to an anesthetic

If you go to a dentist, it is highly likely that you have been used procaine, a local anesthetic, and its "relative" is cocaine, which is well-known as a "drug".

Cocaine, an alkaloid isolated from South American coca leaves, was the earliest local anesthetic used in clinics in 1884. It is very effective on local anesthesia, but highly toxic and can easily lead to addiction and even death. The chemical structure of cocaine is a complex double ring. In 1905, Alfred Einhorn, a chemistry professor at the University of Munich in Germany, simplified the structure of cocaine and synthesized a compound called procaine, which retains only one ring but has better anesthetic effects. Moreover, it is not addictive and will not be abused. This is also the first injectable local anesthetic. From that time on, people realize that the complex structure of natural products can be simplified, with unchanged or even better effects. And the development of new drugs has an additional pathway - simplifying the structure of natural products. This is one of the classic examples of designing and discovering new drugs based on natural compounds.

（赵春贞）

Section 6   The influence of liver function on drug action

[Experimental objective]

(1) Observe the influence of liver function on the effects of propofol.

(2) Understand the importance of the liver in drug metabolism.

(3) Understand the methods for creating models of liver damage.

[Experimental principle]

The liver is the largest solid organ in the human body and serves as the primary organ for drug metabolism. The majority of drugs are metabolized by the liver, their metabolites become inactive. However, a small number of drugs require liver metabolism to convert into active metabolites that exert pharmacological effects. When liver function is impaired, the liver's ability to metabolize drugs decreases, leading to an increase in the parent drug (i.e., increased C_{max}) and prolonged half-life ($t_{1/2}$), which can enhance the drug's effects and increase adverse reactions. Carbon tetrachloride, once it enters hepatocytes, is activated by cytochrome P450 enzymes to produce trichloromethyl free radicals ($.CCl_3$). These free radicals covalently bind to membrane phospholipids and protein molecules, disrupting the structural and functional integrity of the membrane, particularly damaging the mitochondrial membrane structure. This affects metabolic functions and energy synthesis, ultimately leading to hepatocyte degeneration and even necrosis. Therefore, animals poisoned by carbon tetrachloride are often used as animal models of toxic hepatitis to observe the influence of liver function status on drug effects, as well as to screen and test drugs that protect liver function.

Propofol is a rapidly acting, short-acting intravenous general anesthetic used for procedures such as sedation in critically ill patients undergoing mechanical ventilation and for painless artificial abortion surgeries under anesthesia. The mechanism of action of Propofol may involve activating central gamma-aminobutyric acid receptors and modulating the hypothalamic sleep pathway. Propofol has a very high lipo-solubility and a plasma protein binding rate of 96% to 98%. Due to its rapid metabolism and elimination, its anesthetic duration is short, lasting approximately 4 to 6 minutes. Propofol is primarily metabolized and eliminated by the liver, potentially through conjugation with glucuronic acid, and its metabolites are excreted in urine. The functional status of the liver directly affects the strength and duration of its pharmacological effects (Figure 1-6-1).

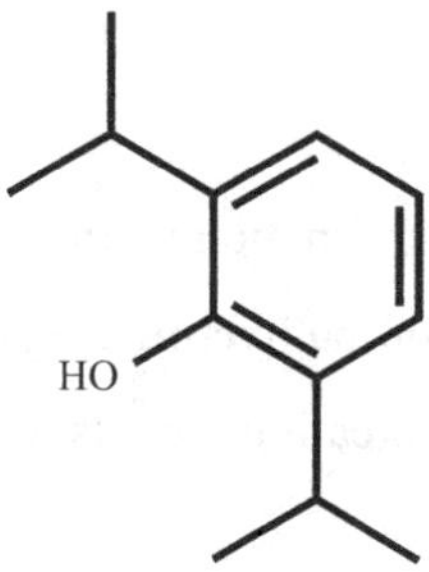

Figure 1-6-1   Molecular structure fo propofol

[Experimental materials]

Electronic balance, beaker, syringe (1 mL), mouse cage, frog board, surgical scissors, forceps.

[Experimental animals]

4 mice (18 ~ 22 g), regardless of gender.

[Experimental reagents]

1% propofol solution, 10% carbon tetrachloride, normal saline, picric acid solution.

[Experimental methods]

The experimental operation steps are as follows, seen in Figure 1-6-2.

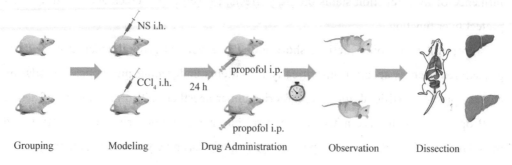

Figure 1-6-2   Schematic diagram of operation steps

1. Grouping and numbering of experimental animals

Select 4 mice with similar body weights and randomly divide them into two groups, Group A and Group B. After weighing, mark each mouse with picric acid for identification and observe their normal activities.

2. Establishment of liver injury model

Twenty-four hours before the experiment, mice in Group A are administered with 10% carbon tetrachloride at a dose of 0.1 mL/10 g via subcutaneous injection to induce liver injury. Mice in Group B receive an equal volume of normal saline as a control.

3. Observation before drug administration

At the beginning of the experiment, perform the righting reflex test on both Group A and Group B mice. Place the mice on their backs on the experimental platform. If they are able to return to their normal position, the righting reflex is present. Otherwise, it is absent.

4. Drug Administration

Inject 1% propofol solution at a dose of 0.1 mL/10 g (dosage of 100 mg/kg, 1 mg/10 g) into the abdominal cavity of mice in both Group A and Group B. Immediately after injection, record the time. The disappearance of the righting reflex serves as the indicator of the onset of anesthesia, and this period is recorded as the anesthesia induction time. Continue observing the mice until the righting reflex returns, recording this period as the anesthesia duration. Other observation indicators include mouse activity, respiratory depth and frequency. Compare the differences in anesthesia duration between the two groups.

5. Dissection and observation

After the mice recover from anesthesia, euthanize them by cervical dislocation. Dissect and observe the liver for morphological differences, comparing liver size, color, and degree of congestion between the two groups. Pay attention to the relationship between liver morphological changes and anesthesia duration.

[Experimental records and results]

Record the experimental results, including the onset time, duration, and liver morphology of anesthesia for each group of mice in Table 1-6-1.

Table 1-6-1　Effect of liver function on the action of propofol

Group	Number	Weight (g)	Dosage (mg/10 g)	Time of anesthesia onset (min)	Duration of anesthesia (min)	Liver morphology
Liver damage group	1					
	2					
Control group	3					
	4					

[Precautions]

(1) It is best to maintain the room temperature at around 25°C. If the temperature falls below 20°C, it is recommended to provide warmth for the anesthetized mice, as hypothermia can slow down their metabolism and make it difficult for them to recover.

(2) Carbon tetrachloride is toxic to humans, so it is important to handle it safely. It is recommended that the establishment of liver injury models be handled uniformly and in advance by the research department.

(3) When establishing liver injury, attention should be paid to the dosage of carbon tetrachloride to avoid excessive doses that could lead to the death of the mice.

(4) The disappearance of the righting reflex refers to the inability of the mouse to spontaneously turn over within 1 minute when placed on its back. If the mouse is able to turn over spontaneously, it is considered to be awake.

[Practice questions]

1. The pathological changes of liver cells caused by carbon tetrachloride poisoning are

_____.

A. hyaline degeneration   B. fatty infiltration

C. calcification   D. fibrinoid necrosis

2. Which statement about the pharmacological characteristics of propofol is incorrect?

A. It has a rapid onset and induces anesthesia smoothly.

B. It can reduce cerebral blood flow, cerebral metabolic rate, and intracranial pressure.

C. It has no respiratory depressant effect.

D. It can cause pain at the injection site and local phlebitis.

3. When patients with impaired liver function take medications that are metabolized

and deactivated by the liver, the dosage should be _____ .

A. increased   B. decreased   C. unchanged   D. forbidden

[Thinking questions]

(1) What is the difference in anesthesia duration between mice with liver damage and normal mice after administering propofol? Why?

(2) What is the guiding significance of liver function status for clinical medication dosage?

[Knowledye expansion]

The liver in the context of traditional Chinese medicine theory

The ancient people's understanding of the liver was primarily based on the theories of traditional Chinese medicine (TCM). The liver is considered one of the five organs and has physiological functions such as regulating blood flow, storing blood, and regulating tendons. In TCM, the liver is intimately connected with emotions, eyesight, digestion, and other aspects. Ancient people believed that the liver is a crucial organ in the human body, playing a vital role in maintaining good health. Furthermore, TCM has formulated theories and treatments related to the liver to regulate the body and treat illnesses.

Huangdi Neijing (*The Yellow Emperor's Inner Classic*): As the foundational work of TCM theory, *Huangdi Neijing* provides profound insights into the functions of the liver and drug metabolism. For instance, the *Suwen* (*Plain Questions*) section mentions, "The liver is the general of the body, where plans and strategies originate," vividly depicting the liver's significant position and role in the human body.

Shanghan Zabing Lun (*Treatise on Cold Damage and Miscellaneous Diseases*): Written by Zhang Zhongjing of the Eastern Han Dynasty, this work not only includes therapeutic prescriptions for various diseases but also implicitly embodies the concept of herbal medicine metabolism and transformation within the human body.

Drug Metabolism Example: Take the traditional Chinese medicine Chaihu (Bupleurum chinense) as an example. According to TCM theory, Chaihu has the effects of soothing the liver and relieving depression, as well as lifting yang qi. Modern research has also discovered that the active ingredients in Chaihu, after being metabolized in the liver, exhibit anti-inflammatory and antiviral pharmacological effects.

In summary, ancient Chinese records regarding the liver and drug metabolism not only reflect the profoundness and comprehensiveness of TCM theory but also provide valuable references and insights for modern research on traditional Chinese medicine.

（童骏森）

Section 7　Effects of different dosage on drug action

[Experimental purpose]

To observe the difference in the effects of drugs with different doses (pentobarbital sodium or chloral hydrate) on mice.

[Experimental principle]

The relationship between drug dosage and clinical pharmacological effects is complex, as the effects of drugs entering the body are influenced by complex regulatory compensatory mechanisms. The relationship between drug concentration and its effect in a carefully controlled *in vitro* experimental system is called dose-response relationship. The drug effect is proportional to the dosage within a certain range.

The size of drug dosage determines the high or low blood concentration of the drug in the body and the strength of the drug's effect. When the dosage of the drug increases, the effect of the drug also increases. However, the increase in this effect is not unlimited. Once the effect reaches a certain level, if the drug concentration or dosage continues to increase, the effect will not continue to strengthen and will remain constant at a certain level. When the dosage of medication is too high, it can lead to poisoning or death.

Sodium pentobarbital and chloral hydrate are both central inhibitory drugs, and their pharmacological effects vary depending on their dosage. The righting reflex is the observation indicator in this experiment. The righting reflex refers to the immediate restoration of normal posture in normal mice by gently lying them on their side or back with hands. The disappearance of the righting reflex is an objective indicator of the sleep effect in mice. If a mouse cannot be corrected by gently lying on its side or back for more than 1 minute, it is considered that the righting reflex has disappeared (Figure 1-7-1).

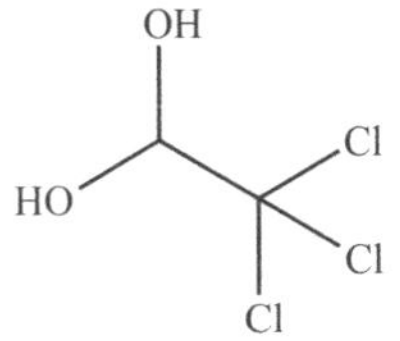

Molecular structute of   3D structure of
hydrated chloral   hydrated chloral

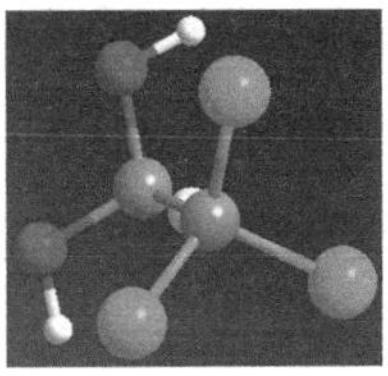

Figure 1-7-1   Molecular structure of chloral hydrate

[Experimental materials]

1 mL syringe, electronic balance.

[Experimental animals]

Mice (18 ~ 25 g), regardless of gender.

[Experimental reagents]

0.3% sodium pentobarbital solution, 2.5% chloral hydrate solution, 4% chloral hydrate solution, 2% picric acid solution, physiological saline solution.

[Experimental methods]

The experimental operation steps are as follows, as shown in Figure 1-7-2.

1. Label and weigh

Take 3 mice, label mice 1, 2, and 3 with picric acid, and observe the normal activity status of the mice such as breathing, activity, and coordination of movements. Weigh and record weight.

2. Drug administration

Calculate the dosage based on the weight of the mice and record it. Rat 1 was intraperitoneally injected with 0.1 mL/10 g of physiological saline. Rat 2 was intraperitoneally injected with 0.1 mL/10 g of 2.5% chloral hydrate solution. And Rat 3 was intraperitoneally injected with 0.1 mL/10 g of 4% chloral hydrate solution. Carefully observe the reaction of mice after administration and record the time of disappearance and recovery of the righting reflex. If the injected drug is 0.3% pentobarbital sodium solution, the administration method is as follows: Rat 1 is intraperitoneally injected with 0.1 mL/ 10 g of physiological saline. Rat 2 is intraperitoneally injected with 0.06 mL/10 g of 0.3% pentobarbital sodium solution. And Rat 3 is intraperitoneally injected with 0.12 mL/10 g of 0.3% pentobarbital sodium solution.

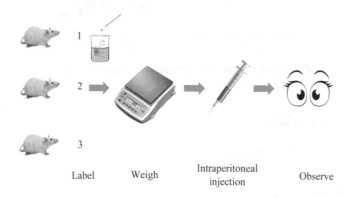

Label　　Weigh　　Intraperitoneal injection　　Observe

Figure 1-7-2　Schematic diagram of operation steps

3. Observe and record experimental results

Carefully observe the reactions of mice before and after administration, and record them truthfully.

[Experimental records and results]

Fill in the experimental records and results in the table, as shown in Table 1-7-1.

Table 1-7-1　Effects of dose on drug action

Number	Weight/g	Dosage/ mL	Route of administration	Disappearance time of righting reflex	Recovery time of righting reflex
1					
2					
3					

[Precautions]

(1) The weight of experimental animals should be uniform to minimize errors.

(2) If the room temperature is below 20 ℃, it is necessary to keep the mice warm, otherwise it may slow down metabolism and be difficult to wake up, affecting experimental observation.

(3) The syringes and needles used for different drugs should be distinguished, and the syringes should be cleaned before each injection to avoid affecting the experimental results.

[Practice questions]

1. Sodium pentobarbital _____.

A. half life exceeding 10 hours

B. possessing dual properties of drug and drug

C. no need to store in the dark

D. belongs to benzodiazepine sedative hypnotic drugs

2. Efficiency refers to _____.

A. effects produced by extreme dosage

B. effects produced by therapeutic dosage

C. maximum effect

D. drug potency

3. Which of the following statements about chloral hydrate is correct _____.

A. non irritating to gastric mucosa

B. can be converted into stronger trichloroethanol

C. no anticonvulsant effect

D. used orally only

[Thinking questions]

(1) What insights does this experiment provide for pharmacological experiments and clinical medication?

(2) What are the differences between the mechanisms pentobarbital sodium and chloral hydrate induced sleep in mice?

[Knowledye expansion]

Euthanasia and pentobarbital sodium

Currently, only a few countries in the world have decriminalized active euthanasia. In China, euthanasia is opposed and prohibited. The medication chosen for euthanasia abroad, whether orally or intravenously, is pentobarbital sodium. The active ingredient of pentobarbital sodium is pentobarbital, the sodium salt form of pentobarbital, chemically known as pentobarbital sodium. Sodium pentobarbital has anesthetic, sedative, and hypnotic effects and belongs to the barbiturates class of sedative and hypnotic drugs. In China, pentobarbital is listed as the second category of psychotropic drugs in the Catalogue of Psychotropic Drugs. In China, euthanasia of animals can be legally carried out by rapid intravenous injection of high concentration pentobarbital sodium. If intravenous injection is difficult for young animals, the same dose can be administered intraperitoneally. Deep anesthesia causes loss of consciousness, respiratory center depression, and respiratory arrest, leading to cardiac arrest.

（赵春贞）

Section 8　Effects of different administration routes on the action of magnesium sulfate

[Experimental purpose]

To observe the effect of different administration routes on the action of magnesium sulfate.

[Experimental principle]

There are multiple ways for drugs to enter the human body. Different treatment needs, physicochemical properties and biological characteristics of drugs, patient safety and compliance, and other factors determine administration method to use.

The administration route is an important factor affecting the drug's effect. Different administration routes result in different rates of drug absorption, distribution, etc., which can affect the strength and speed of drug action, and even alter the properties of drug action. The different routes of administration can directly affect the speed and strength of drug effects (Figure 1-8-1). According to the time of onset of drug efficacy, the order is: intravenous injection, inhalation administration, sublingual administration, intramuscular injection, subcutaneous injection, oral administration, and dermal administration.

The magnesium sulfate used in this experiment has four administration routes in clinical practice: oral administration, intravenous injection, intramuscular injection, and external application. Different administration routes correspond to different indications and therapeutic effects.

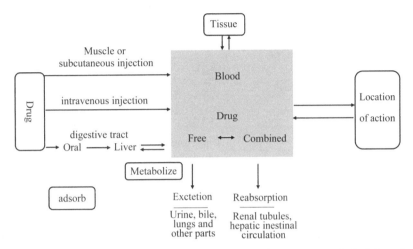

Figure 1-8-1 Metabolism of drugs in vivo through different routes of administration

[Experimental materials]

1 mL syringe, electronic balance, mouse gavage needle.

[Experimental animals]

Mice (18 ~ 22 g), with similar weight.

[Experimental reagents]

15% magnesium sulfate solution.

[Experimental methods]

The experimental operation steps are as follows, as shown in Figure 1-8-2.

1. Label

Take 4 mice, numbered 1, 2, 3, and 4 with picric acid, and observe their normal activity statusbreathing, activity, and coordination of movements.

2. Weigh

Weigh with an electronic balance and record the weight.

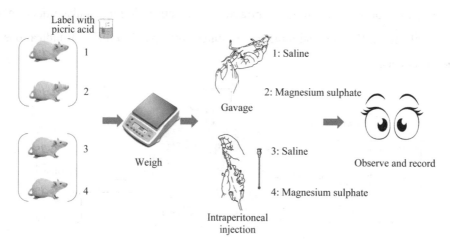

Figure 1-8-2　Schematic diagram of operation steps

3. Drug administration

Calculate the dosage based on the weight of the mice and record it. Rat 1 was intraperitoneally injected with 0.2 mL/10 g of physiological saline. Rat 2 was intraperitoneally injected with 0.2 mL/10 g of 15% magnesium sulfate solution. Rat 3 was orally administered with the same dose of saline solution at 0.2 mL/10 g. And rat 4 was orally administered with the same dose of 15% magnesium sulfate solution (0.2 mL/10 g).

4. Observe and record

Place the mice in a cage, observe the performance of each group of mice, and keep records.

[Experimental records and results]

Fill in the experimental records and results in the table, as shown in Table 1-8-1.

Table 1-8-1　The effect of administration route on the action of magnesium sulfate

Number	Weight/g	Drug	Dose/mL	Route of administration	Performance before administration	Performance after administration
1						
2						
3						
4						

[Precautions]

(1) When administering gastric lavage, it is important not to accidentally enter the trachea or puncture the esophagus, as this can lead to animal suffocation or even death.

(2) After injection of medication, the effect is rapid and requires careful observation

(3) Before oral administration, animals should generally undergo a period of fasting and avoid drinking water.

[Practice questions]

1. Apart from vascular administration, the fastest absorption method of administration is _____.

    A. inhalation

    B. sublingual ingestion

    C. rectal administration

    D. subcutaneous injection

2. The medicine bottle should be clearly labeled. What kind of label should be affixed on the outside of oral medication bottles?

    A. Red border.

    B. Black border.

    C. Blue border.

    D. Yellow border.

3. What is the mechanism of magnesium sulfate's anticonvulsant effect?

    A. Reduce the effect of blood calcium.

    B. Increase the effect of blood magnesium.

    C. Combined effect of increasing blood magnesium and decreasing blood calcium.

    D. Competitive inhibition of calcium action, reduce the release of acetylcholine from motor nerve endings.

[Thinking questions]

(1) What are the differences in the effects of magnesium sulfate administered by gavage and intraperitoneal injection?

(2) Analyze the mechanisms by which different routes of administration leading to different drug effects. What clinical guidance significance does this have for clinical medication?

[Knowledye expansion]

What do you know about febrile seizures in children?

The report of the 20th National Congress of the Communist Party of China pointed out that prioritizing the protection of people's health and improving policies to promote people's health should be given strategic importance. Children are the future of the country and the hope of the nation, and their health is an important guarantee for sustainable economic and social development. Febrile convulsion is one of the common neurological diseases in childhood, and its incidence rate varies from country to region, about 5% ~ 6% in China. The first onset of febrile seizures is more common between 6 months and 5 years old, occurring in a febrile state (anal temperature $\geq$ 38.5 ℃, axillary temperature $\geq$ 38℃), with no evidence of central nervous system infection or other causes of seizures, and no history of febrile seizures. Some children with febrile seizures may start as seizures, and fever may not be detected before the seizure, but fever may appear immediately after or during the seizure. Clinically, attention should be paid to avoid misdiagnosis as the first seizure of epilepsy. Febrile seizures usually occur within 24 hours after the onset of fever. If the fever persists for more than 3 days, seizures may occur. Pay attention to finding other causes of seizures. Convulsive seizures are often brief self-limiting episodes, and parents should remain calm. However, there is currently a lack of high-quality clinical research evidence on seizures in domestic children. With the accumulation of clinical evidence on various febrile seizures in children, their prevention, diagnosis, treatment, as well as health education and long-term management, will become more scientific and standardized.

（赵春贞）

Section 9　Determination of IC$_{50}$ of drugs *in vitro*

[Experimental objective]

(1) Learn the detecting method of IC$_{50}$ of anti-tumor drugs on tumor growth inhibition

using MTT Methods.

(2) Understand the significance of calculating the IC_{50} of drugs in vitro.

[Experimental principle]

The 50% inhibitory concentration (IC_{50}) refers to the concentration of the inhibitor at which the "reaction" is inhibited by half. Here, the reaction can be an enzyme catalyzed reaction, an antigen antibody reaction, or an apoptosis reaction of tumor cells against tumor drugs. In terms of apoptosis, it can be understood as a certain concentration of a drug inducing 50% apoptosis of tumor cells. This concentration is called the 50% inhibitory concentration, which is the concentration corresponding to the ratio of apoptotic cells to the total number of cells being equal to 50%. The IC_{50} value can be used to measure the ability of a drug to induce apoptosis, that is, the stronger the induction ability is, the lower the value is. And of course, it can also indicate the tolerance of a certain cell to the drug in reverse.

MTT (methyl thiazolyl tetrazolium) is a yellow compound that can detect cell survival and growth. The detection principle is that succinate dehydrogenase in live cells mitochondria can reduce exogenous MTT to insoluble purple formazan crystals deposited in the cells. The amount of formazan crystals is proportional to the number of live cells (succinate dehydrogenase disappears in dead cells and cannot reduce MTT). Dimethyl sulfoxide can dissolve formazan in cells. The light absorption value can be detected at a wavelength of 490 nm using an enzyme-linked immunosorbent assay detector, which indirectly reflects the number of live cells. The higher the absorption value is, the more live cells there are (Figure 1-9-1).

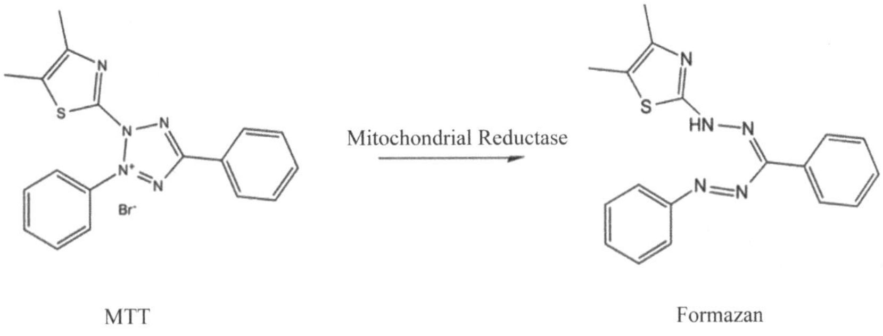

MTT   Mitochondrial Reductase   Formazan

Figure 1-9-1   The principle of MTT method

[Experimental materials]

Carbon dioxide cell incubator, ultra clean workbench, desktop centrifuge, enzyme-linked immunosorbent assay detector, microscope, 25 cm² sterile culture bottle, sterile 96 well culture plate, micropipette, sterile pipette tip (1 mL, 200 μL, 10 μL), test tube rack.

[Cell line]

Human non-small cell lung cancer cell line A549.

[Experimental reagents]

Paclitaxel, DMEM medium, fetal bovine serum, trypsin, 100 U/mL penicillin, 100 U/mL streptomycin, 5 mg/mL MTT solution, dimethyl sulfoxide.

[Experimental methods]

1. Preparation before the experiment

Before the experiment, prepare to clean the ultra clean table and the outer packaging of the pipettes, test tube racks, culture bottles, and culture plates required for the experiment with 75% alcohol. Turn on the ultraviolet sterilization lamp and irradiate for at least 30 minutes for sterilization treatment.

2. Cell culture

A549 cells are commonly used cell lines in lung cancer research, with epithelial morphology and polygonal adherent growth. A549 cells with exponential growth were selected for the experiment and cultured in DMEM medium containing 10% fetal bovine serum. Penicillin and streptomycin were added to the medium to prevent bacterial infection. When the cell density in the culture bottle reaches 80% ~ 90%, digest the cells with trypsin to suspend them, collect the cell suspension, adjust the density to 5×10^4 cells/mL, and plant it into a 96 well culture plate with a volume of 100 μL per well. Cultivate the culture plate in a 37 °C incubator containing 5% CO_2.

3. Drug treatment

After 24 hours, the cells were divided into 8 groups with 6 replicates in each group. Each group was treated with paclitaxel at final concentrations of 1 nmol/L, 2 nmol/L, 4 nmol/L, 8 nmol/L, 16 nmol/L, 32 nmol/L, and 64 nmol/L, with a final volume of 100 μL per well. Add equal amount of DMEM medium to the negative control group. Continue to culture the cells for 48 hours.

4. MTT assay

After 48 hours, MTT assay was performed by adding 20 μL of MTT at a concentration of 5 mg/mL to each well. Continue to culture in the incubator for 4 hours, and then under the microscope, purple crystals can be seen depositing inside the cells. Be careful to discard the culture medium in the wells, add 100 μL of dimethyl sulfoxide to each well, shake for 5 minutes to completely dissolve the purple crystals.

5. Absorbance measurement

Use an enzyme-linked immunosorbent assay detector to detect the absorbance values of each well at of 490 nm wavelength.

6. IC_{50} calculation

Based on the principle that the absorbance value is proportional to the number of cells, the relative number of cells treated with different concentrations of paclitaxel can be obtained, and the inhibition rate of paclitaxel on lung cancer cell growth at different concentrations can be calculated. The formula is as follows:

GI (growth inhibition rate)=[1– (OD value in drug treated group / OD value in negative control group)] × 100%

According to the inhibition rates of each experimental group, the IC_{50} value of paclitaxel on A549 cells after 48 hours was calculated using SPSS software (using logit method).

[Experimental records and results]

Record the experimental results and calculate the inhibition rate of different concentrations of paclitaxel on A549 cell viability according to the formula. Please refer to Table 1-9-1 for details. Based on the inhibition rate, calculate the IC_{50} value of paclitaxel on A549 cells for 48 hours and plot it.

Table 1-9-1   Inhibition rates of paclitaxel at different concentrations on A549 cell viability

Group	Negative control	1 nmol/L paclitaxel	2 nmol/L paclitaxel	4 nmol/L paclitaxel	8 nmol/L paclitaxel	16 nmol/L paclitaxel	32 nmol/L paclitaxel	64 nmol/L paclitaxel
Inhibition rate(%)								

[Precautions]

(1) During cell culture, attention should be paid to aseptic operation, as bacterial infection can affect cell growth.

(2) The dosage of drug added should be accurate.

(3) MTT is sensitive to light, and attention should be paid to avoiding light when adding MTT.

(4) MTT reagent and dimethyl sulfoxide reagent are toxic, please wear gloves when operating.

[Practice questions]

1. What is the anticancer mechanism of paclitaxel?

A. Affects protein synthesis and function.

B. Directly disrupting DNA structure.

C. Interference with nucleic acid biosynthesis.

D. Interference with alkaloid synthesis.

2. What are the targets of paclitaxel?

A. Microtubule   B. Mitochondria   C. Cell nucleus   D. Telomeres

[Thinking questions]

Is the IC_{50} value of a drug fixed and unchanging? What is the guiding significance for clinical medication?

[Knowledye expansion]

Discovery of paclitaxel

Paclitaxel is the world's best-selling natural anti-tumor drug, with advantages such as high efficiency, low toxicity, and broad spectrum. It comes from the precious endangered gymnosperm plant Taxus chinensis. It was first isolated from the bark of the short leaved Chinese yew and its molecular structure was confirmed by X-ray diffraction and nuclear magnetic resonance in 1971. However, the extraction yield of paclitaxel is very low, only 0.004%. At the same time, the rare and protected plant Taxus chinensis is rare in quantity and grows slowly, which greatly limits the application of paclitaxel.

In January 2024, a research team from the Shenzhen Institute of Agricultural Genomics, Chinese Academy of Agricultural Sciences, successfully identified key missing enzymes in the biosynthesis pathway of paclitaxel, revealed a novel mechanism for the formation of oxetane structures in plant cells, and established the shortest biosynthesis pathway of paclitaxel to date. This research marks China's world leading position in the theory and technology of paclitaxel synthetic biology, representing a milestone new height achieved by a group of young and middle-aged scientists in the field of synthetic biology after nearly 20 years of exploration and struggle, paving the way for the green and sustainable production of paclitaxel.

（王琳琳）

Chapter 2 Pharmacology of efferent nervous system

Section 1 Dose-effect relationship of acetylcholine

[Experimental objective]

(1) To understand the dose-effect relationship of acetylcholine (Ach).

(2) To grasp the methods of measuring dose-effect relationship and drawing dose-effect curve.

[Experimental principle]

The pharmacological effects are proportional to the dosage within a certain range, which is known as the dose-effect relationship. The dose-response curve is plotted as a straight hyperbolic curve with the strength of the effect as the vertical axis and drug dose or concentration as the horizontal axis. If the logarithmic values of drug concentration was used as the horizontal axis, a typical symmetrical S-shaped curve is formed, which is commonly known as the dose-effect curve.

ACh acts on skeletal muscles to induce muscle contraction, and its pharmacological effects are positively correlated with the dosage within a certain dosage range. Plotting the logarithm of acetylcholine concentration on the x-axis and muscle contraction effect on the y-axis yields an S-shaped dose-response curve.

[Experimental materials]

1 set of surgical instruments, frog board, probe, suture, 1 mL syringe, smooth muscle baths, ventilation hooks, muscle transducers, air bladder, and BL-422 biological function experiment system.

[Experimental animals]

Toad.

[Experimental reagents]

ACh solution, Ren's solution.

[Experimental methods]

The main steps of the experiment are as follows, as shown in Figure 2-1-1.

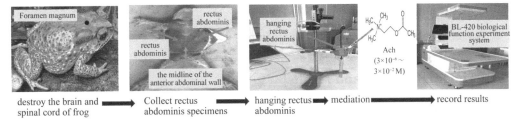

destroy the brain and ➡ Collect rectus ➡ hanging rectus ➡ mediation ➡ record results
spinal cord of frog   abdominis specimens   abdominis

Figure 2-1-1   Schematic diagram of experimental steps

1. Instrument preparation

Brush the smooth muscle bath dish, ventilate the air bladder, turn on the BL-422 biological function experimental system software and set relevant parameters.

2. Preparation of isolated rectus abdominis muscle specimens

Use a probe to destroy the toad brain and spinal cord, and fix the toad in a supine position on a frog board. The abdominal skin was cut to expose the rectus abdominis muscles. Peel off a 2 ~ 3 cm long and 0.5 ~ 0.8 cm wide rectus abdominis muscle from the pubic and sternum ends on one side of the abdominal white line, ligate both ends with sutures, and cut them off. Be careful not to excessively stretch the rectus abdominis muscle.

3. Suspension of specimens

Fix one end of the rectus abdominis specimen on a ventilation hook and immerse it in a smooth muscle bath containing 30 mL of Ren's solution (adjust the length of the line to fully immerse the rectus abdominis into Ren's solution), and introduce air into Ren's liquid. The other end is connected to the muscle strength transducer and BL-422 biological function experimental system.

4. Medication and observation

The rectus abdominis muscle is stabilized in a smooth muscle bath for 10 minutes. The normal contraction curve is recorded and the muscle tension value at this time is recorded. ACh solution can be added in sequence according to the dosage (concentration) shown in Table 2-1-1 for the experiment. Using cumulative administration method, add acetylcholine solution at low concentration → high concentration. The signal recording speed should be slow. 2 ~ 3 minutes after each dose of medication, wait until the muscle contraction response no longer increases and record this tension value. Add the next dose and continue until the maximum effect occurs, then record the tension value at that time.

5. Data Calculation

Effect percentage of each dose=Effect of each dose / Maximum effect × 100%

6. Draw a dose-effect curve

Automatically drawn by yourself or a computer.

[Experimental records and results]

Record the effects of each dose and calculate the percentage response of each dose. Plot a dose-effect curve using the effect percentage as the vertical axis and the negative logarithm of ACh dose as the horizontal axis.

Table 2-1-1　Dose and effects of Acetylcholine

		Original records		Record after organization	
Ach(M)	Dosage (mL)	Bath concentration	Effect/g	LgC	Effect/g
3×10^{-6}	0.1	1×10^{-8}		−8	
	0.2	3×10^{-8}		−7.5	
3×10^{-5}	0.1	1×10^{-7}		−7	
	0.2	3×10^{-7}		−6.5	
3×10^{-4}	0.1	1×10^{-6}		−6	
	0.2	3×10^{-6}		−5.5	
3×10^{-3}	0.1	1×10^{-5}		−5	
	0.2	3×10^{-5}		−4.5	
3×10^{-2}	0.1	1×10^{-4}		−4	
	0.2	3×10^{-4}		−3.5	

[Precautions]

(1) The bath must be thoroughly cleaned before and after the experiment.

(2) Inject 1 ~ 2 bubbles of air per second.

(3) Ren's solution should be maintained at $26 \pm 0.5°C$.

(4) The connection between the isolated rectus abdominis specimen and the transducer should not touch the wall of the bath vessel.

(5) The dosage should be accurate each time, and do not drip onto the line or bath tube wall during dosing, otherwise it will affect the experimental results.

[Practice questions]

1. The receptor types activated by acetylcholine include _____.

A. α receptors   B. $β_1$ receptors   C. M, N receptors   D. α, β receptors

2. Which of the following meanings of the dose-response curve is incorrect?

A. Compare the strength of drug efficacy.

B. Reflect the absorption range of the drug.

C. Provide reference values for clinical drug dosage.

D. Evaluate drug safety.

3. The parameter that cannot be observed from the dose-response curve is _____.

A. minimum effective dose   B. maximum effect

C. potency intensity   D. median lethal dose

[Thinking questions]

(1) Based on the experimental results, analyze the relationship between drug dosage and effect, and what is the pattern of this relationship? What issues should be noted during the application of drugs?

(2) What is the relationship between dose-effect curves and intrinsic activity and affinity, and how to compare the intrinsic activity and affinity of drugs from dose-response curves?

[Knowledye expansion]

Discovery of acetylcholine

Acetylcholine (ACh) is the first neurotransmitter discovered by humans, acting on the pre-ganglionic fibers of all sympathetic and parasympathetic nerves, motor nerves, post ganglionic fibers of all parasympathetic nerves, and a small number of post ganglionic fibers of sympathetic nerves. ACh has the effects of relaxing blood vessels, reducing myocardial contractility, stimulating gastrointestinal smooth muscle, and causing skeletal muscle contraction.

The discovery of ACh can be traced back to the classic double frog heart perfusion experiment conducted by German scientist Otto Loewi. Through this experiment, Loewi speculated that when the vagus nerve is excited, it releases a certain chemical substance that is transmitted through liquid and can affect the heart activity of another frog. Loewi initially identified this chemical substance as ACh in 1926. Subsequent research, particularly in 1930, led by British scientist Dale, further confirmed this chemical substance and officially named it ACh. Together with Otto Loewi, they were awarded the 1936 Nobel Prize in Physiology or Medicine. Professor Zhang Xijun, the founder of modern physiology in China, first measured acetylcholine crystals in the spleen of mammals, opening up avenues for studying the physiological mechanisms of acetylcholine. The discovery of acetylcholine further unveiled the mystery of neurotransmitters. Its discovery tells us that as long as we keep thinking and exploring tirelessly, inspiration will come knocking on our hearts, and success will belong to us.

（潘瑞艳）

Section 2　The effect of efferent nervous system drugs on isolated intestinal smooth muscle

[Experimental objective]

(1) To understand the agonism effect of cholinergic neurotransmitter Acetylcholine (ACh) on M-choline receptor in intestinal smooth muscle and the blocking effect of their receptor antagonist atropine.

(2) To learn the preparation and perfusion of isolated small intestinal smooth muscle.

[Experimental principle]

Gastrointestinal smooth muscle, like skeletal muscle and myocardium, has characteristics similar to muscle tissue, such as excitability, conductivity, and contractility.

However, the excitability of smooth muscle in the digestive tract is low, with slow contraction, rich extensibility, tension, automatic rhythm, and sensitivity to chemical, temperature, and mechanical stretching stimuli. By providing isolated intestinal muscles with a suitable environment similar to in vivo conditions, the smooth muscle of the digestive tract can still maintain physiological characteristics.

The smooth muscles of the gastrointestinal tract, bladder, and other organs are dominated by cholinergic nerves. Low doses or concentrations of ACh can stimulate the M cholinergic receptor, producing a similar effect to the excitation of postganglionic cholinergic nerve, and stimulating the smooth muscles of the gastrointestinal tract. Atropine binds to choline receptors without producing or producing less cholinergic effects, thus block the binding of cholinergic neurotransmitters or cholinergic drugs to receptors, thereby producing anticholinergic effects.

[Experimental materials]

Maxwell bath、thermostatic smooth muscle tank、tension transducer、BL-422 biological function experiment system, HW-200S *in vitro* intestinal tube and hot plate test constant temperature device、air bladder、petri dish、1 mL syringe、a set of surgical instruments、suture、and mallet.

[Experimental animals]

Guinea pig, weighing 200 ~ 250 g, either gender.

[Experimental reagents]

10^{-2} g/L acetylcholine chloride, 1 g/L atropine sulfate, Tyrode's solution.

[Experimental methods]

The main steps of the experiment are as follows, as shown in Figure 2-2-1.

1. Experimental preparation

Add a fixed amount of Tyrode's solution to the Maxwell bath, and adjust the temperature of the HW-200S *in vitro* intestinal tube and hot plate test constant temperature device to stabilize the temperature inside the Maxwell bath at 37±0.5°C. The Submarine snorkel is connected to pipeline of oxygen supporting with a screw clamp to adjust the gas flow rate and the amount of oxygen supply should be regulated at bubble-by-bubble release into the bath. The tension transducer is fixed on an iron pillar, and the output line of the transducer is connected to a microcomputer biological signal processing system. Click on the BL-422 biological function experiment system and set the relevant experimental parameters.

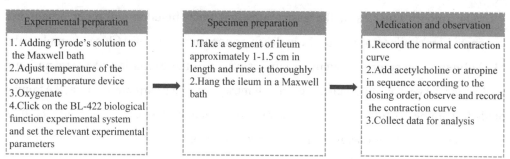

Experimental perparation	Specimen preparation	Medication and observation
1. Adding Tyrode's solution to the Maxwell bath 2.Adjust temperature of the constant temperature device 3.Oxygenate 4.Click on the BL-422 biological function experimental system and set the relevant experimental parameters	1.Take a segment of ileum approximately 1-1.5 cm in length and rinse it thoroughly 2.Hang the ileum in a Maxwell bath	1.Record the normal contraction curve 2.Add acetylcholine or atropine in sequence according to the dosing order, observe and record the contraction curve 3.Collect data for analysis

Figure 2-2-1　Schematic diagram of experimental steps

2. Specimen preparation

(1) Take a guinea pig and strike its occipital area with a mallet to death. Immediately cut the abdominal cavity, find the ileocecal part, and then cut it 1 cm away from the ileocecal part, take out a section of the ileum about 10 cm, place it in a culture dish containing preheated Tyrode's solution, and continue to oxygenate. Separate the mesentery along the intestinal wall, rinse the intestinal contents with Tyrode's solution, and then cut the ileum into several small sections (approximately $1 \sim 1.5$ cm each), replacing them with fresh Tyrode's solution for later use. Be careful not to pull the intestinal segment during operation to avoid affecting the contraction function.

(2) Take a section of the ileum that has been processed as described above, thread it through the diagonal walls at both ends with a sewing needle, and tie a knot. Pay attention to keeping the intestinal tract unobstructed and not sealing it. One end of the intestinal tube is connected to the fixed hook of the bath, and then placed in a 37°C Maxwell bath. The other end of the intestinal tube is connected to the cantilever beam of the tension transducer, and the muscle tension is adjusted to 2 g.

3. Medication and observation

After stabilizing the isolated ileum for 10 minutes, record a normal contraction curve, and then drip the following drugs to the Maxwell bath in sequence. After adding a drug solution, observe for $2 \sim 3$ minutes and record the changes in the contraction amplitude of the intestinal tract, and then rinse it three times continuously with Tyrode's solution until the baseline returns to the level before medication. Then record a baseline and add the second drug solution. Note that the capacity of the bath liquid should be equal.

(1) Add 0.2 mL of 10^{-2} g/L ACh, observe and record its contraction curve, and change the solution.

(2) Add 0.2 mL of 10^{-2} g/L Ach. When the effect is significant or the contraction reaches its peak, add 0.2 mL of 1g/L atropine and observe the contraction curve. At this time, do not change the solution. After the curve drops to baseline or stabilizes, add the same amount of ACh and observe and record the contraction curve.

[Experimental records and results]

Record the experimental results on the experimental report paper, mark the administration for analysis.

[Precautions]

(1) The animals fasted for 24 hours before the experiment, unable to resist water and kept their intestines free of feces.

(2) When making isolated intestinal specimens, the movements should be gentle and agile, avoiding repeated pulling.

(3) When adding medicine to the Maxwell bath, do not touch the connecting wire or drop the medicine onto the tube wall.

(4) The connection between the intestinal tube and the transducer should not be too tight, nor should it come into contact with the bath wall.

(5) Throughout the entire experiment, pay attention to continuous oxygen supply and maintaining a constant temperature.

[Practice questions]

1. Which type of smooth muscle does atropine have the strongest effect on?

A. Gastrointestinal smooth muscle.　　B. Bronchial smooth muscle.

C. Smooth muscle of biliary tract.　　D. Smooth muscle of uterus.

2. Intramuscular injection of atropine to treat colic and cause dry mouth is called

_____.

A. therapeutic effect　　　　　　　B. allergic reactions

C. side effect　　　　　　　　　　D. after effects

3. The therapeutic dose of atropine can cause _____.

A. gastrointestinal smooth muscle spasm

B. central inhibition

C. reduced salivary gland secretion

D. pupil dilation and decreased intraocular pressure

[Thinking questions]

(1) What receptors are present on the smooth muscles of the gastrointestinal tract? What are the effects of excitement and inhibition?

(2) What are the different effects of atropine on different visceral smooth muscle?

[Knowledye expansion]

The discovery history and effects of atropine

Atropine is an M receptor blocker and a white crystalline racemic hyoscyamine extracted from plants in the Solanaceae family, such as *atropa belladonna, datura stramonium, datura metel, or Hyoscyamus niger*. Currently, it can also be artificially synthesized. The discovery of atropine can be traced back to the 4th century BC, when the ancient Greek scientist Theophrasus recorded that *datura stramonium* could treat pain, gout, and insomnia. Germany chemist Ferdinand Runge was the first person to study the dilating effect of atropine. In 1831, Germany pharmacist Mein successfully purified toxic atropine pure crystals from plants. It was not until 1894 that Germany organic chemist Richard Wilstet elucidated the chemical structure of atropine and first synthesized it artificially in 1901. Atropine not only inhibits smooth muscle spasms in the gastrointestinal tract, but also has antiarrhythmic effects, suppresses glandular secretion, dilates pupils, increases intraocular pressure, anti-shock effects, and rescues acute organophosphate pesticide poisoning. It is one of the commonly used drugs in the clinic.

（潘瑞艳）

Section 3   The effect of efferent nervous system drugs on the pupil of rabbits

[Experimental objective]

(1) To observe the effects of anticholinergic drugs (atropine) and sympathomimetic drugs (phenylephrine) on the pupil and analyze their mechanisms of action.

(2) To study rabbit eye drops and pupil measurement methods.

[Experimental principle]

Vision is the main way for people to obtain information from the outside world, and the eye is the peripheral sensory organ that causes vision, including the eyeball, visual pathway, and accessory organs of the eye. The eyeball is composed of the eyeball wall and contents, among which the eyeball wall includes the outer membrane, middle membrane, and inner membrane. The iris is the anterior part of the middle membrane, a round disc-shaped film, with a round hole in the center called the pupil. The functions of the pupil include regulating the amount of light reaching the retina, reducing chromatic aberration and spherical aberration caused by peripheral incompleteness of the cornea and lens optical system, and increasing the field of view. The diameter of the normal human pupil is between 1.5 ~ 8.0 mm, and the size of the pupil is closely related to visual quality. The reflex of the pupil constricting in strong light and dilating in weak light is called the light reflex of the pupil. It is an adaptive function of the eye, the significance of which is to regulate the amount of light entering the eye, so that the retina will not be damaged due to excessive light intensity, nor will vision be affected due to insufficient light intensity.

The diameter of the pupil is influenced by the double effect of the sphincter pupillae and dilator pupillae muscles. The sphincter pupillae muscle mainly distributes M receptors, and the dilator pupillae muscle mainly distributes α receptors. After the application of cholinergic receptor agonist eye drops, the M receptors on the sphincter pupillae muscle can be excited, causing the pupil to constrict. After the application of M cholinergic receptor antagonist eye drops, the M receptors on the sphincter pupillae muscle can be blocked, causing the sphincter pupillae muscle to relax, making the function of the adrenergic nerve-innervated dilator pupillae muscle dominant, causing the pupil to dilate. After the application of phenylephrine eye drops, the α receptors on the dilator pupillae muscle can be excited, causing the pupil to dilate (Figure 2-3-1).

The process of the light reflex is as follows: when strong (or weak) light stimulates the retina, the impulse generated is transmitted along the optic nerve to the pretectal area of the midbrain to change neurons, and then reaches the bilateral oculomotor nerve constrictor pupillae nucleus, and then along the parasympathetic fibers in the oculomotor nerve to the ciliary ganglion, and finally the ciliary nerve controls the sphincter pupillae muscle, causing the pupil to constrict (or dilate). The central nervous system of the light reflex is located in the midbrain, and it is often used as an index to judge the depth of anesthesia and the severity of the disease in the clinic. In addition, it is clinically used to evaluate the visual input of the retina, optic nerve, and anterior visual pathway, which is helpful for the diagnosis and monitoring of visual efferent system diseases.

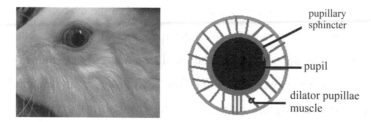

Figure 2-3-1　The diagram of rabbit pupil and pupil regulation

[Experimental materials]

Surgical scissors, dropper, rabbit cage, ruler, flashlight.

[Experimental animals]

Rabbit, weighing 2 ~ 3 kg.

[Experimental reagents]

1% atropine sulfate solution, 1% hydrochloric deoxyepinephrine.

[Experimental methods]

(1) Take one healthy rabbit, place it in the rabbit fixation box, cut off the eyelashes,

measure and record the normal pupil diameter (mm) and light reflex on both sides under natural light, and then administer 4 ~ 5 drops each in the following order.

Left eye: 1% atropine sulfate solution.

Right eye: 1% hydrochloric deoxyepinephrine.

When administering the drops, pull the lower eyelid into a cup shape and press the nasolacrimal duct with your finger to keep it in the eyelid for 1 minute, then gently release your hand and let it drain naturally.

(2) 15 minutes after administering the drops, measure and record the size of each eye's pupils and light reflex again under the same intensity of light.

[Experimental Records and results]

Record the experimental results and organize them into Table 2-3-1.

Table 2-3-1   The effect of autonomic nervous system drugs on the pupil of rabbits

Eye	Drug	Pupil diameter(mm)		light reflex	
		Before	After	Before	After
Left	Atropine				
Right	deoxyepinephrine				

[Precautions]

(1) When measuring the pupil, do not stimulate the cornea, otherwise it will affect the size of the pupil.

(2) When administering the drops, press the nasolacrimal duct at the inner corner of the eye to prevent the medicine from entering the nasal cavity and being absorbed through the nasal mucosa.

(3) The amount of drops administered to each eye must be accurate and the time they remain in the eye should be consistent to ensure the medicine is fully effective.

(4) The conditions for measuring the pupil must be consistent before and after medication, such as the intensity of the light, the angle of the light source, etc.

(5) When observing the reflection of light, the surrounding ambient light should not be too strong or too weak.

[Practice questions]

1. Which of the following statements is incorrect when measuring the pupil?

A. Before measuring, the eyelashes need to be trimmed.

B. During measurement, the ruler should be pressed tightly against the cornea of the rabbit.

C. The intensity of light before and after administration of the drug should be the same.

D. The angle of the light source before and after administration should be the same.

2. The purpose of pressing the nasolacrimal duct of the rabbit after eye drops is _____.

A. to prevent the drug from draining through the nasolacrimal duct

B. to reduce the stimulation of the pupil by drugs

C. to increase corneal absorption of the drug

D. to increase aqueous humor production

3. The pharmacological action of atropine on the eyes does not include _____.

A. dilating pupils   B. accommodation spasm

C. increasing intraocular pressure   D. accommodation paralysis

[Thinking questions]

(1) What is the light reflex of the pupil? What is the significance of detecting the light reflex of patients in the clinic?

(2) What is the effect of the drugs used in this experiment on the pupil? What are the clinical applications?

(3) What drugs can be used to treat glaucoma?

[Knowledye expansion]

The effect of atropine in myopia control among children

On March 5, 2024, the National Medical Products Administration approved the marketing of 0.01% atropine sulfate eye drops, used to alleviate the progression of nearsightedness in children aged 6 ~ 12. This drug is the first domestically approved drug to delay the progression of myopia in children.

Atropine is an M-cholinergic receptor blocker, which has a high affinity for M-cholinergic receptors, can block the binding of Ach or cholinergic receptor agonists to the receptor, and antagonize their excitatory effect on M receptors. Atropine can block the M receptors on the pupil sphincter muscle, causing the pupil sphincter muscle to relax, making the function of the adrenergic nerve-controlled dilator muscle dominant, and the pupil dilates. At the same time, due to the dilation of the pupil, the iris retreats to the surrounding edges, blocking the flow of aqueous humor, leading to an increase in intraocular pressure. In addition, it can also block the M receptors on the ciliary muscle, making the lens flattened, reducing the refractive power, leading to blurred vision of near objects and clear vision of far objects (i.e., accommodation paralysis). Early studies found that high-concentration atropine can significantly inhibit the growth of the anterior and posterior diameters of the eye, slow down the progression of myopia, and its control efficiency for myopia can reach 60% ~ 96%. However, it has adverse reactions such as photophobia, facial redness, increased heart rate, and decreased vision, as well as rebound effects after drug withdrawal. Clinical studies have found that 0.01% atropine (low concentration) has a significant effect in slowing down the progression of myopia, with a myopia control efficiency of 27% ~ 83%, and has a cumulative effect, but no serious systemic adverse reactions have been found, with small adverse reactions and rebound effects after drug withdrawal. However, this drug cannot prevent myopia, let alone treat myopia, it only slows down the progression of myopia in children, and the control effect is different for different individuals. Therefore, the prevention and control of myopia in children and adolescents should also be emphasized from the aspects of eye hygiene habits and living and learning environment.

（李成檀）

Section 4   Inhibition of atropine on smooth muscle in mice

[Experimental objective]

(1) To observe the inhibitory effect of atropine on the peristalsis of smooth muscle in mice.

(2) To understand the neural regulation mechanism of gastrointestinal smooth muscle movement.

[Experimental principle]

The intestine, a vital component of the human digestive system, extends from the pylorus of the stomach to the anus, being the longest and most functionally significant segment of the digestive tract. The mammalian digestive tract comprises the small intestine and large intestine. The small intestine, coiled within the abdominal cavity, connects the stomach via the pylorus and the large intestine via the cecum. The cecum, a pouch-like structure, marks the beginning of the large intestine, which extends from the cecum to the anus. The intestines are suspended and fixed by the mesentery. The small intestine has a relatively thin wall and a smooth surface (Figure 2-4-1).

Smooth muscle in the digestive tract shares common characteristics of muscle tissue, including excitability, conductivity, and contractility. It also possesses unique functional features such as low excitability, slow contraction, spontaneous rhythmicity, a certain degree of tone, and significant extensibility, enabling propulsive movements. While insensitive to electrical stimulation, cutting, and burning, intestinal smooth muscle is highly responsive to mechanical stretch, temperature changes, and chemical stimuli. Its activity is further regulated by neural and humoral factors. The gastrointestinal smooth muscle is innervated by both the parasympathetic and sympathetic nerves. When the parasympathetic nerve is activated, its terminals release the neurotransmitter acetylcholine (ACh), which binds to M receptors on smooth muscle, causing excitation and subsequent intestinal muscle contraction. In contrast, when the sympathetic nerve is stimulated, most postganglionic fibers release noradrenaline (NA), which binds to α and β receptors on smooth muscle membranes, inhibiting motility and weakening gastrointestinal motility. Certain drugs, including adrenaline, neostigmine, and atropine, can alter the contractile activity of gastrointestinal smooth muscle, affecting its rhythm, intensity, speed, and tonic contraction.

Atropine, an antagonist of acetylcholine M receptors, competitively binds to M-cholinergic receptors, thereby blocking the effects of ACh. Upon atropine inhibition, gastrointestinal smooth muscle relaxes, resulting in decreased amplitude and frequency of peristalsis. Consequently, atropine is highly effective in relieving gastrointestinal smooth muscle spasms and alleviating gastrointestinal colic. Apart from treating various visceral colics, high doses of atropine can relieve microvascular spasms, improve microcirculation, inhibit glandular secretion, lift vagal inhibition on the heart, increase heart rate, dilate pupils, elevate intraocular pressure, stimulate the respiratory center, and relieve respiratory depression. It is also used in conditions such as sinus bradycardia, atrioventricular block, arrhythmia, septic shock, and organophosphorus poisoning.

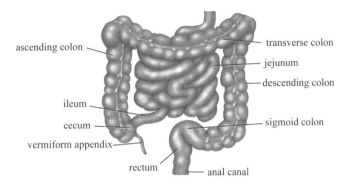

Figure 2-4-1   Diagram of intestinal system

[Experimental materials]

Electronic balance, bealcer, syringe (1 mL), mouse cage, frog board, surgical scissors, forceps, ruler.

[Experimental animals]

2 mice (18 ~ 22 g), either gender.

[Experimental reagents]

0.05% atropine sulfate solution, normal saline, ink.

[Experimental methods]

The experimental operation steps are as follows, seen in Figure 2-4-2.

1. Hunger treatment

Take 2 mice with similar body weights, weigh and mark them using picric acid. Subject the mice to fasting for 12 to 24 hours with free access to water.

2. Intragastric administration

Administer medication to the fasted mice. Mouse A is given 0.1 mL/10g (Dosage of

5 mg/kg, 0.05 mg/10 g) of 0.05% atropine sulfate solution intragastrically, while Mouse B is given 0.2 mL of saline solution intragastrically.

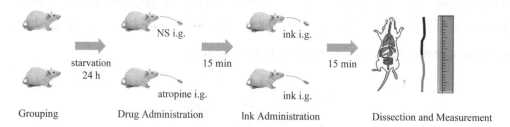

Figure 2-4-2   Schematic diagram of operation steps

3. Ink administration

After 15 minutes, administer 0.2 mL of ink intragastrically to both Mouse A and Mouse B.

4. Dissection

After another 15 minutes, euthanize both mice by cervical dislocation and immediately perform a laparotomy. Remove one end of the small intestine from the pylorus of the stomach and the other end from the cecum. Isolate the entire small intestine, place it on a frog board, and moisten it with a small amount of saline. Use tweezers and surgical scissors to dissect the mesentery and gently lay the intestine in a straight line on the frog board without stretching it.

5. Measurement of ink movement distance

Starting from the pylorus as the origin and the cecum end as the terminus, use a ruler to measure and record the total length of the small intestine. Simultaneously, measure the distance that the ink has moved within the intestinal lumen, starting from the pylorus.

6. Calculation of gastrointestinal propulsion rate

Calculate the gastrointestinal propulsion rate by dividing the distance traveled by the ink within the intestinal lumen by the total length of the small intestine and multiplying by 100%. This represents the percentage of the total length of the small intestine covered by the movement of ink in the mouse.

[Experimental records and results]

Record the experimental results and calculate the propulsion rate of ink in the intestines of different mice according to the formula. See the table below in Table 2-4-1.

Table 2-4-1   Inhibition of atropine on smooth muscle in mice

Group	Weight (g)	Drugs	Drug volume (mL)	Total length (cm)	Distance of ink traveled (cm)	Propulsion rate (%)
A		atropine sulfate solution				
B		normal saline				

[Precautions]

(1) The volume of ink administered intragastrically must be precise.

(2) The time interval between ink administration and euthanasia must be accurate.

(3) In this experiment, 1% carmine solution can be used as an alternative to ink.

(4) When removing the gastrointestinal tract or measuring the small intestine, avoid stretching the intestinal tube to prevent affecting the accuracy of the measured length. Keep the intestine moist after removal by adding some saline solution to prevent it from sticking to the experimental bench.

[Practice questions]

1. The effect of neostigmine on intestinal smooth muscle movement should be

_____.

A. enhanced movement   B. reduced movement

C. no effect   D. cause spas

2. The purpose of hunger treatment for experimental mice is _____.

A. to enhance gastrointestinal motility   B. to weaken the mice

C. to empty the intestines   D. to enhance drug efficacy

3. Which of the following does not belong to the clinical applications of atropine?

A. To rescue organophosphate poisoning

B. To treat motion sickness

C. To relieve visceral spasms

D. For ophthalmological pupillary dilation examination

[Thinking questions]

(1) What receptors are present on intestinal smooth muscle, and what effect does their activation have on intestinal smooth muscle movement?

(2) How does neostigmine affect intestinal smooth muscle, and how does it differ from acetylcholine?

(3) What is the effect of adrenaline (epinephrine) on intestinal smooth muscle activity? How do propranolol and phentolamine influence the changes in intestinal smooth muscle contraction caused by adrenaline? Why?

[Knowledye expansion]

Anticholinergic drug "654-2" from Chinese unique plant Anisodus tanguticus

654-2, with the scientific name of Raceanisodamine, is an anticholinergic drug similar in mechanism of action to atropine, exhibiting significant peripheral anticholinergic effects. Anisodamine is an alkaloid first extracted by Chinese scientists from the solanaceous plant *Anisodus tanguticus*, an achievement accomplished in April 1965, hence its code name "654." *Anisodus tanguticus*, unique to China, is also known as Zhangliu, Tangchuannabao, and Tangut Anisodus, and is primarily distributed in Gansu, Yunnan, Qinghai, and other regions. Its natural form, designated "654-1," is a dextrorotatory isomer, while the product synthesized artificially is known as "654-2," a recemate. Both share the same mechanism of action, yet 654-2 exhibits higher potency. Currently, "654-2" is widely used in the clinic.

Similar to atropine, 654-2 exerts peripheral anticholinergic receptor effects, relieving acetylcholine-induced smooth muscle spasms. It relaxes gastrointestinal smooth muscle, inhibiting its peristalsis, albeit with slightly weaker effects compared to atropine. Furthermore, it can relieve microvascular spasms, improving microcirculation. Its inhibition of salivary gland secretion and mydriasis is relatively weak, about 1/20 to 1/10 of atropine's effects. Since it does not easily cross the blood-brain barrier, its central nervous system effects are also weaker than atropine's, rarely causing central excitatory symptoms.

Clinically, 654-2 is frequently used for antispasmodic and analgesic treatments, with indications including septic shock due to infections, smooth muscle spasms, circulatory disorders resulting from vascular spasms and embolisms, ocular fundus diseases, various neuralgias, organophosphate poisoning, sudden deafness, vertigo, and other conditions.

（童骏森）

Section 5　Poisoning and rescue of organophosphorus pesticides

[Experimental objective]

(1) To observe the M-like symptoms, N-like symptoms and central symptoms of organophosphorus pesticide poisoning.

(2) To observe the effect of the M receptor blocker atropine on the M-like symptoms and the cholinesterase reactivation drug pralidoxime on the N-like symptoms and central symptoms.

[Experimental principle]

Organophosphorus pesticides are a class of irreversible cholinesterase inhibitors with high fat solubility and easy absorption through digestive tract, respiratory tract and even skin to cause poisoning. Phosphoryl group contained in organophosphorus pesticides can irreversibly combine with acetylcholinesterase (AChE) to form phosphorylation AChE, which makes AChE lose the activity of acetylcholine (ACh) hydrolysis (Figure 2-5-1). Resulting in a large amount of ACh accumulation in the synaptic gap or neuromuscular junction, causing cholinine-like poisoning symptoms. After organophosphorus pesticide poisoning, it can be manifested as the excitatory effect of M receptor (such as cardiac depression, increased secretion of superficial glands, contraction and spasm of visceral smooth muscle, etc.) and the excitatory effect of N receptor (such as increased muscle tension and even muscle tremor). In severe poisoning, it can also be manifested as the toxic reaction of central excitation and then inhibition.

The M receptor blocker atropine can selectively block the cholinergic M receptor and effectively relieve the symptoms of M-like poisoning. Pralidoxime (PAM), a cholinesterase reactivator, can compete with phosphacylated AChE for phosphoryl groups, generate phosphacylated PAM and revive AChE, and quickly relieve the symptoms of muscle tremor and central symptoms in acute poisoning of organophosphate pesticides (Figure 2-5-2).

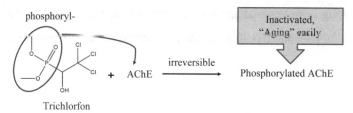

Figure 2-5-1   Mechanism of organophosphorus pesticide poisoning

Figure 2-5-2   Mechanism of pralidoxime reactivating cholinesterase

[Experimental materials]

Rabbit fixator, scale, syringe (1 mL, 2.5 mL, 5 mL, 10 mL), pupil measuring scale.

[Experimental animals]

Rabbit, weighing 1.5 ~ 2.5 kg, either gender.

[Experimental reagents]

5% refined trichlorphon solution, 0.2% atropine sulfate solution, 2.5% proxime iodide solution.

[Experimental methods]

1. Experimental preparation

1 rabbit was taken, weighed and recorded, the dosage was calculated according to the weight, and the medicine was taken for use.

2. Observation before administration

Rabbits were placed on the experimental table to observe their activity, respiration, salivation, excretion and muscle tension, etc., and pupil diameter was measured with pupil scale.

3. Observe the symptoms of organophosphate pesticide poisoning

Rabbits were given 5% purified trichlorfon solution of 4mL/kg by intraperitoneal injection, and the changes of rabbit activity, respiration, salivary secretion, urine and feces, pupil size and muscle tension (whether there is muscle tremor) were closely observed, and the manifestations of convulsion were also observed. At the same time, according to the weight of the rabbit, the rescue drug was drawn for use.

4. Observe the relief of M-like symptoms administrated with atropine

After the obvious symptoms of rabbit poisoning were observed (pupil shrank to the size of mung bean and muscle tremor was obvious), 0.2% atropine sulfate solution of 1 mL/kg was injected into the ear vein immediately, and then the changes of various symptoms of rabbit poisoning were closely observed (pay attention to which symptoms were relieved and which symptoms were not relieved?).

5. Observe the relief of N-like symptoms and central symptoms administrated with pralidoxime

After the M-like symptoms of rabbits were relieved (the pupil was basically restored to before poisoning), the ear vein was continued to be injected with 2.5% pralidoxime iodides solution 2mL/kg, and then the changes of various poisoning symptoms of rabbits were closely observed (whether the symptoms that were not relieved after atropine were relieved?).

[Experimental Records and results]

Record the changes in various indicators of rabbits before and after administration in the table. Please refer to Table 2-5-1 for details.

Table 2-5-1   organophosphorus pesticide poisoning and rescue observation

	Activity	Breathing	Pupil	Salivation	Urinary and bowel movement	Muscle tension	muscle tremor	Convulsion
Before dosing								
After giving trichlorfon								
After giving atropine								
After giving pralidoxime								

[Precautions]

(1) The changes of poisoning symptoms should be closely observed after the rabbit is given trichlorfon solution. If the rabbit has obvious muscle tremor or central excitation symptoms, even if the M-like symptoms have not reached the standard of severe poisoning at this time, atropine solution should be injected into the ear vein immediately to rescue, otherwise it is easy to cause death of the rabbit.

(2) Trichlorfon solution is an organophosphorus pesticide, which is highly toxic. Attention should be paid to protection when drawing and using. If the skin comes into contact with the trichlorphon solution, it should not be cleaned with alkaline substances.

(3) The pupil measurement before and after giving trichlorfon and after rescue must be carried out in the same side and the same position, so as to avoid the experimental error caused by the influence of different eyes and different light on the pupil self-regulation.

(4) If the intraperitoneal injection of trichlorfon does not appear obvious symptoms of poisoning after 15 to 20 minutes, 1/3 of the amount can be added.

[Practice questions]

1. What kind of odor does the patient have in their breath when considering organophosphate pesticide poisoning?

A. Rotten apples.　　B. Garlic.　　　　C. Ammonia.　　　　D. Fishy odor.

2. Symptoms of organophosphorus pesticide poisoning are not included _____.

A. blurred vision　　　　　　　　B. incontinence

C. slowed breathing rate　　　　　　D. excessive sweating and salivation

3. The nicotinoid symptom of organophosphorus pesticide poisoning is _____.

A. hyperhidrosis　　　　　　　　B. salivation

C. nausea and vomiting　　　　　　D. muscle tremor

[Thinking questions]

(1) Why should rescue in time when organophosphorus pesticide poisoning?

(2) What are the principles of atropine and pralidoxime used in clinic to rescue organophosphorus pesticide poisoning? Why?

[Knowledye expansion]

Environment friendly pesticides

There are many varieties of pesticides, which can be divided into organochlorine, organophosphorus, organic nitrogen, organic sulfur, carbamate, pyrethroids, amide compounds, etc., according to their chemical structure. Organochlorinated insecticides chlorobenzene structure is stable, not easy to be degraded by organisms, disappear slowly in organisms. The half-life in water can reach 20 years, and the half-life in the soil is mostly 1 ~ 12 years, which has a significant impact on the ecological environment and has been listed as banned pesticides in production. Organophosphorus insecticides produce different degrees of residues in crops, and the toxicity of each variety is different, most of them are medium and high toxicity, a few are low toxicity. The harm to the human body is mainly acute toxicity, mostly caused by a series of neurotoxicity after large doses or repeated contact, such as sweating, salivation, blurred vision, tremor, confusion, speech disorders, etc. Severe cases will appear respiratory paralysis and even death. Organophosphorus insecticides have ever been widely used in China's agriculture, but are not conducive to the construction of ecological civilization, and some varieties have been banned (such as parathion, methamidophos, methylparathion, fossamine, monocrotophos). Pyrethroids have low toxicity to human beings, mainly including cypermethrin (permethrin), deltamethrin (decks), and fungicide ester (fenvalerate) etc. They have a wide insecticidal spectrum and good effect, but they are highly toxic to aquatic organisms and are not conducive to the ecological environment. Diamide insecticides are the latest type of insecticides, with outstanding advantages and high safety for human beings, and have become the focus of insecticide research and development at present. The development of insecticides is in the direction of high efficiency, low toxicity, environment and ecological friendliness, which is also in line with the strategic decision of the Party Central Committee to vigorously promote the construction of ecological civilization, reflecting the scientific decision of the Party Central Committee on the construction of ecological civilization.

（王舒舒）

Chapter 3　Central nervous system pharmacology

Section 1　Analgesia experiment of drugs

[Experimental objective]

(1) Observe the analgesic effects of pethidine and rotundine.

(2) Understand commonly used analgesic experimental methods and master the analgesic experimental method of twisting body method.

[Experimental principle]

Pain is one of the common clinical conditions, which is a painful sensation caused by actual or potential tissue damage. Severe pain not only brings emotional reactions such as pain and anxiety to patients, but can also cause physiological dysfunction and even trigger shock.

The methods for creating animal pain models include chemical stimulation, mechanical stimulation, electrical stimulation, etc. Chemical stimulation is a method of inducing pain reactions in animals by injecting or subcutaneous injection of chemical substances into their bodies. For example, intraperitoneal injection of acetic acid solution or potassium antimony tartrate solution in mice can cause twisting reactions. Mechanical stimulation refers to the application of pressure or mechanical force to the body parts of animals to induce pain responses, such as by applying a certain amount of pressure to the tail tip of rats, causing them to produce a neighing response due to pain. The pressure level at which the neighing response occurs in rats is used as the pain threshold, and the smaller the pain threshold, the weaker the analgesic effect of the drug. Electric stimulation method refers to the use of electrical stimulation on animal body parts to produce pain effects, such as by stimulating the tail of rats to produce pain, using the rat's neigh response as a pain indicator, and using the magnitude of the electrical stimulation generated by the rat's neigh response as a pain threshold. The smaller the pain threshold, the weaker the analgesic effect of the drug. In addition, there are other methods such as hot plate method by placing mice on a hot plate and using the temperature of the hot plate corresponding to their jumping or licking behavior as the pain threshold, the smaller the pain threshold is, the weaker the analgesic effect of the drug is.

The experimental method used in this experiment is twisting body method. The peritoneum of mice has a wide distribution of sensory nerves. Injecting acetic acid into the abdominal cavity can quickly cause pain reactions in mice, manifested as abdominal concavity, hind leg extension, and hip lifting, collectively known as the twisting response. Using the number of twisting reactions as a pain indicator, the more twisting reactions occur, the stronger the pain experienced by the mouse.

[Experimental materials]

1mL syringe, squirrel cage, electronic balance.

[Experimental animals]

Mice weighing 18 ~ 22 g, either gender.

[Experimental reagents]

0.6% glacial acetic acid solution, normal saline, 0.2% pethidine solution, 0.2% rotundine solution, and picric acid solution.

[Experimental methods]

The experimental operation steps are as follows, as shown in Figure 3-1-1.

1. Weigh and label

Take 3 healthy mice weighing 18 ~ 22 g, and randomly divide them into three groups named as A, B, and C. Weigh and record, mark with picric acid.

2. Drug administration

Group A mice were intraperitoneally injected with 0.2% pethidine at the dosage of 20 mg/kg, Group B mice were intraperitoneally injected with 0.2% rotundine at the dosage of 20 mg/kg, and Group C mice were intraperitoneally injected with normal saline at the dosage of 0.1 mL/10 g.

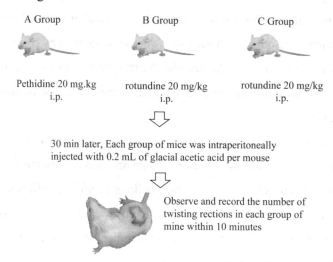

Figure 3-1-1   Schematic diagram of operation steps

3. Establishment of pain model

After 30 minutes of administration, mice in groups A, B, and C were simultaneously intraperitoneally injected with 0.6% acetic acid at the dosage of 0.2 mL per mouse. Acetic acid can hurt the peritoneum of mice and cause pain.

4. Observe and record

After injecting glacial acetic acid, observe and record the number of twisting reactions that occur in each group within 10 minutes. The specific manifestation of twisting reaction is abdominal concavity, hind leg extension, and hip lifting.

5. Calculation

Collect the experimental results of the entire class, calculate the percentage of drug inhibition of twist reaction. The specific calculation formula is as follows:

$$\text{Percentage of twisting reaction inhibition} = \frac{\begin{array}{c}\text{Number of twisting reactions in the experimental group}\\ -\text{ Number of twisting reactions in the control group}\end{array}}{\text{Number of twisting reactions in the control group}} \times 100\%$$

[Experimental records and results]

Record the experimental results and calculate the percentage of drug inhibition of twisting reactions according to the formula. Please refer to Table 3-1-1 for details.

Table 3-1-1　Analgesic effects of pethidine and rotundine

Group	Drug	Number of torsional reactions								Twisting body reaction percentage(%)
		1	2	3	4	5	6	7	8	
A	Pethidine									
B	Rotundine									
C	Normal saline									

[Precautions]

(1) It is advisable to prepare a new solution of 0.6% acetic acid solution before use, as prolonged storage can weaken its effectiveness.

(2) Mice have a light body weight and a low frequency of twisting reactions, so the weight difference between groups of mice should not be too large.

(3) The appropriate room temperature is 20°C, and the number of body twists in mice decreases at low temperatures.

(4) The pain response of animals varies greatly among individuals, so the more animals used in the experiment, the more reliable the results will be.

[Practice questions]

1. Which one is the function of pethidine?

A. Analgesia, sedation, cough suppression.　B. Analgesia, respiratory excitation.

C. Analgesia, euphoria, antiemetic.　D. Analgesia, tranquilizer, mydriasis.

2. The main reason why morphine should not be used for chronic dull pain is _____.

A. poor effect on dull pain　B. addiction

C. can cause constipation　D. causes orthostatic hypotension

3. What is the main reason why pethidine is more commonly used than morphine?

A. Strong analgesic effect

B. Strong gastrointestinal smooth muscle effect

C. Less addictive than morphine

D. Slow action and longer duration of maintenance

4. Which of the following is not included in the main clinical applications of pethidine?

A. Analgesia.　B. Cardiogenic asthma.

C. Nausea, vomiting, constipation.　D. Medication administered before anesthesia.

[Thinking questions]

(1) What are the differences in analgesic characteristics between pethidine and rotundine? What are its main clinical uses?

(2) What are the differences in the mechanisms between pethidine and rotundine?

[Knowledye expansion]

The "credit" and "disadvantage" of morphine

Morphine comes from the plant poppy. When the immature fruit of the poppy is cut open, white juice seeps out from the wound. The juice is collected and dried to form a brown gel, which is called opium in China. Since BC, opioids have been used as anesthetics. The Ming Dynasty's *Yi Lin Ji Yao* recorded the earliest method of producing and using opium in China, and at that time opium was commonly referred to as "A Fu Rong". In 1803, German pharmacist Zertina isolated and extracted morphine from opioids, enhancing their analgesic effects. During World War Ⅱ, morphine successfully alleviated the pain of the wounded and became an important medical material. At the same time, due to the fact that morphine produces both analgesic and euphoric effects, a large number of wounded soldiers became addicted to morphine after the war. After becoming addicted to morphine, it poses a huge threat to health, causing users to lose their ability to work. At the same time, addiction can lead to family bankruptcy, divorce, and even illegal activities, posing great harm. The struggle between the state and drugs has never stopped since Lin Zexu destructed opium at Humen, which shows that the Chinese nation has the heroic spirit and fighting spirit to dare to fight against aggression. At the same time, we should clarify the definition of drugs, use central analgesic drugs such as morphine reasonably, strengthen medical ethics and conduct education, and practice medicine in accordance with laws and regulations.

（王琳琳）

Section 2   The effect of chlorpromazine on electric stimulation-induced agitation in mice

[Experimental objective]

To observe the effect of chlorpromazine on the response to electrical stimulation in mice.

[Experimental principle]

Chlorpromazine is an antipsychotic drug that mainly inhibits the central nervous system by blocking the D2 receptors of the midbrain limbic and midbrain cortical pathways, also known as neuroprotective effects.

After continuous exposure to weak current or low voltage stimulation on the feet of mice, they may exhibit provocative behaviors such as avoidance, fighting, and mutual biting. Chlorpromazine counteracts the anger response caused by electrical stimulation in mice.

[Experimental materials]

YLS-9A multi-purpose pharmacological and physiological instrument, electric stimulation-induced agitation box, 1mL syringe, balance.

[Experimental animals]

Mice, weighing 18 ~ 22 g, either gender.

[Experimental reagents]

0.1% chlorpromazine solution, saline, picric acid.

[Experimental methods]

The experimental operation steps are as follows, as illustrated in Figure 3-2-1.

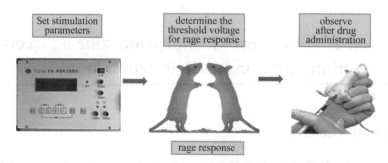

Figure 3-2-1   Schematic diagram of operation steps

1. Set stimulation parameters

Utilize the YLS-9A multi-functional pharmacological and physiological instrument and select the "continuous wave output" mode for stimulation.

2. Determine the threshold voltage for rage response

Take 4 mice, weigh and mark them, and group them in pairs. Take 2 mice each time and place them in the electrical stimulation and stimulation box. Turn on the power switch of the pharmacological and physiological multi-purpose device and adjust the stimulation voltage from low to high until the mice exhibit an electrical stimulation response (such as lifting their forelimbs off the ground, standing upright, facing each other, or even hissing and biting each other). At this point, the voltage is the threshold voltage required for the group of mice to exhibit electrical stimulation response.

3. Drug administration and observation

One group of mice was intraperitoneally injected with 0.1% chlorpromazine at a dose of 0.15 mL/10 g, while the other group of mice was intraperitoneally injected with physiological saline at a dose of 0.15 mL/10 g as a control. After 20 minutes of administration, mice were stimulated with threshold voltage before administration in each group, and the differences in response to electrical stimulation between the two groups of mice before and after administration were observed.

[Experimental records and results]

Record the experimental results as detailed in Table 3-2-1.

Table 3-2-1　Effect of Chlorpromazine on Electrical Stimulation-Induced Rage Response in Mice

Mouse No.	Drug	Weight (g)	Dose (mg/kg)	Threshold voltage (V)	Rage Response	
					Before Drug	After Drug
1	0.1%Chlorpromazine					
2	0.1%Chlorpromazine					
3	Normal Saline					
4	Normal Saline					

[Precautions]

(1) The stimulation voltage should be set from small to large. If it is too low, it is not easy to cause mouse anger reaction, and if it is too high, it is easy for mice to escape.

(2) Apply the same threshold voltage to mice before and after administration, and compare the similarities and differences in mouse responses.

(3) Mouse urine and feces on the conductive copper wire plate should be removed at all times to avoid short circuits.

[Practice questions]

1. The effect of chlorpromazine on normal individuals is _____.

A. restlessness　　　　　　　　　B. elevated mood

C. tension and insomnia　　　　　　D. emotional indifference

2. The primary mechanism of chlorpromazine's antipsychotic effect is _____.

A. blocking α-receptors　　　　　　B. blocking M-receptors

C. blocking D2 receptors in the tuberoinfundibular system

D. blocking D2 receptors in the mesolimbic and mesocortical systems

3. Which of the following adverse reactions of chlorpromazine can be exacerbated by cholinergic receptor blockers?

A. Parkinsonism.　　　　　　　　　B. Tardive dyskinesia.

C. Akathisia.　　　　　　　　　　　D. Orthostatic hypotension.

[Thinking questions]

(1) What are the dopamine neurotransmitter pathways in the central nervous system? How does chlorpromazine affect these dopamine neurotransmitter pathways?

(2) How does this experiment prove that chlorpromazine has a sedative effect?

[Knowledye expansion]

Ruixintuo—the independently developed new anti-schizophrenia drug in China, has been approved for market launch

Ruixintuo which is an independently developed new anti-schizophrenia drug in China, has been approved for market launch.

Schizophrenia is a chronic and persistent disease that recurs repeatedly. The main difficulty in treating schizophrenia is the recurrence of the condition caused by patients interrupting treatment or reducing medication on their own. Data statistics show that 60% of patients with first-time attacks have poor medication adherence, and the recurrence rate within 5 years exceeds 80%. Repeated relapses lead to a prolonged course of the disease, increasing the difficulty and burden of treatment.

In 2021, China's independently developed new anti-schizophrenia drug named Ruixintuo was officially launched. This is Chinese first innovative microsphere formulation with independent intellectual property rights and global registration, as well as the first domestically developed second-generation antipsychotic long-acting injection, bringing new hope for about 10 million schizophrenia patients in China to reintegrate into society. At present, Ruixintuo has been included in the national medical insurance drug catalog.

（房春燕）

Section 3　Effects of aspirin and chlorpromazine on body temperature

[Experimental objective]

(1) To observe the cooling effects of aspirin and chlorpromazine in different environments.

(2) To grasp the cooling characteristics of aspirin and chlorproma-zine and compare their differences.

[Experimental principle]

Homothermal animals have a perfect body temperature regulation mechanism. When the ambient temperature changes, the thermoregulatory center maintains a relatively constant body temperature by regulating the process of heat production and heat dissipation. Chlorpromazine, also known as hibernation, is a blocking agent of dopamine receptor D_2 in the midbrain-limbic system and midbrain-cortical pathways, so it is generally used clinically as a central nervous system inhibitor and plays an antipsychotic pharmacological role. Chlorpromazine has a strong inhibitory effect on the hypothalamic thermoregulatory center. The body temperature changes with the ambient temperature, and with the coordination of physical cooling, the normal body temperature can be lowered below the normal level.

Aspirin, also known as acetylsalicylic acid, is a typical example of non-steroidal anti-inflammatory drugs. The mechanism is to inhibit prostaglandin synthase, reducing the ability of arachidonic acid to be converted into prostaglandins, thereby causing the body temperature of febrile individuals to decrease or return to normal levels. Aspirin has no effect on the body temperature of normal individuals.

[Experimental materials]

Electronic balance, anal thermometer, 1 mL syringe, ice maker or refrigerator (ice cube), beaker.

[Experimental animals]

Mice weighting 22 ~ 25 g, either gender.

[Experimental reagents]

0.08% chlorpromazine hydrochloride solution, 1% aspirin solution, normal saline, 10% yeast suspension, liquid paraffin.

[Experimental methods]

1. Experimental preparation

Mice were randomly divided into groups, weighed, and numbered. This experiment consists of two parts: antipyretic experiment and low-temperature experiment, with 6 mice in each experiment. The mice in each experiment were divided into three groups, A, B, and C, with 2 mice in each group. The activity of the mice was observed before the experiment.

2. Body temperature measurement

Fix the mouse with one hand, and gently insert the rectal thermometer with liquid paraffin coated at the end of the temperature probe into the mouse's anus with the other hand about 1 cm away. After 3 minutes, remove it and read the value as the normal body temperature of the mouse.

3. Antipyretic experiment

Dry yeast induced fever in mice: 10% yeast suspension was injected subcutaneously, and mouse body temperature was measured 3 h later. The experiment started when the body temperature increased by more than 0.8°C. Mice in group A, group B and group C were intraperitoneally injected 0.08% chlorpromazine hydrochloride solution, 1% aspirin solution and normal saline (0.1 ml/10 g), and their body temperature was measured once after 30 min and 60 min respectively. The activities of the mice were observed and recorded (Figure 3-3-1).

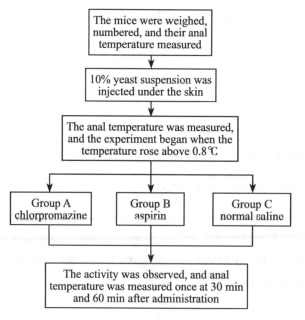

Figure 3-3-1   Flow chart of antipyretic experiment

4. Low-temperature experiment

Mice in group A, B and C were intraperitoneally injected with 0.08% chlorpromazine hydrochloride solution, 1% aspirin solution and normal saline (0.1 mL/10 g) respectively.

After medication, the three mice (A1, B1, C1) were placed in a beaker and the beaker was placed in an ice bath. Mice A2, B2 and C2 were placed under normal temperature. Anal temperature of mice in each group was detected again at 30 min and 60 min respectively, and the activity of mice was observed (Figure 3-3-2).

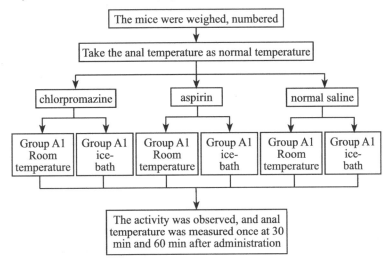

Figure 3-3-2　Flow chart of low temperature experiment

[Experimental records and results]

The results of antipyretic experiment were recorded in Table 3-3-1. For low temperature experiment, the results were recorded in Table 3-3-2.

Table 3-3-1　Effects of chlorpromazine and aspirin on body temperature in mice

Groups	Drugs	Environment	Body temperature			Activities	
			Before treatment	After treatment 30 min	After treatment 60 min	Before treatment	After treatment
A	Chlorpromazine	Room temperature					
B	Aspirin	Room temperature					
C	Saline	Room temperature					

Table 3-3-2　Effects of chlorpromazine and aspirin on body temperature in mice

Groups	Drugs	Environment	Body temperature			Activities	
			Before treatment	After treatment 30 min	After treatment 60 min	Before treatment	After treatment
A1	Chlorpromazine	Room temperature					
A2	Chlorpromazine	Ice-bath					
B1	Aspirin	Room temperature					
B2	Aspirin	Ice-bath					
C1	Saline	Room temperature					
C2	Saline	Ice-bath					

[Precautions]

(1) Room temperature affects the experimental results. It is best to conduct the experiment at around 20 ~ 25℃ and keep the room temperature constant.

(2) Put the beaker in the ice bath for the experiment.

(3) Apply a little liquid paraffin at the end of the thermometer to reduce resistance when measuring anal temperature.

(4) When taking the temperature, fix the mouse and do not stir too much. Keep the thermometer inserted at the same depth and time each time, and ensure that each animal uses the same thermometer on a fixed basis.

[Practice questions]

1. Which is misdescribed about the pharmacological action of chlorpromazine ?

A. Antipsychotic.　　　　　　　　　　B. Emetic action.

C. Sedative effect.　　　　　　　　　　D. Cooling effect.

2. Which one is wrong about the pharmacological effects of aspirin?

A. Abirritation.　　　　　　　　　　　B. Antiinflammation.

C. Antipyretic effect.　　　　　　　　　D. Sedative effect.

3. The main pathway of action of antipsychotics is _____.

A. nodular-funnel system　　　　　　　B. ascending reticular system

C. nigro-striatum system　　　　　　　D. mesencephalic limbic system

[Thinking questions]

(1) How is the cooling effect of chlorpromazine different from the antipyretic effect of aspirin?

(2) According to the action characteristics of aspirin and chlorpromazine, describe the clinical application of aspirin and chlorpromazine.

[Knowledye expansion]

A good medicine for psychiatry

Before the discovery of chlorpromazine, the treatment of psychiatric patients can be described as "no medicine available", and has experienced medieval exorcism treatment, heat therapy, psychosurgical treatment, electroconvulsive therapy and other stages, but had little effect. Until 1950, Rona Planck originally found anti-malarial drugs from antihistamines, synthetic products such as chlorpromazine, one of which was sold by the company under the name "promethazine". In the same year, Henri Laborit, a surgeon in Paris, observed that patients treated with promethazine appeared very calm and relaxed. Based on this, Laborite published a clinically recorded observation with no data. Coincidentally, it was quickly picked up by Rhone-Planck, who immediately began to shift antihistamines to developing drugs that acted on the central nervous system. In 1952, Laborit suggested that chlorpromazine could be used in the treatment of mental illness. And clinical findings that chlorpromazine could significantly reduce the illusions and delusions of psychiatric patients caused a stir in the medical community. The discovery of chlorpromazine gave birth to the "antipsychotic drug" this new drug variety. Countless psychiatric patients have been liberated, achieving a revolution in the history of psychiatric medicine. Therefore, some people refer to chlorpromazine as the "penicillin" of psychiatry.

（韩　雪）

Section 4　Comparison of the effects of pancuronium bromide and succinylcholine on muscle relaxation in rabbits

[Experimental objective]

(1) To learn the head-drooping experimental method of muscle relaxants in rabbits.

(2) To observe the differences between the effects of depolarizing and non-depolarizing muscle relaxants.

[Experimental principle]

Muscle relaxants act on the neuromuscular junction, binding to N_2 cholinergic receptors and blocking the transmission of excitation between nerves and muscles, thereby producing muscle relaxation. They can be categorized into two major groups: depolarizing and non-depolarizing muscle relaxants. Depolarizing muscle relaxants, such as succinylcholine, are N_2 receptor agonists. Non-depolarizing muscle relaxants, like pancuronium bromide, are N_2 receptor antagonists, and their muscle relaxant effects can be antagonized by anticholinesterase drugs. Both types of drugs can block the neuromuscular junction, but they differ in their modes of blockade and characteristics of action.

Succinylcholine, a representative of depolarizing muscle relaxants, is also known as a non-competitive muscle relaxant. Its characteristics include: ① Prolonged depolarization after binding to N_2 receptors, rendering the receptors unresponsive to ACh and resulting in skeletal muscle relaxation. ② Resistance to hydrolysis by cholinesterase. Anticholinesterase drugs not only fail to antagonize succinylcholine's effects but may enhance its muscle relaxation, thus overdose cannot be treated with neostigmine.

Pancuronium bromide is a non-depolarizing muscle relaxant, also known as a competitive muscle relaxant. Its characteristics include: ① Competing with acetylcholine for N_2 receptors at the neuromuscular junction without activating them, competitively blocking ACh's depolarizing effect and causing skeletal muscle relaxation. ② Its muscle relaxant effects can be antagonized by anticholinesterase drugs, allowing for treatment of overdose with appropriate doses of neostigmine.

[Experimental materials]

2 mL syringe, infant scale.

[Experimental animals]

Rabbits, weighing 2.0 ~ 3.0 kg, either gender.

[Experimental reagents]

0.008% pancuronium bromide solution, 0.05% succinylcholine solution, 0.05% neostigmine sulfate solution, 0.05% atropine solution.

[Experimental methods]

Follow the experimental operation steps as shown in Figure 3-4-1.

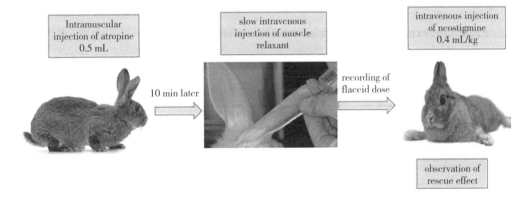

Figure 3-4-1   Schematic diagram of operational steps

1. Take 2 rabbits, weigh and label them

Observe their respiration, posture, and muscle tone of the neck and limbs. Inject atropine solution intramuscularly at a dose of 0.5 mL per rabbit and wait for approximately 10 minutes.

2. Rabbit A

Administer 0.008% pancuronium bromide solution intravenously at a slow rate of 0.5 mL/min (push-stop-push-stop-push...), with a total dose of 0.5 mL/kg. Pause and closely observe upon the onset of muscle relaxation, paying attention to the degree of relaxation. If the rabbit shows a tendency to droop its head, immediately stop the injection and gently tap its head. If the rabbit fails to lift its head, record the amount of drug already injected, which represents the head-drooping dose for that rabbit (approximately half the total dose). Resume the injection slowly with approximately double dose of pancuronium bromide solution and observe changes in limb muscle tone, respiration, and posture. Immediately inject 0.05% neostigmine sulfate solution intravenously at a dose of 0.4 mL/kg and observe the rabbit's response.

3. Rabbit B

Using the same method, administer 0.05% succinylcholine solution intravenously at a dose of 0.5 mL/kg and observe for signs such as muscle fasciculations, head drooping, or generalized paralysis. Upon the onset of muscle relaxation, immediately inject 0.05% neostigmine sulfate solution intravenously at a dose of 0.4 mL/kg and observe the rabbit's response. Compare the changes observed in Rabbit B with those in Rabbit A.

[Experimental records and results]

Record the experimental results as detailed in Table 3-4-1.

Table 3-4-1　Comparison of muscle relaxant effects of pancuronium bromide and succinylcholine on rabbits

Rabbit ID	Weight(kg)	Drug	Dosage	Post-drug manifestations
A		Pancuronium bromide		
		Neostigmine		
B		Succinylcholine		
		Neostigmine		

[Precautions]

(1) Inject the muscle relaxant slowly and at a constant rate of approximately 0.5 mL/min to accurately determine the head-drooping dose and observe its effects on the rabbit.

(2) Administer neostigmine promptly after the rabbit exhibits muscle relaxation to avoid difficulties in reversal. If the reversal effect is inadequate, increase the dosage of neostigmine.

[Practice questions]

1. Which of the following drugs can enhance the muscle relaxant effect of succinylcholine?

　A. Atropine.　　　　B. Epinephrine.　　　C. Neostigmine.　　　D. Pilocarpine.

2. The mechanism of action of succinylcholine in relaxing skeletal muscles is _____.

A. causing persistent depolarization of skeletal muscle motor endplates

B. blocking N_2 receptors

C. blocking N_1 receptors

D. blocking M receptors

3. Which of the following drug intoxications can be treated with neostigmine?

　A. Pancuronium bromide　　　　　　B. Pilocarpine

　C. Succinylcholine　　　　　　　　D. Physostigmine

[Thinking questions]

(1) What are the differences between depolarizing and non-depolarizing muscle relaxants?

(2) How does neostigmine differ in its effects on rabbits when used to reverse the toxicity of these two types of muscle relaxants in the experiment? Why?

[Knowledye expansion]

The clinical application of succinylcholine

　　Amidst the vast expanse of medical knowledge, skeletal muscle relaxants shine like brilliant stars, illuminating the path of surgical procedures and emergency rescues. Among them, succinylcholine, as the earliest discovered depolarizing muscle relaxant, stands out in medical history with its unique pharmacological effects and widespread applications.

　　Since its discovery in 1942, succinylcholine has swiftly become a vital tool in the hands of anesthesiologists. It induces rapid relaxation of all skeletal muscles within mere seconds, providing invaluable support for endotracheal intubation, mechanical ventilation, and complex surgical operations. This discovery marks a significant breakthrough in anesthesiology and a vivid illustration of medical technological advancement. The development and application of succinylcholine are testaments to the courage and innovation of researchers. They remind us that in today's rapidly evolving technological landscape, only continuous innovation can propel the sustainable development of medical science.

In the operating room, the application of succinylcholine is not only a demonstration of technology, but also a manifestation of humanistic care. It facilitates surgeries that would otherwise be hindered by muscle tension, allowing for smoother procedures and securing precious treatment time for patients. Furthermore, in emergency rescue situations, succinylcholine serves as a life-saving weapon. It swiftly alleviates respiratory muscle spasms in patients, buying time for subsequent interventions. In medical practice, healthcare professionals consistently prioritize patients' safety and well-being. The use of succinylcholine vividly exemplifies this commitment, emphasizing the need to focus on patients' needs and feelings throughout diagnostic and therapeutic processes.

Succinylcholine plays a pivotal role in the medical field, but its administration carries inherent risks. Improper usage can lead to severe complications such as hyperkalemia and arrhythmias. Therefore, healthcare professionals must strictly adhere to operational protocols and medication principles when administering succinylcholine to ensure patient safety. Medical work necessitates professionalism, rigorousness, and a profound sense of responsibility. When handling high-risk medications like skeletal muscle relaxants, utmost vigilance and caution are paramount.

（房春燕）

Section 5　Anticonvulsant effect of phenobarbital sodium in mice

[Experimental objective]

(1) Learn the methods of electrical stimulation-induced and drug-induced seizure model in mice.

(2) Observe the anticonvulsant effect of phenobarbital sodium and master its mechanisms.

[Experimental principle]

Convulsions are involuntary contractions of the whole body or local skeletal muscles caused by varying degrees of abnormal neuronal firing in the brain tissue. Animal convulsion models are commonly used in research, including electrical stimulation-induced and drug-induced seizure model in mice. In the electrical stimulation-induced seizure model, the currents generated by an instrument stimulate the brain through the electrodes clamped to the ears of mice, resulting in generalized tonic convulsions that manifest as flexion of the forelimbs and straightening of the hind limbs. In the drug-induced seizure model, some convulsive agents such as pentylenetrazol, nikethamide, etc. are often used to directly excite the central nervous system by high-dose intraperitoneal or subcutaneous injection, resulting in convulsive seizures in mice that manifest as a generalized tonic-clonic seizures. Both of these models can be used for the pharmacodynamic evaluation of anticonvulsant drugs and the screening of compounds with potential anticonvulsant activity.

Phenobarbital sodium is a barbiturate, and its mechanism of action is mainly through agonism of $GABA_A$ receptor, prolonging the time of Cl^- channel opening, increasing GABA-mediated Cl^- inward flow, causing hyperpolarized inhibitory synaptic effects, thus producing obvious inhibitory effects on the central nervous system. As the dose is increased, the central inhibitory effect is progressively enhanced. Anticonvulsant effects appear when the dose is higher than the hypnotic dose (Figure 3-5-1).

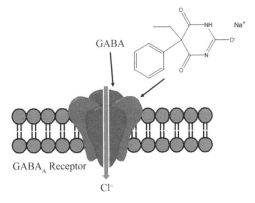

Figure 3-5-1　The structure of phenobarbital sodium and its binding site to the $GABA_A$ receptor

[Experimental materials]

YSD-4G pharmaco-physiological multi-purpose instruments (or electrical stimulator), guidewires and alligator clips, mouse experimental cage, cotton balls, syringe (1 mL), electronic balance.

[Experimental animals]

ICR mice, weight 22 ~ 25 g, available for either gender.

[Experimental reagents]

0.5% phenobarbital sodium solution, normal saline, 0.5% pentylenetrazol solution.

[Experimental methods]

1. Electrical stimulation-induced seizure model

1) The seizure threshold stimulation method

(1) The tips of the alligator clips at the front end of the output wires were wrapped with saline moistened cotton balls and clamped at the root of both ears of a mouse respectively. The parameters of the YSD-4G pharmaco-physiological multi-purpose instrument (or electrical stimulator) were set to the stimulation mode "single sinusoidal pulse", the stimulation frequency "50 Hz", and the stimulation time "0.2 s". The stimulation current intensity started from 7 mA and was increased by 1 mA every 1 min until a tonic response appeared in the hind limbs of the mouse, and the current intensity was recorded as the seizure threshold of the mouse. The seizure thresholds of six mice were determined by the above method.

(2) Six mice were weighed, labeled, and randomly divided into two groups, A and B, with three mice in each group. The mice in group A were injected intraperitoneally with 0.5% phenobarbital sodium solution at the dose of 15 mg/kg, while the mice in group B were injected with an equal amount of normal saline as a control.

(3) 30 min after administration, the mice were electrically stimulated again using the seizure threshold of each mouse measured above as the stimulation current, with the remaining parameters as above. The seizure stage of the mice was recorded. No response was recorded as stage 0, the anterior and posterior limb clonus was recorded as stage 1, the anterior

limb tonus was recorded as stage 2, and the posterior limb tonus was recorded as stage 3.

(4) The data with each mouse were recorded in Table 3-5-1.

2) The fixed current intensity stimulation method

(1) Six mice were weighed, labeled, and randomly divided into two groups, A and B, with three mice in each group. Mice in group A were injected intraperitoneally with 0.5% phenobarbital sodium solution at the dose of 50 mg/kg, while mice in group B were injected with an equal amount of normal saline as a control. After 30 min of drug administration, electrical stimulation test was performed.

(2) The tips of the alligator clips at the front end of the output wires were wrapped with saline moistened cotton balls and clamped at the root of both ears of a mouse respectively. The parameters of the YSD-4G pharmaco-physiological multi-purpose instrument (or electrical stimulator) were set to the stimulation mode "single sinusoidal pulse", the stimulation frequency "50 Hz", the stimulation time "0.2 s" and the current intensity "25 mA". Each mouse was stimulated and the seizure stage was recorded. No response was recorded as stage 0, the anterior and posterior limb clonus was recorded as stage 1, the anterior limb tonus was recorded as stage 2, and the posterior limb tonus was recorded as stage 3.

(3) The data with each mouse were recorded in Table 3-5-2.

2. Drug-induced seizure model

(1)Two mice were weighed, labeled and injected intraperitoneally with 0.5% phenobarbital sodium solution at the dose of 50 mg/kg and an equal amount of normal saline respectively.

(2) After 10 min, both mice were injected subcutaneously with 0.5% pentylenetrazol solution at the dose of 50 mg/kg. Then, the latency of seizure (the duration between the administration of pentylenetrazol and the first appearance of clonic seizure) and mortality of mice were recorded in 30 min.

(3) The data with each mouse were recorded in Table 3-5-3.

[Experimental records and results]

Depending on the methods used to induce convulsions, the results of the experiments were recorded in the corresponding tables. Specifically, see Table 3-5-1, Table 3-5-2 and Table 3-5-3.

Table 3-5-1　Anticonvulsant effect of phenobarbital sodium on electrical stimulation-induced seizure (the seizure threshold stimulation method) in mice

Group	No.	Weight	Seizure threshold	Drug and delivery Volume	Seizure stage
A					
A					
A					
B					
B					
B					

Table 3-5-2　Anticonvulsant effect of phenobarbital sodium on electrical stimulation-induced seizure (the fixed current intensity stimulation method) in mice

Group	No.	Weight	Drug and delivery Volume	Seizure stage
A				
A				
A				
B				
B				
B				

Table 3-5-3　Anticonvulsant effect of sodium phenobarbital on drug-induced seizure in mice

Group	No.	Weight	Drug and delivery Volume	The latency of seizure	Seizure or not	Death or survival
A						
B						

[Precautions]

(1) There are individual differences in the response of mice to electrical stimulation. To avoid the death of a large number of mice caused by excessive current, the seizure threshold stimulation method is recommended when using the electrical stimulation-induced seizure model in mice.

(2) When using the electrical stimulation-induced seizure model, please take care to ensure that the experimenter's hands do not touch the metal part of the alligator clips or the metal guide wires and the two alligator clips are not allowed to contact with each other while the equipment is energized.

(3) The dose of the drug should be administered accurately and the results should be

observed and recorded promptly and exactly.

(4) In this experiment, 0.1% diazepam solution can be used instead of 0.5% phenobarbital sodium solution; while 5% nikethamide solution can also be used instead of 0.5% pentylenetrazol solution in the drug-induced seizure method.

[Practice questions]

1. The binding sites of barbiturates as sedative-hypnotic drugs are located at _____.

A. NMDA receptor   B. GABA receptor

C. 5-HT receptor   D. DA receptor

2. Which description of the role and application of barbiturates is incorrect?

A. The extent of its inhibitory effect on the central nervous system increases gradually with increasing dose.

B. Barbiturates can produce anticonvulsant effect at higher than hypnotic doses.

C. Barbiturates are still used as the first line of clinical sedative-hypnotic drugs.

D. The velocity of drug onsct is rclatcd to fat solubility.

3. Which description of the operation of subcutaneous injection in mice is correct?

A. It can be operated by only one person, instead of by two people.

B. The injection site is usually subcutaneous on the back and the neck of mice.

C. The absorption velocity of subcutaneous injections in mice is faster than that of intravenous injections.

D. There is no limit to the volume of subcutaneous injections in mice.

[Thinking questions]

(1) What are the drugs with anticonvulsant effects? What are the differences in their anticonvulsant mechanisms?

(2) What are the causes of convulsions?

[Knowledye expansion]

Translation of non-therapeutic and therapeutic effects of drugs

Phenobarbital is a barbiturate sedative-hypnotic drug that was first marketed and used in 1912 and was used until the 1960s. Phenobarbital has significant residual effect, is susceptible to tolerance and dependence, and acute toxicity is more likely to occur. In addition, the drug is a strong hepatic enzyme inducer, inducing elevated activity or increased amounts of a variety of hepatic enzymes, leading to accelerated metabolism and decreased effect of other drugs combined with phenobarbital. Due to the above adverse effects, the use of phenobarbital has been limited, gradually replaced by later marketed benzodiazepines and so on. It is no longer routinely used as a sedative-hypnotic drug. However, its hepatic enzyme-inducing effect has been found to have new clinical applications. The principle is that phenobarbital can induce a kind of hepatic enzyme called glucuronosyltransferase, which can promote the binding of glucuronic acid to bilirubin in the blood, thereby accelerating the metabolism of bilirubin. Therefore, phenobarbital can reduce the concentration of bilirubin through its hepatic enzyme-inducing effect, and treat hyperbilirubinemia and cholestatic jaundice. This example of "drug repurposing" shows that the role of drugs often have advantages and disadvantages, but is a unity of opposites, the non-therapeutic effects of drugs can be converted into therapeutic effects under certain conditions. This suggests that we should have a comprehensive understanding of the role of drugs, which not only helps us to understand the complexity of the role of drugs, but also provides useful guidance for us to develop a scientific and rational treatment program in clinical practice.

（钟　恺）

Section 6　The effect of drugs on resisting nikethamide-induced convulsions

[Experimental objective]

(1) Observe the preventive effect of diazepam against convulsions induced by nikethamide in mice.

(2) Learn the experimental methods for preparing animal convulsion models using drugs.

[Experimental principle]

Convulsion is a symptom of excessive excitation in the central nervous system caused by various reasons, manifested as involuntary twitching of the whole body or local muscles. The mechanism of convulsion occurs due to an imbalance between inhibitory and excitatory neurotransmitters in the brain, leading to abnormal discharge of cerebral motor neurons. The duration of a convulsive episode is mostly between 3 to 5 minutes, and it can sometimes recur repeatedly, presenting a persistent state. Common symptoms include twitching of limbs and facial muscles, rolling up of eyeballs, frothing at the mouth, purple or bluish complexion, loss of consciousness, and apnea.

Nikethamide (also known as Coramine), a respiratory stimulant, can directly stimulate the respiratory center in the medulla oblongata at therapeutic doses. It can also stimulate the chemoreceptors in the carotid bodies and aortic bodies, causing a reflex excitation of the respiratory center. However, at toxic doses, it can significantly increase the excitability of the entire central nervous system, leading to convulsion symptoms in the body, which may even progress to irreversible central inhibition, ultimately resulting in animal death.

Diazepam (trade name "Valium"), a long-acting benzodiazepine, enhances the efficacy of gamma-aminobutyric acid (GABA), which is the primary inhibitory neurotransmitter in the brain. It exhibits sedative, hypnotic, anxiolytic, anticonvulsant, and central skeletal muscle relaxant effects. It is also used to treat alcohol withdrawal symptoms and as a premedication for anesthesia. Diazepam is effective against convulsions caused by various reasons, such as eclampsia, tetanus, and febrile seizures in children. Compared to barbiturate hypnotics, diazepam has a high therapeutic index, minimal respiratory effects, virtually no impact on rapid eye movement (REM) sleep, no effect on hepatic enzymes, and does not induce anesthesia even at high doses. It is one of the most commonly used hypnotics in clinical practice. Its anticonvulsant effect is very potent, being 10 times stronger than chlordiazepoxide. With a plasma half-life of 20 to 50 hours, diazepam is considered a long-acting medication.

Molecular structures of Nikethamide and Diazepam, seen in Figure 3-6-1.

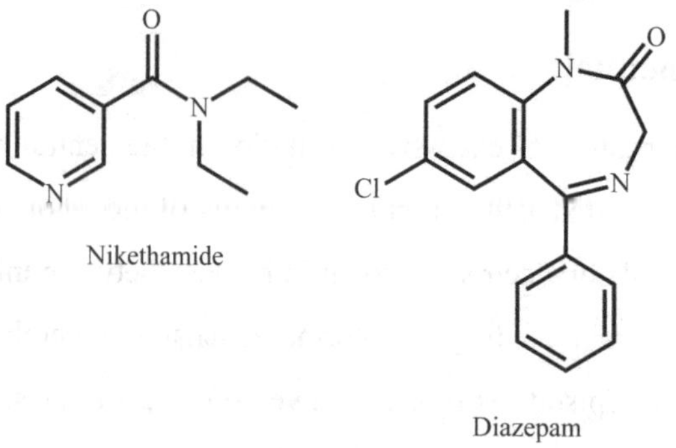

Nikethamide

Diazepam

Figure 3-6-1 Molecular structures of Nikethamide and Diazepam

[Experimental materials]

Mouse cage, electronic balance, beaker, syringe (0.25 mL).

[Experimental animals]

2 mice (18 ~ 22 g), either gender.

[Experimental reagents]

0.5% Diazepam, 2% Nikethamide, physiological saline, picric acid.

[Experimental methods]

The experimental operation steps are as follows, see Figure 3-6-2.

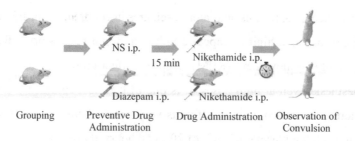

Figure 3-6-2 Schematic diagram of operation steps

(1) Animal Grouping Take 2 mice, weigh and label the number with picric acid.

(2) Drug Administration Administer an intraperitoneal injection of 0.5% Diazepam at a dose of 0.017 mL/10 g (equivalent to 8.5 mg/kg) to Mouse A. Administer an intraperitoneal injection of physiological saline at a dose of 0.017 mL/10 g to Mouse B.

(3) Drug-induced convulsion After 15 minutes, administer an intraperitoneal injection of 2% Nikethamide at a dose of 0.1 mL/10 g (equivalent to 200 mg/kg) to both mice.

(4) Observation of convulsion phenomena Observe whether convulsions (using clonic convulsions or abnormal jumping as an indicator) occur in both mice. Record the occurrence of convulsions, their intensity, and any deaths that may occur.

[Experimental records and results]

Record the experimental results, including whether convulsions occurred in the mice, the intensity of convulsions, and any deaths, seen in Table 3-6-1.

Table 3-6-1　The effect of drugs on resisting Nikethamide-induced convulsions

Group	Weight (g)	Preventive Drug	Drug volume (mL)	Dosage of Nikethamide (mg/10 g)	Time of convulsion occurrence (min)	Intensity of Convulsion and Phenomena	Whether death occurred
A		Diazepam					
B		Normal Saline					

[Precautions]

(1) After administering nikethamide, the prodromal symptoms of convulsion can manifest as tail-raising, jumping, screaming, and teeth-grinding.

(2) When performing intraperitoneal injections, attention should be paid to proper technique to avoid injuring internal organs.

[Practice questions]

1. The angle between the mouse and the syringe during intraperitoneal injection in mice should be _____.

A. 0°　　　　　　　　B. 15°　　　　　　　　C. 45°　　　　　　　　D. 90°

2. Which of the following statements about diazepam is incorrect ?

A. It is a class II psychotropic drug and is a prescription medication.

B. It can produce sedative and hypnotic effects.

C. It does not have addictive properties.

D. It acts on the cerebral cortex, inhibiting the excitability of the central nervous system.

3. Which of the following is not an indication for nikethamide?

A. Carbon monoxide poisoning.

B. Asthma.

C. Morphine poisoning.

D. Heart failure.

[Thinking questions]

(1) What is the mechanism of diazepam's antagonism against the convulsive effects induced by nikethamide in mice?

(2) What are the common categories of anticonvulsant drugs? What are the similarities and differences in their primary actions and uses?

(3) What is the mechanism of convulsion occurrence caused by an overdose of nikethamide?

[Knowledye expansion]

Diazepam—a drug with long history

Penicillin, aspirin, and diazepam are recognized as the three drugs that have contributed the most to human health, leaving an indelible mark in human history. Among them, diazepam has opened a new chapter in sedative-hypnotic medications. Developed by Dr. Leo Sternbach, a Swedish chemist who is considered one of the founders of modern pharmacology in the late 1950s, diazepam is commercially known as "Valium." In 1959, 2,000 physicians treated 20,000 patients with it, yielding remarkable results. Currently, diazepam is widely used in the treatment of symptoms such as anxiety disorders, epilepsy, convulsions, insomnia, and acute alcohol withdrawal syndrome. Its remarkable efficacy has made it the first "blockbuster" drug to surpass sales of $1 billion, highlighting its significant position in the history of medicine. Its development ushered in a golden age of benzodiazepine sedative-hypnotics. Although diazepam exhibits significant clinical efficacy, it also carries a certain degree of drug dependence. Long-term use of diazepam may lead to psychological and physical dependence in patients, and withdrawal may result in discontinuation reactions. Diazepam and similar drugs, such as clonazepam and alprazolam, are classified as Class II psychotropic drugs, which are strictly controlled by the state. Prescriptions for

Class II psychotropic drugs generally should not exceed a seven-day supply, and the prescriptions must be kept for at least two years. Medicines should be used rationally, normatively, and safely, without self-medication or arbitrarily increasing the dosage or extending the course of treatment.

（童骏森）

Section 7   Anxiolytic effects of diazepam

[Experimental objective]

(1) Learn to evaluate anxiety-like behavior of mice using the elevated plus-maze (EPM) test.

(2) Observe the anxiolytic effect of diazepam and analyze its mechanisms and clinical significance.

[Experimental principle]

Anxiety disorder is one of the neuropsychiatric disorders characterized by persistent tension, worry, fear, or episodic panic attacks, which seriously affect the quality of life of patients and easily lead to many physical and mental diseases and social problems. Animal behavioral assessment methods are widely used in the study of anxiety disorders, which are characterized by relatively easy availability, strong operability, and fewer ethical and moral issues, and have become an important method of efficacy evaluation in the study of anxiolytic drugs.

EPM test is one of the most effective and widely used behavioral assessment methods for anxiety disorders, with the advantages of simple design, economical and practical, free for long-term training, and bi-directional sensitivity to drugs, etc. The EPM, which is approximately 0.5 m above the ground, consists of two symmetrical open arms, two closed arms and a central zone. The open arms of EPM have both novelty and threat to animals, causing anxiety reactions while generating curiosity for exploration. The animals were initially placed in the central zone of the EPM. Then their behavioral activities were observed for a certain period of time, and their movement trajectories were recorded, as well as the duration and number of times they entered the open and closed arms respectively. If the animal mainly retreated into the closed arm, it indicated that its anxiety level was high. On the contrary, it indicated that its anxiety level was low.

Currently, the main therapeutic agents for anxiety disorders are benzodiazepines, selective 5-hydroxytryptamine reuptake inhibitors, and selective 5-hydroxytryptamine and norepinephrine reuptake inhibitors. Diazepam is a benzodiazepine, and its mechanism is related to binding to the benzodiazepine binding site on the GABA$_A$ receptor complex, inducing a change in receptor conformation, promoting the binding of GABA to the GABA$_A$ receptor, increasing the frequency of Cl$^-$ channel opening, enhancing the GABA-mediated Cl$^-$ influx, and then exerting a pronounced central inhibitory effect. Thus a small dose of diazepam can produce anxiolytic effects (Figure 3-7-1).

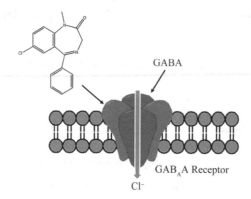

Figure 3-7-1　Diagram of diazepam structure and its binding site to GABA$_A$ receptor

[Experimental materials]

EPM, camera, video analysis software, mouse cage, electronic balance, syringe (1 mL).

[Experimental animals]

ICR mice, weight 22 ~ 25 g, either gender.

[Experimental reagents]

0.1% diazepam solution, normal saline.

[Experimental methods]

(1) Before starting the experiment, place the mice in the laboratory where the elevated cross maze is located to adapt to the environment for 1 hour.

(2) Take 2 mice that have adapted to the environment, weigh and number them, and assign them to group A and group B respectively. Group A mice were intraperitoneally injected with 10 mL/kg of 0.1% diazepam solution, while Group B mice were intraperitoneally injected with an equal amount of normal saline as a control.

(3) After 30 min, the mice were respectively placed in the central zone of the EPM, with their heads facing the open-arm zone, and the activities of the mice within 5 min were recorded by vertical shooting with the camera. The video analysis software was used to analyze the movement trajectories of the mice and calculate the indexes such as the number of the accesses to the open arm, the duration inside the open arm, the distance inside the open arm, and the corresponding percentage. All of the data were recorded in Table 3-7-1.

(4) Collect the raw data of all groups in the class, tabulate them for statistical processing, find out the mean and standard deviation of the indicators of groups A and B, and conduct statistical tests on the differences of the indicators.

[Experimental records and results]

Record the results of the experiment in Table 3-7-1, in which the indicators of the number of the accesses to the open arm, the duration inside the open arm, the distance inside the open arm were generally derived directly by the software, and the percentage indicators were calculated by the following formula: Percentage of the number of the accesses to the open arm = the number of the accesses to the open arm / (the number of the accesses to the open arm + the number of the accesses to the closed arm) × 100%. Percentage of the duration in the open arm = the duration in the open arm / (the duration in the open arm + the duration in the closed arm) × 100%. Percentage of the distance in the open arm = the distance in the open arm / total distance of mice within the EPM × 100%.

Tabel 3-7-1　Anxiolytic effect of diazepam on the EPM test in mice

Group	Weight	Drug and delivery Volume	the number of the accesses to the open arm	percentage of the number of the accesses to the open arm	the duration in the open arm	percentage of the duration in the open arm	the distance in the open arm	percentage of the distance in the open arm
A								
B								

[Precautions]

(1) 3 days before the experiment, the experimenter can put the mice on the hand and touch them for 5 min every day to eliminate the nervousness and fear of the mice.

(2) The experiments should be conducted in a quiet environment with moderate light intensity (the lowest brightness that can distinguish the subtle activities of mice at a distance of 1.5 m) and stable light in the laboratory to minimize extraneous stress stimuli.

(3) At the end of each mouse test, the excreta in the EPM should be removed in a timely manner, and the maze should be wiped with 75% alcohol to eliminate odors and to reduce the influence of these factors on mice in subsequent experiments.

(4) In this experiment, 1.25% buspirone solution can be used instead of 0.1% diazepam solution.

[Practice questions]

1. What is the mechanism of benzodiazepines in causing central inhibition?

A. Increasing Na^+ channel opening.　　B. Increasing K^+ channel opening.

C. Increasing Ca^{2+} channel opening.　　D. Increasing Cl^- channel opening.

2. Which of the following descriptions of diazepam is false?

A. No specific antagonist available for emergency treatment of acute diazepam poisoning.

B. Status epilepticus can be treated with high doses of diazepam.

C. Diazepam has anxiolytic effects in small doses, while moderate doses of diazepam have sedative-hypnotic effects.

D. The inhibitory effect of diazepam on the central nervous system increases progressively with increasing dose.

3. Which description of the EPM is correct?

A. EPM needs to be more than 1.5 m above the ground.

B. When the mice mainly activate within the closed arms, it indicated that their anxiety levels were low.

C. When the mice mainly activate within the open arms, it indicated that their anxiety levels were low.

D. When the mice mainly activate within the open arms, it indicated that their anxiety levels were high.

[Thinking questions]

(1) What are other methods of animal behavioral evaluation of anxiolytic drugs?

(2) Why is diazepam less commonly used in clinics for the treatment of anxiety disorders?

[Knowlcdye expansion]

The discovery of diazepam, the classic drug created by an experimental error

In the 1950s, the main sedative-hypnotic drugs on the market at that time were still barbiturates, but they had already shown a number of intolerable adverse reactions in clinical application. As a result, many pharmaceutical companies and research institutes set up specialized research groups and began to search for new sedative-hypnotic drugs. The research group led by Leo Sternbach, a researcher at Roche, was one of them. However, none of the 40 new compounds synthesized by the group showed significant sedative-hypnotic activity in pharmacological tests. Thus, Roche decided to give up and disband Leo's group. While they were cleaning up the lab, someone noticed a compound that had been accidentally synthesized earlier, Ro-50690. Due to a feeding error, Ro-50690 was then considered an experimental error and was not tested for pharmacological activity. When Leo learned of this, he sent the compound for testing, even though he felt it was unlikely to be effective, since it was the last compound that could be sent for testing before the group disbanded. A few days later, the head of the pharmacology department called to say that the results were amazing. And the compound not only had sedative, anti-anxiety, and muscle relaxant effects, but also was more effective than any commercially available barbiturate at the time. Therefore, Roche decided to restart the research with Ro-50690 as the lead compound, and subsequently synthesized 3,000 related compounds, and finally obtained diazepam in 1959, which was successfully marketed in 1963. After its availability, diazepam quickly became one of the best-selling drugs in the history of medicine, because of its precise efficacy and fewer adverse reactions. It is considered as one of the three classic drugs in the history of medicine.

（钟　恺）

Section 8　Rescue effect of nikethamide on morphine induced respiratory depression

[Experimental objective]

(1) To observe the effects of morphine overdose on breathing.

(2) To observe the rescue effect of nikethamide on morphine indcued respiratory depression.

(3) To learn and master the respiration rate measurement and observation methods of rabbits.

[Experimental principle]

Nikethamide is a respiratory stimulant that can selectively stimulate the medullary respiratory center, and can also reflexively stimulate the respiratory center through carve and aortic body chemical receptors to deepen and accelerate breathing. When the respiratory center is suppressed, its excitement is more obvious. Morphine is a powerful analgesic, but it also has side effects that inhibit breathing. This experiment was observed by injecting morphine into rabbits to cause respiratory depression, and then injecting nikethamide to observe its relief effect on respiratory inhibition.

[Experimental materials]

Syringe, Malley's air drum, nasal cannula, timer, experimental table, electronic scale, iron support, rabbit fixing box, tape, respiratory frequency monitor.

[Experimental animals]

Domestic rabbit.

[Experimental reagents]

1% morphine hydrochloride solution, 5% nikethamide solution, 0.5% diazepam solution.

[Experimental methods]

(1) Rabbits were weighed and placed on the test bench. Fix the head and limbs, and connect the respiratory frequency monitor.

(2) Record the normal breathing frequency of rabbits.

(3) Slowly inject 1% morphine hydrochloride solution into the ear vein (calculated dose based on rabbit's weight, 0.5 ~ 1.0 mL/kg) to observe changes in rabbit's respiratory frequency and pores.

(4) When the rabbit's breathing frequency is significantly reduced (such as falling below 50% of the normal value), immediately inject 5% nikethamide solution (0.5 mL/kg based on the rabbit's body weight) to observe the recovery of breathing frequency and changes in the pores.

(5) If the rabbit has a convulsive reaction (such as facial muscle spasm, limb twitching, etc.), immediately inject 0.5% Diazepam solution into the ear vein for relief.

(6) Record data such as changes in respiratory frequency, injection time, rescue time, etc (Figure 3-8-1).

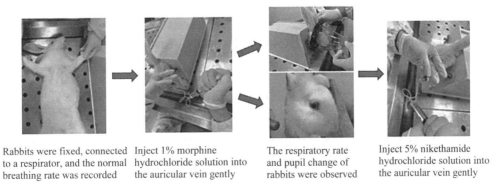

| Rabbits were fixed, connected to a respirator, and the normal breathing rate was recorded | Inject 1% morphine hydrochloride solution into the auricular vein gently | The respiratory rate and pupil change of rabbits were observed | Inject 5% nikethamide hydrochloride solution into the auricular vein gently |

Figure 3-8-1   Diagram of experimental procedure

[Experimental records and results]

(1) The changes of respiratory frequency in rabbits during the experiment were recorded and the curves of respiratory frequency changes were drawn.

(2) The pupil changes of rabbits after morphine and nikethamide injection were recorded.

(3) Record the respiratory frequency changes and rescue time, and then fill in Table 3-8-1.

Table 3-8-1　Effect of nikethamide on respiratory depression of morphine

Record item	Control	after morphine injection	after nikethamide injection
Pupil change			
Respiratory rate (times /min)			
Rescue time			

[Thinking questions]

(1) Analyze the rescue effect of nikethamide on morphine respiratory depression and possible adverse reactions (such as convulsion).

(2) Discuss the pharmacological mechanism of nikethamide as a respiratory stimulant, as well as possible problems and precautions in practical application.

(3) Analyze the causes of convulsive reactions in the experiment and rescue measures.

[Precautions]

(1) Rabbits should be kept in a quiet state during the experiment to avoid external interference.

(2) When injecting drugs, the dose should be accurately calculated to avoid to be excessive or insufficient.

(3) The drug should be injected slowly and steadily to avoid leakage of the liquid or rapid injection.

(4) In the experiment, we should pay close attention to the respiratory changes and possible adverse reactions of rabbits, and take timely rescue measures.

(5) Rabbits should be properly handled after the experiment to avoid harming experimental animals.

[Practice questions]

1. What type of drugs is nikethamide mainly used to rescue respiratory depression caused by?

　　A. Pethidine.　　　　　B. Morphine.　　　C. Phenobarbital.　　　　D. Chlorpromazine.

2. How did the respiratory frequency and amplitude of rabbits change after injection of morphine in this experiment?

　　A. The breathing rate increases and the amplitude increases.

　　B. The respiratory rate is slowed down and the amplitude is reduced.

　　C. There were no significant changes in respiratory rate and amplitude.

　　D. The breathing rate increases and the amplitude is reduced.

3. What is the mechanism of Nikethamide against morphine-induced respiratory depression?

　　A. Inhibits central opioid receptors.　　　　B. Excitatory of central medulla receptor.

　　C. Inhibits central dopamine receptors.　　　D. Excitatory central dopamine receptors.

[Thinking questions]

What are the possible complications and corresponding treatment measures of Nikethamide in rescuing morphine respiratory depression?

[Knowledye expansion]

Coramine - a stimulant for refreshing and invigorating the mind

Coramine, also known as Niketamide, is a relatively rare stimulant. Coramine is the hydrochloride salt of lobelanine extracted from the North American plant lobelia, which is now mostly chemically synthesized. Mountain stem vegetables are found throughout the North American continent and are a herbaceous plant used by Native Americans to treat asthma. Moderate intake of this substance is safe, but excessive use can cause vomiting, spasms, high blood pressure, epilepsy, and may even be fatal. Research has shown that coramine has significant effects on physiological activities such as sleep, emotions, and mood, and was once known as a wake-up medicine. At the 1972 Munich Olympics, two cyclists from the Netherlands and Spain won bronze medals in both the team and individual road races. However, their medals were cancelled after a positive doping test for coramine.

（周　倩）

Section 9　Local and systemic effects of procaine

[Experimental objective]

(1) To understand the excitatory and inhibitory effects, local and systemic effect of drugs.

(2) To observe the anticonvulsant effect of thiopental sodium.

[Experimental principle]

Procaine is a commonly used local anesthetic. After local injection, it can block the flow of sodium ions in nerve cell membrane, block the generation and conduction of action potential, and temporarily block the conduction of pain and motor function. If procaine enters the blood circulation from the site of administration, it will have an absorption effect, block the flow of sodium ions in the cell membrane of the cardiovascular system, inhibit cardiovascular excitability, and lead to the toxic reaction of circulation inhibition. In addition, procaine absorption will also have an impact on the central nervous system, leading to the central first excitation and then inhibition of toxic reactions.

In this experiment, procaine was injected into the sciatic nerve of rabbits to produce ipsilateral hind limb pain and movement disorders. The local effect was observed, that is, the effect of blocking pain and movement function. And further observe its absorption effect by intramuscular injection of procaine. The experiment can observe the central first excitation and then inhibition of the toxic reaction, that is the first convulsion. If the rescue is not timely, it can appear death. Thiopental sodium is an inhibitory drug for the central nervous system, which can combat convulsion caused by intramuscular injection of procaine.

[Experimental materials]

Rabbit fixator, scale, syringe (2.5 mL, 5 mL, 10 mL), medical gauze.

[Experimental animals]

Domestic rabbit, weighing 1.5 ~ 3.0 kg, either gender.

[Experimental reagents]

5% procaine solution, 2.5% thiopental sodium solution.

[Experimental method]

1. Experiment preparation

Take a rabbit, weigh it, and observe the normal activities such as standing and walking posture of limbs. The pain reflex was measured by needling the hind limb.

2. Observation of local effects

Inject 1 mL/kg (50 mg/kg) of 5% procaine solution around the sciatic nerve on one side (the rabbit was placed in a natural prone position, and a concavity was found between the ischial crest and the femoral head in the tail), and observe whether there were movement and sensory disorders in the ipsilateral hind limb (Figure 3-9-1).

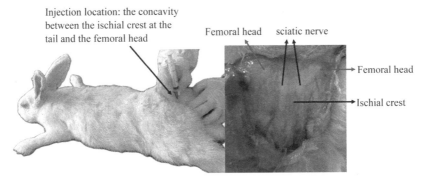

Figures 3-9-1　Schematic diagram of injection around sciatic nerve in rabbits

3. Observation of systemic effect

After the local effect was obvious (2-3 minutes), 1 mL/kg of 5% procaine solution was injected into the muscle of the other side of the rabbit hind limb, and the corresponding dose of thiopental sodium was prepared according to the weight of the rabbit, and the rabbit reaction was closely observed to appear toxic symptoms (convulsion).

4. Poisoning rescue

After convulsion was observed in rabbits, 2.5% sodium thiopental solution was slowly injected through the ear vein immediately until muscle relaxation (about 0.5 mL/kg).

[Experimental records and results]

Observe and record the experiment results. Fill in Table 3-9-1.

Table 3-9-1 Local and absorption effect of procaine

Animals	Weight (kg)	Observation phase	Activity and performance of rabbits
Rabbits		Before dosing	
		After an injection of procaine around the sciatic nerve	
		After intramuscular injection of procaine	
		After an intravenous injection of thiopental sodium	

[Precautions]

(1) Test the pain reflex by needling the ankle joint of the hind limbs, mild and moderate.

(2) When determining the location of the sciatic nerve, straighten the hind limbs and feel a depression between the ischial crest and the femoral head. The injection site should be as close to the femoral head as possible, and the needle tip should be slightly retracted when inserted into the iliac bone.

(3) Procaine injected around the sciatic nerve can cause conduction block, and excessive dosage or accidental entry into blood vessels can lead to poisoning. The main manifestations include central excitation followed by inhibition, such as restlessness, convulsions, coma, respiratory depression, etc.

[Practice questions]

1. Procaine is not generally used for _____.

A. surface anesthesia   B. infiltration anesthesia

C. conduction anesthesia   D. lumbar anesthesia

2. The purpose of ephedrine for lumbar anesthesia is _____.

A. prevent anaphylactic shock   B. prevent dilation of blood vessels

C. to prevent the lowering of blood pressure during anesthesia

D. to prolong the duration of local anesthetic action

3. What is the local anesthetic method of procaine injection around sciatic nerve of

rabbit?

    A. Infiltration anesthesia.

    C. Surface anesthesia.

    B. Conduction anesthesia.

    D. Lumbar anesthesia.

[Thinking questions]

(1) What adverse reactions will occur to patients after local anesthetics that are absorbed into the blood? How to reduce or avoid the absorption of local anesthetics clinically?

(2) What are the selective effects of procaine? What are the therapeutic effects? What are the adverse effects?

[Knowledye expansion]

Herbal anesthetic

It is reported that the earliest anesthetic in the world was invented by the famous medical scientist Hua Tuo in the late Eastern Han Dynasty. His invention was more than 1600 years earlier than the successful invention of ether anesthesia by the American dentist Moreton (1846). However, due to Cao Cao's suspicion, Hua Tuo was sent to prison and tortured to death in his later years. His medical book was lost, and Ma Fei SAN naturally disappeared into history. According to future research, the main components of Mafei SAN may be Datura flower (yellow flower) and scopolamine. According to research conducted by scientists outside Japan, Mafei SAN is composed of one liter of Datura flower, four coins each for raw aconite, Angelica, Angelica, Chuanxiong and one for fried South star. The atropine substances contained in Datura flower have the effects of relieving asthma, dispelling wind, anesthetizing and relieving pain. It can be used as an anesthetic for surgical operations. Caowu is a medicine for dispelling wind and dampness, which can be used to treat wind cold dampness syndrome, cold pain in the heart and abdomen, and can also be used for traumatic injuries and anesthesia pain relief. It contains aconitine that has obvious anti-inflammatory and analgesic effect, highly toxic. Angelica dahurica has the effect of dispelling wind and relieving pain, while ligusticum chuanxiong horn has the effect of promoting blood circulation and relieving pain. After The Three Kingdoms, doctors also developed different anesthesis. The Song Dynasty's *Bian Que New Book* used "sleeping holy powder" made of mandala flowers and marijuana flowers. In the early Ming Dynasty, after the publication of the Ming Dynasty's *Puji Recipe*, "Caowusan" became the most common anesthetic. The book stipulated strict dosages for the use of drugs, and anesthesia was already relatively safe at this time. Wang Kentang, a doctor in the Ming Dynasty, successfully completed local anesthesia by mixing anesthetic drugs with wine. There is a large number of records in the way of local anesthesia to complete all kinds of surgical operations in Wu Qian's *Medical King Golden Kam*. Every step of the research and development of anesthetics has considerable risks. Behind this rapid development of anesthesia technology, generations of famous doctors have tried drugs with their own bodies and almost spent their lives in practice. The Chinese medical sages left behind exquisite medical skills, practical and safe medical books and prescriptions, but also left us the stubborn figure of searching up and down and the spirit of exploring without fear of difficulties and excellence.

（王舒舒）

Chapter 4　Cardiovascular system pharmacology

Section 1　Effect of efferent nervous system drugs on blood pressure in rabbits

[Experimental objective]

(1) To observe the effects of epinephrine, norepinephrine and phentolamine on the blood pressure of rabbits, and to analyze the interactions and mechanisms of drug action.

(2) Proficiency in the basic operations of the house rabbit experiment.

[Experimental principle]

Blood pressure is related to three basic factors: ventricular ejection, vascular resistance, and circulating blood volume, and is maintained through the neuro humoral regulatory mechanism. Efferent nervous system drugs stimulate or block adrenergic and acetylcholine receptors distributed in the cardiovascular system, affecting myocardial contractility, the degree of vasodilation and vasoconstriction of blood vessels, thereby increasing or decreasing blood pressure.

Adrenaline, used for severe respiratory distress due to bronchospasm, can quickly relieve anaphylaxis caused by drugs, etc., can also be used to prolong the effect of infiltration anesthesia drugs. There are both α-receptor and β-receptor agonistic effects. α-receptor agonists causes vasoconstriction of the skin, mucous membranes, viscera, while β-receptor agonists causes coronary vasodilatation, skeletal muscle, myocardial excitation, heart rate increase, bronchial smooth muscle. The effect of adrenaline on blood pressure is related to the dosage. The commonly used dose makes the systolic blood pressure rise while the diastolic blood pressure does not rise or falls slightly. The high dose makes the systolic blood pressure and diastolic blood pressure rise. There is a significant first-pass effect after oral administration.

Noradrenaline is an alpha adrenergic receptor agonist. It is used as an adjunctive drug to replenish blood volume in emergency situations in order to restore blood pressure. It is also used for hypotension during intravertebral block and blood pressure maintenance after resuscitation from cardiac arrest. Norepinephrine has a significant excitatory effect on alpha receptors, but is slightly weaker than adrenaline and has no selectivity for α_1 and α_2 receptors. This product mainly acts on α receptors, causing blood vessels to contract, leading to an increase in systolic and diastolic blood pressure, accompanied by a reflex bradycardia. In clinics, intravenous infusion is generally used. After intravenous administration, the effect is rapid, and the duration of action is maintained for $1 \sim 2$ minutes after stopping the infusion.

Phentolamine is an alpha Adrenaline receptor blocker. It can antagonize the effects of adrenaline and norepinephrine in the blood circulation, reduce peripheral vascular resistance by vasodilatation, antagonize the effect of catecholamines, and is used in the diagnosis and treatment of pheochromocytoma, but has little effect on the blood pressure in normal people or patients with essential hypertension. It can reduce the peripheral vascular resistance, reduce the cardiac afterload, lower the left ventricular end-diastolic pressure and the pulmonary arterial pressure, and increase the volume of the cardiac output, so it can be used in the treatment of heart failure.

[Experimental materials]

Rabbit table, arterial clips, tissue scissors, hemostatic forceps, arterial cannula, pressure transducer, ophthalmic scissors, forceps, glass minute needles, BL-422 bidogical function experimental system, 1 mL, 10 mL syringes, silk thread.

[Experimental animals]

One rabbit, weighing $2.0 \sim 3.0$ kg.

[Experimental reagents]

0.002% adrenaline, 0.002% norepinephrine, 2.5% phentolamine, saline, 25% urethane, heparin solution.

[Experimental Method]

The experimental procedure is as follows, seen in Figure 4-1-1.

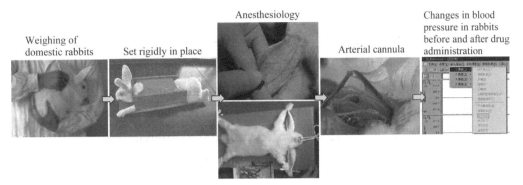

Figure 4-1-1   Schematic diagram of operation steps

1. Weighing, fixation and anesthesia

One rabbit was weighed (catch and hold method, lifting the back and buttocks) and recorded to calculate the dose to be administered. Fixation was done and anesthesia was given by intravenous injection at the ear margins with 25% urethane 4 mL/kg. Push slowly 2/3rd of the volume and observe the responses such as respiration, heartbeat, tone and corneal reflexes.

2. Arterial intubation

Fix in supine position, make a 4 cm incision in the middle of the neck, detach the muscle, expose the trachea, make a T incision in the second subglottic ring to insert the tracheal tube, and then ligate and fix it. The common carotid artery was separated and ligated distally, and the blood flow was blocked by a proximal arterial clip, and a small "V"-shaped incision was cut near the ligature line. The arterial cannula was filled with heparin saline solution and inserted into the common carotid artery in a cardiac direction, ligated and secured, and the other end of the arterial cannula was connected to the pressure transducer.

3. Administer and record

Open the arterial clip and record the normal blood pressure curve (BL-422 system-input signal-channel 1-pressure, with the paper walking speed set to the slowest). The marginal ear vein was administered separately in the following order, the blood pressure curve was recorded immediately, and the next drug was added after each administration when the blood pressure returned to normal.

(1) Group Ⅰ Drugs: (Purpose: To carefully observe the differences in the effects of epinephrine and norepinephrine on the blood pressure of rabbits respectively, with emphasis on the effect of phentolamine on the action of norepinephrine)

① Saline 0.5 mL;

② 0.002% Adrenaline 0.25 mL/kg; (add ③ after blood pressure stabilization)

③ 0.002% norepinephrine 0.25 mL/kg; (add ④ after blood pressure stabilization)

④ 2.5% Phentolamine 0.3 mL/kg; (observe blood pressure changes, add ⑤ after 5 ~ 10 min)

⑤ 0.002% norepinephrine 0.25 mL/kg. (observe for blood pressure changes)

(2) Drug Group Ⅱ: (objective: to scrutinize the differences in the effects of norepinephrine and epinephrine on blood pressure in rabbits respectively, with emphasis on the effect of phentolamine on the action of epinephrine)

① Saline 0.5mL;

② 0.002% norepinephrine 0.25 mL/kg; (added after blood pressure stabilization ③)

③ 0.002% epinephrine 0.25 mL/kg; (add ④ after blood pressure stabilization)

④ 2.5% Phentolamine 0.3 mL/kg; (observe blood pressure changes, add ⑤ after 5 ~ 10 min)

⑤ 0.002% epinephrine 0.25 mL/kg. (observe for changes in blood pressure)

[Experimental records and results]

Record the experimental results, depict the blood pressure change curves of rabbits before and after the administration of the drug, and analyze the mechanisms of the blood pressure change, as shown in Table 4-1-1, taking the first group as an example.

Table 4-1-1　Effects of arterial blood pressure in rabbits

Subgroup on drug handling	Plotting arterial blood pressure in rabbits
Adrenaline 0.25 mL/kg	
Norepinephrine 0.25 mL/kg	
Phentolamine 0.3 mL/kg	
Norepinephrine 0.25 mL/kg	

[Precautions]

(1) Insulation measures are taken to prevent the body temperature of rabbits from dropping after anesthesia.

(2) Skin, subcutaneous, and muscle, in that order, are separated by layers.

(3) During operation, do not contaminate, squeeze, injure or pull with force.

(4) The liquid is ready for use, and the dosage is accurately grasped.

(5) Anesthesia should not be too deep.

(6) Rabbits were executed by overdose of anesthetic drugs at the end of the experiment. And the end of the experiment, euthanize the rabbit by air embolism.

[Practice questions]

1. In the experiment of drug regulation of blood pressure in rabbits, heparin saline was injected for the purpose of _____.

A. anticoagulation to prevent blockage of arterial cannulas

B. blood volume supplementation

C. elevated blood pressure

D. decrease blood pressure

2. In the experiment of regulating blood pressure in rabbits with drugs, which statement is incorrect?

A. Anesthetizing an animal should be based on the principles of shallow rather than deep and slow rather than fast.

B. Separation of vascular nerves should avoid excessive traction.

C. The carotid artery incision should be close to the cardiac tip.

D. The pressure transducer is at the same level as the position of the rabbit heart.

3. The difference between the effects of norepinephrine and adrenaline on cardiovascular system is _____.

A. orthostatic muscle action

B. raise blood pressure

C. diastolic coronary vascularization

D. negative frequency effect

[Thinking questions]

(1) What are the effects of epinephrine, norepinephrine, and phentolamine, respectively, on blood pressure in rabbits?

(2) How does phentolamine affect the action of epinephrine and norepinephrine? Is there any difference? Try to analyze it in terms of the receptor doctrine.

[Knowledye expansion]

Traditional Chinese medicine and modern medicine —building a healthy defense

The idea of "treating the disease before it occurs" in the *Yellow Emperor's Classic of Internal Medicine* reminds us that prevention is better than cure. In the face of hypertension which is a global health problem, the combination of Chinese medicine and modern medicine is particularly important. Hypertension, as a manifestation of cardiovascular syndrome, is as important to prevent as it is to treat. Chinese medicine regards hypertension as a sign of imbalance in the body and emphasizes timely adjustment to restore balance. Just as the body naturally returns to normal after putting down a heavy object, so does blood pressure. However, the stress of modern life often causes people to ignore this natural law. Prolonged stress leads to a prolonged recovery time for blood pressure, which may eventually lead to hypertension. This is where modern medical testing and treatment tools become especially important. Combining the lifestyle adjustments of Chinese medicine and the scientific treatments of modern medicine, we can effectively prevent and control hypertension. Reasonable diet, moderate exercise and good mood are all preventive measures recommended by traditional Chinese medical science. Meanwhile, modern medicine provides drugs and treatments to help patients stabilize their blood pressure and reduce complications. Through the wisdom of Chinese medicine and the science of modern medicine, we build a health defense that not only guards personal health, but also contributes to the public health of society. Let's join hands, use wisdom and science to guard our health and create a harmonious society.

（方　辉）

Section 2　The effect of lidocaine on arrhythmia induced by electrical stimulation

[Experimental objective]

(1) Observe the antagonistic effect of lidocaine on arrhythmia caused by electrical stimulation.

(2) Learn how to induce arrhythmia through electrical stimulation.

[Experimental principle]

Electrical stimulation refers to the application of electrical stimulation to the vagus nerve of animals to increase the release of acetylcholine. Acetylcholine that acts on M-cholinergic receptors, can slow down heart rate, reduce conduction, decrease myocardial contractility, and inhibit conduction in the sinoatrial and atrioventricular nodes. The difficulty of inducing animal models through electrical stimulation is relatively low, the operation is simple, and the controllability is strong. It has a certain degree of reversibility. Lidocaine which is a class I b antiarrhythmic drug can inhibit Na^+ influx into Purkinje fibers and ventricular myocytes, promoting K^+ efflux. It can also reduce self-discipline, shorten the duration of action potential duration and effective refractory period, thereby exerting an anti-arrhythmic effect.

[Experimental materials]

Equipment BL-422 biological functional system, stimulation electrode, 1mL syringe, regular scissors, surgical scissors, tweezers, frog board, pushpin, frog heart clip, iron frame, etc.

[Experimental animals]

One toad.

[Experimental reagents]

0.2% lidocaine, Ren's solution.

[Experimental methods]

1. Sample preparation

Take a toad, destroy its brain and spinal cord, fix it in an upright position on the frog board with a pushpin. Then cut the abdominal wall along both sides, find the superficial vein of the abdominal wall that flows back to the liver near the gallbladder. Tie it with a thread here, cut it below the knot, turn the abdominal wall downwards. Then open the chest along the sternum, lift the pericardium with tweezers, carefully cut the pericardium, expose the entire heart. Use a frog heart clip with a long thread tied to one end, clamp the apex of the heart, and connect the thread to the transducer of the recorder.

2. Record a normal electrocardiogram

Activate the BL-422 biological function experimental system, and firstly record a segment of normal cardiac contraction curve.

3. Inducing arrhythmia

Place the stimulation electrode on the surface of the ventricular muscle near the interventricular septum. Parameter setting: coarse voltage, continuous single stimulation, stimulation frequency 10 times/s, voltage intensity 1 ~ 10 V, stimulation time 30 s. Observe and record changes in arrhythmia.

4. Medication administration

Immediately inject 0.4 ~ 0.6 mL of 0.2% lidocaine slowly from the superficial abdominal vein after significant irregularity in heart rhythm (ventricular fibrillation) occurs After 3 ~ 4 minutes of medication, stimulate for another 30 seconds with the same intensity and frequency, and observe the results (Figure 4-2-1).

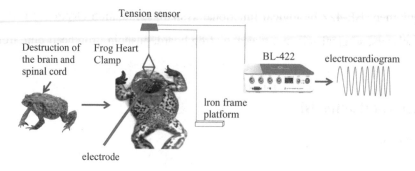

Figure 4-2-1　Schematic diagram of experimental operation process

[Experimental records and results]

Draw a curve graph and observe and record the changes in toad heart electrocardiogram before and after administration of lidocaine.

Observe and record the changes in heart electrocardiogram of toads before and after lidocaine administration. Draw a curve.

[Precautions]

(1) The room temperature should be maintained at around 25°C. As too low a temperature can affect the experimental results.

(2) The exposed heart should be regularly moistened with Ren's solution.

(3) The electrode should not be placed too tightly on the ventricular muscle to avoid affecting the heartbeat.

[Practice questions]

1. The mechanism of action of lidocaine against arrhythmia is _____.

A. to enhance myocardial autonomy

B. to block the action of β receptors

C. to inhibit K^+ efflux

D. to change conduction velocity in the lesion area

2. Clinical applications that do not belong to lidocaine are _____.

A. ventricular arrhythmia caused by acute myocardial infarction

B. ventricular arrhythmia caused by cardiac catheterization examination

C. ventricular arrhythmia caused by digitalis poisoning

D. paroxysmal rapid atrial fibrillation

3. Which of the following does not belong to the clinical application of lidocaine ?

A. Sodium chloride.   B. Potassium chloride.

C. Calcium chloride.   D. Sodium hydroxide.

4. The electrode should be placed in _____.

A. atria   B. ventricles

C. interventricular septum   D. apex

[Thinking questions]

(1) What are the methods to induce arrhythmia?

(2) How to choose drugs for the treatment of rapid arrhythmia?

[Knowledye expansion]

The history of lidocaine
Lidocaine, as a class I antiarrhythmic drug, was widely used for the treatment and prevention of ventricular arrhythmias twenty years ago. The results of the Cardiac Arrhythmia Suppression Trial (CAST) and subsequent CAST2 trials in 1989 showed that class I antiarrhythmic drugs, such as Enkanib, Flukanib, and Imathiazide, were effective in treating ventricular premature beats after myocardial infarction, but increased the overall mortality rate of patients. Since then, the use of all class I antiarrhythmic drugs has rapidly decreased.

（孙志朋）

Section 3　The therapeutic effect of antiarrhythmic drugs on BaCl$_2$-induced arrhythmia

[Experimental objective]

(1) To learn the method of inducing arrhythmia in rabbits using barium chloride.

(2) To observe the anti-arrhythmic effect of lidocaine.

[Experimental Principle]

Barium chloride can facilitate the influx of Na^+ into Purkinje fibers while inhibiting the efflux of K^+, promoting phase 4 automatic depolarization, thereby increasing autorhythmicity and inducing ventricular arrhythmias. Additionally, it can inhibit the Na^+-K^+-ATPase enzyme, leading to a decrease in intracellular K^+ and a reduction in the maximum diastolic potential. The increase of intracellular Na^+ leads to an increase in Ca^{2+} through Na^+-Ca^{2+}

exchange, resulting in an increase in oscillatory potential and triggering activity, thereby increasing autorhythmicity. It also increases the excitability of the myocardial sympathetic nerves, resulting in ectopic rhythms manifested as ventricular premature beats, bigeminy, trigeminy, and ventricular fibrillation, among others. It is commonly used as a model for various types of ventricular arrhythmias. This arrhythmia model is relatively simple to produce, has good stability, and a high success rate. This model has differences in the occurrence of human related diseases, but it is more objective in studying the mechanism of arrhythmia and the expression regulation of related indicators. The barium chloride induced arrhythmia model is currently one of the commonly used rapid arrhythmia models.

Lidocaine is an antiarrhythmic drug of class Ib, which can block the activated and inactivated states of sodium channels. The blocking effect is rapidly reversed when the channel returns to its resting state. Therefore, lidocaine has a strong effect on depolarized tissues and effectively inhibits arrhythmias caused by depolarization due to ischemia or digitalis toxicity. This medication restrains the small influx of Na^+ involved in phase 2 of the action potential's repolarization, shortening or having no effect on the action potential duration in Purkinje fibers and ventricular muscles. It reduces the depolarization slope during phase 4 of the action potential, raises the excitation threshold, and decreases automaticity, thereby exerting its effect against rapid ventricular arrhythmias (Figure 4-3-1).

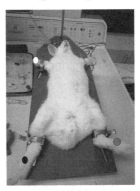

Figure 4-3-1   Schematic diagram of electrode connections for

lead Ⅱ electrocardiogram (ECG) in rabbits

[Experimental materials]

BL-422 biological signal acquisition and analysis system, surgical scissors, rabbit operating table, syringes, intravenous injection needles, cotton balls.

[Experimental animals]

One rabbit, weighing 2 ~ 3 kg.

[Experimental reagents]

Barium chloride solution 0.4%, Lidocaine hydrochloride injection 0.5%, Urethane 20%, saline.

[Experimental methods]

(1) Take one rabbit, weigh it, and inject 20% uranyl acetate 4 ~ 5 mL/kg through the ear marginal vein anesthesia, fix it on the rabbit operating table.

(2) Insert needle electrodes into the subcutaneous tissue of the distal limbs of the rabbit, connect the BL-422 biological signal acquisition and analysis system, select standard II lead, record normal electrocardiogram (standard voltage 1 mV corresponds to 10 mm, paper speed 25 mm/s).

(3) Inject 0.4% $BaCl_2$ solution 0.5 mL/kg through the ear marginal vein, and then inject 0.5 mL/kg of saline, immediately record the electrocardiogram to observe whether arrhythmia occurs.

(4) After the arrhythmia occurs, immediately inject 0.5% lidocaine 1 mL/kg (i.e. 5 mg/kg) through the ear marginal vein, record the electrocardiogram, and observe whether the drug can immediately stop arrhythmia and the duration of maintaining normal electrocardiogram.

[Experiment records and results]

Record the experimental results, including the onset time and duration of lidocaine treatment. Select normal ECG, typical ECG of arrhythmia caused by barium chloride, and typical ECG after lidocaine treatment, and print.

[Precautions]

(1) Lidocaine can rapidly antagonize the arrhythmia induced by barium chloride. Therefore, ECG recording can begin during lidocaine injection to observe the transformation process.

(2) The lead wires must be well contacted to reduce interference from alternating current. The needle electrodes should not be inserted into the muscles of the limbs to avoid electromyographic interference.

(3) When the room temperature is low, pay attention to the animal's warmth to avoid muscle tremors affecting the recording.

(4) The anesthesia level of rabbits should be appropriate to avoid anesthesia that is too shallow or too deep, which may even lead to death.

[Practice questions]

1. In a normal ECG, what does the P wave represent?

A. Atrial depolarization.　　　　　　B. Atrial-to-ventricular conduction time.

C. Ventricular depolarization.　　　　D. Ventricular repolarization.

2. When lidocaine is used to treat arrhythmias caused by barium chloride, an electrocardiogram should be _____.

A. recorded the electrocardiogram of the rabbit while injecting lidocaine

B. recorded the electrocardiogram of the rabbit after injecting lidocaine

C. recorded the electrocardiogram of the rabbit 1 ~ 2 minutes after injecting lidocaine

D. recorded the electrocardiogram of the rabbit 5 minutes after injecting lidocaine

3. What type of arrhythmia is typically caused by barium chloride?

A. Bradyarrhythmia.　　　　　　　　B. Tachyarrhythmia of ventricular type.

C. Atrial tachyarrhythmia.　　　　　　D. Atrioventricular block.

[Thinking questions]

(1) What are the characteristics of lidocaine antiarrhythmic drugs? What are the clinical uses?

(2) What are the commonly used antiarrhythmic drugs in clinics? How should drugs be selected for the treatment of rapid ventricular arrhythmias?

[Knowledge expansion]

Pharmacological effects of lidocaine

Lidocaine is an aminoamide local anesthetic that was introduced in 1948 and works by blocking Na$^+$ channels. It is a commonly used local anesthetic in clinics due to its rapid onset, strong and long-lasting effect, strong penetration, and large safety margin, with almost no irritation to tissues. It is used for various forms of local anesthesia and is known as a "universal anesthetic." In addition, the drug is also used to treat arrhythmias, primarily for the treatment of various types of ventricular arrhythmias, such as tachycardia or ventricular fibrillation caused by acute myocardial infarction or digitalis toxicity. Recent studies have found that lidocaine has some analgesic effects. For postherpetic neuralgia, 5% lidocaine gel patch is a first-line analgesic, recommended for use on unbroken skin to cover the most severe pain area. Peripheral neuropathy caused by diabetes can also be treated with this dosage form. Intravenous injection of lidocaine can reduce the amount of opioid drugs used during the perioperative period, reduce the release of inflammatory cytokines (such as IL-6, IL-8, IL-1, TNF-a) during the perioperative period, and promote the release of anti-inflammatory factors (such as IL-10). In addition, lidocaine can also inhibit the proliferation of tumor cells, activate cell apoptosis pathways, and exert antitumor effects. Lidocaine not only inhibits the metastasis of breast cancer cells but also increases the antitumor effect of cisplatin.

（李成檀）

Section 4 The effect of cardiac glycosides on the relaxation and contraction of detached frog hearts

[Experimental objective]

(1) Learn how to make detached frog hearts.

(2) Observe the effect of drugs on the contraction intensity and rhythm of isolated frog hearts.

[Experimental principle]

Cardiotonic glycoside drugs can bind to Na$^+$; K$^+$-ATPase on the myocardial cell membrane, inhibit the activity of Na$^+$; K$^+$-ATPase, and suppress the transport of Na$^+$ and K$^+$. The intracellular Na$^+$ gradually increases and K$^+$ gradually decreases. The Na$^+$-Ca^{2+}

exchange system on the cell membrane exchanges Na^+ with Ca^{2+}, increasing Na^+ efflux and Ca^{2+} influx, thereby increasing intracellular Ca^{2+}. Ca^{2+} acts on cardiac contractile proteins, increasing myocardial contractility. Its positive muscle strength and negative frequency effects are more pronounced in heart failure caused by calcium deficiency.

[Experimental materials]

A set of surgical instruments, frog board, probe, Si's frog heart tube, frog heart clip, iron bracket, beaker, dropper, pushpin, cotton thread, BL-422 biological signal acquisition system, tension transducer, etc.

[Experimental reagents]

Cedilanid injection (or 5% digitalis solution, 0.1% Forsythin G solution), Ringing solution (pH 7.0), low calcium Ringing solution (including $CaCl_2$, with a content of 25% of conventional Ringing solution) or calcium free Ringing solution, 1% calcium chloride solution.

[Experimental animals]

Frog or toad.

[Experimental Methods]

1. Preparation of frog heart

Take one frog, insert a probe into the foramen magnum, destroy the brain and spinal cord, and fix it in an upward position on the frog board with a needle. Cut the chest skin and cartilage to fully expose the heart (Figure 4-4-1) .

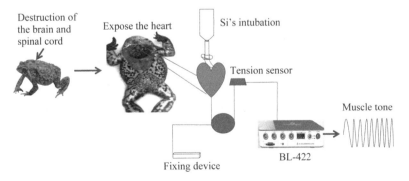

Figure 4-4-1   Schematic diagram of experimental steps

2. Snail frog heart catheterization

Thread a line under the left aorta and tie a flexible knot. Lift the ligature line on the aorta with your left hand, and use an ophthalmic scissors to cut an oblique incision on the arterial wall below the ligature line in the centripetal direction with your right hand. Select a frog heart trocar of appropriate size, and then insert a small amount of Ringer's fluid into the opening of the Slender frog heart trocar. When the tip of the trocar reaches the base of the arterial cone, the trocar should be slightly retracted to push the tip towards the back and lower part of the arterial cone and the direction of the heart apex. It should be inserted into the ventricular cavity through the aortic valve, but not too deeply to avoid the ventricular wall blocking the trocar opening. At this time, blood can be seen rushing into the trocar, causing the liquid level to move up and down with the heartbeat. Use a dropper to draw blood from the sleeve and replace it with fresh Ringer's solution. After stabilizing the sheath, gently lift the spare thread and tightly tie the left and right aorta together with the inserted sheath with double threads. Then fix the knot on the small glass hook of the sheath and cut the blood vessel above the ligature. Gently lift the catheter and heart, see the position of the venous sinus clearly, cut off the involved tissue below the venous sinus, and only retain the connection between the venous sinus and the heart, allowing the heart to detach. Rinse the residual blood in the ventricle repeatedly with Ringer's solution to ensure that there is no residual blood in the perfusion fluid inside the trocar, and maintain the same liquid level inside the trocar before conducting the experiment.

3. Connect the biological signal acquisition system

Fix the frog heart sleeve on the iron frame with a test tube clamp, clamp the apex of the heart with the frog heart clamp during diastole, connect it to the transducer and the biological signal acquisition system, and start recording after the contraction is stable.

4. Medication administration and recording

Record the normal cardiac activity curve, then add medication reagents in the following order to record the amplitude of contractions and changes in heart rate. ① Change into low calcium Ringer's solution. ② When the cardiac contraction is significantly weakened, add 0.2 mL of cedilanid injection, 5% digitalis solution, or 0.1% Forsythrin G solution 0.2 mL into the trocar.

[Experimental records and results]

Evaluate the cardiotonic effect of drugs by observing the amplitude of cardiac contractions and changes in heart rate before and after administration. Record the observation data and fill in the table below after calculating the results of the experimental group (Table 4-4-1).

Table 4-4-1   The cardiotonic effect of cardiac glycosides on frog heart ($\bar{\chi} \pm S$)

Group	Number in each group (n)	Heart frequency (times/min)	Amplitude (mm)
control group			
low calcium Ringer's solution group			
drug group			

[Precautions]

(1) It is better to use frog hearts in this experiment, as toad hearts are less sensitive to cardiac glycoside drugs.

(2) The best frog weight is between 50 ~ 200 g. If it is too large, the catheter may easily detach from the ventricle.

(3) During the entire experiment, the liquid level inside the sleeve should be kept constant to ensure a fixed load on the heart.

(4) To prevent blood clotting from blocking the frog heart opening, an appropriate amount of heparin anticoagulant can be added to Ringer's solution. The general dosage is to add 2 mL heparin injection solution to 1000 mL Ringer's solution.

(5) Avoid veins during the ceremony.

[Practice questions]

1. The most common arrhythmia caused by cardiac glycoside is _____.

A. ventricular premature beats   B. sinus bradycardia

C. ventricular tachycardia   D. atrioventricular block

2. Adverse reactions of cardiac glycoside do not include _____.

A. gastrointestinal reactions   B. endocrine system response

C. atrioventricular block   D. sinus bradycardia

3. When cardiac conduction block is caused by cardiac glycosides, in addition to discontinuing cardiac glycosides and potassium excretion drugs, it is better to choose _____.

    A. atropine   B. potassium chloride   C. lidocaine   D. propranolol

[Thinking questions]

(1) What are the characteristics of cardiac glycosides enhancing myocardial contractility?

(2) What is the impact of perfusion volume on cardiac activity during the experiment?

[Knowledge expansion]

Action potential duration of myocardial cells

1. Depolarization process (phase 0)

When myocardial cells receive a suprathreshold stimulus, the intramembrane potential depolarizes and reverses from –90mV in the resting state to+20 ~ +30 mV, forming the rising phase of the action potential, known as phase 0. When ventricular muscle cells are stimulated and excited, a small amount of Na^+ ions first flow in, causing local depolarization of the membrane. When depolarization reaches the threshold potential level (–65 mV), Na^+ ions flow inward, further depolarizing the membrane.

2. Repolarization process

When the depolarization of ventricular myocytes reaches its peak, the repolarization process begins. According to the shape of the membrane potential change curve and the different ion mechanisms formed, it can be divided into four periods:

(1) Early stage of rapid repolarization (Phase 1): The membrane potential rapidly decreases from +30 mV to around 0 mV. The instantaneous outflow of K^+ causes rapid repolarization in the initial stage of membrane potential.

(2) Platform phase (phase 2): manifested as small changes in membrane potential, with a potential close to 0 mV level, lasting for 100 ~ 150 ms. The influx of Ca^{2+} ions and the efflux of K^+ result in.

(3) Late stage of rapid repolarization (stage 3): After the plateau phase, the rate of cell membrane repolarization accelerates, and the membrane potential gradually

decreases from 0 mV to a resting potential level of –90 mV. After $100 \sim 150$ ms, the outward flow of K^+ gradually increases, surpassing the inward flow of Ca^{2+}.

(4) Resting phase (phase 4): Membrane repolarization is completed, and membrane potential recovers and stabilizes at a resting potential level of –90 mV. Through the Na^+-K^+ pump and Na^+-Ca^{2+} exchange, the influx of Na^+ and Ca^{2+} is expelled from the membrane, while the efflux of K^+ is transported into the membrane, restoring the distribution of intracellular and extracellular ions to their resting state, thereby maintaining the normal excitability of myocardial cells.

（孙志朋）

Section 5   Effects of propranolol on hypoxia tolerance in mice

[Experimental objective]

(1) To learn the methods of hypoxic models in mice.

(2) To evaluate the effects of isoproterenol and propranolol on hypoxia tolerance in mice and analyze their mechanisms.

[Experimental principle]

Isoproterenol, a β adrenergic receptor agonist, stimulates the β_1 receptor on myocardial cells to increase the heart rate and the myocardial contractility, to speed up the heart conduction, to elevate the myocardial oxygen consumption. Propranolol, a non-selective β-antagonist, blocks the effects of isoproterenol on the heart by reducing heart rate, weakening myocardial contractility, slowing cardiac conduction, and decreasing myocardial oxygen consumption. It enhances the tolerance to hypoxia in mice. Isoproterenol can be utilized to establish an animal model with high oxygen consumption for studying the effects of propranolol on improving hypoxia tolerance in mice.

[Experimental materials]

Hypoxia device, stopwatch, mouse cage, electronic weigher, syringe (1 mL).

[Experimental animals]

ICR mice, weight 22 ~ 25 g, either gender.

[Experimental reagents]

0.05% isoproterenol solution, 0.1% propranolol solution, saline, vaseline (optional).

[Experimental methods]

(1) Before the experiment, the mice were allowed to adapt the laboratory environment for 1 hour.

(2) Three mice that have completed adaptation to the environment will be weighed and numbered. After observing their normal behavior, they will be randomly divided into three groups: group A, group B, and group C. The administration route, dosage, and administration time are shown in the table below (Table 4-5-1).

Table 4-5-1　The dosage, method and time of administration schedule

Group	Administration for the first time (0.2 mL/10 g)	Administration for the second time after 15 min (0.2 mL/10 g)
A	0.05% isoproterenol solution, subcutaneous injection	0.1% propranolol solution, intraperitoneal injection
B	0.05% isoproterenol solution, subcutaneous injection	saline, intraperitoneal injection
C	saline, subcutaneous injection	saline, intraperitoneal injection

(3) After the second administration, the mice were placed individually in hypoxia bottles (100 mL) and the activity, the respiration were observed, which the respiratory arrest was as an indicator of mortality. The survival time was recorded. The device of hypoxia bottle was seen as Figure 4-5-1.

(4) The survival time in every group was collected and conducted statistical analysis (Table 4-5-2).

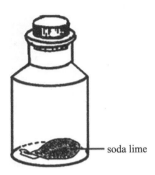

soda lime

Figure 4-5-1　Oxygen device schematic

[Experimental records and results]

Table 4-5-2　The effects of propranolol on hypoxia tolerance in mice

Group	Body weight (g)	Administration for the first time		Administration for the second time		Survival time (min)
		Drug	Volume (mL)	Drug	Volume (mL)	
A						
B						
C						

[Precautions]

(1) Hypoxia bottles must be hermetically sealed, and the bottle closure can be coated with vaseline if necessary.

(2) Accurately grasp the locations and techniques for intraperitoneal injection and subcutaneous injection to avoid the impacts of drug absorption.

(3) When monitoring the survival time of mice, shaking the hypoxia bottle is strictly prohibited to prevent additional oxygen consumption in mice.

[Practice questions]

1. Isoproterenol belongs to _____.

A. α_1 receptor agonist

B. α, β receptor agonist

C. β_1 receptor agonist

D. β receptor agonist

2. Which was the main mechanism of propranolol to improve the hypoxia tolerance?

A. By blocking β_1 receptor to inhibit the heart and reduce the myocardial oxygen consumption.

B. By blocking β_2 receptor to constrict the coronary vessels and the decrease the oxygen consumption.

C. By blocking β_2 receptor to constrict the bronchus and decrease the oxygen consumption.

D. By blocking M receptor to relax the gastrointestinal smooth muscle and reduce the oxygen consumption.

3. Which was the role of sodium lime in the hypoxia bottle?

A. To absorb the water.

B. To absorb CO_2 and to make the environment in hypoxia condition.

C. To remove the odor in the hypoxia bottle.

D. To absorb O_2 and prevent inhaling too much O_2 of mice.

[Thinking questions]

(1) What is the mechanism of isoproterenol increases myocardial oxygen consumption?

(2) What are the advantages and disadvantages of propranolol in enhancing hypoxia tolerance in the body?

[Knowledye expansion]

Propranolol—discovery of a β receptor blocker

Following the conclusion of World War II, Dr. James W. Black (1924—2010), a young lecturer at the University of Glasgow, was employed as the first drug researcher for British Imperial Chemical Industries Group (ICI). He collaborated with Dr. Raymond P Alqvist to explore the hypothesis of two adrenaline receptors such as α and β receptors in the body. The research started on β blockers from 1952. Over a decade, he investigated the interaction between epinephrine, norepinephrine, and their receptors using chemical information. In 1962, Blake and his colleagues successfully synthesized the first beta receptor blocker-pronethalol, but unfortunately it caused thymoma in mice and could not be used clinically. But Blake did not give up and finally synthesized propranolol, a drug that is not only more effective than pronethalol, but also avoids carcinogenic phenomena and does not have "intrinsic sympathetic activity". After using propranolol, it can slow down heart rate, reduce myocardial contractility and cardiac output, decrease coronary blood flow, significantly reduce myocardial oxygen consumption, and lower blood pressure. Nowadays, propranolol has been widely used in the treatment of diseases such as hypertension, angina and myocardial infarction, arrhythmia, chronic congestive heart failure, and hyperthyroidism. However, due to its ability to effectively slow down heart rate and alleviate anxiety, it was listed as a banned substance for athletes by the International Olympic Committee in 1986.

（叶夷露）

Chapter 5   Hormonal visceral pharmacology

Section 1   Antagonistic effect of protamine sulfate on heparin anticoagulant activity

[Experimental objective]

(1) To observe the antagonistic effect of protamine sulfate on heparin's anticoagulant activity.

(2) To learn the method of blood sampling from the retrobulbar vein in mice.

(3) To learn the capillary tube method for measuring clotting time.

[Experimental principle]

Heparin is strongly acidic and carries a large number of negative charges. It enhances the affinity between antithrombin Ⅲ (AT-Ⅲ) and coagulation factors, resulting in the inactivation of multiple coagulation factors. This leads to rapid and potent anticoagulant effects both *in vivo* and *in vitro*, thereby prolonging clotting time. When blood comes into contact with a capillary tube, the extrinsic coagulation system is activated, and fibrils will appear at the broken end of the capillary tube after a certain period.

Protamine sulfate is strongly alkaline and carries a large number of positive charges. In the body, it can bind with heparin to form a stable complex, rendering heparin incapable of anticoagulation. Each 1.0 to 1.5 mg of protamine sulfate can neutralize 100 units of heparin.

[Experimental materials]

1mL syringe, capillary tubes with an inner diameter of 1 mm, balance, mouse cage, stopwatch.

[Experimental animals]

Mice, weighing 18 ~ 22g, either sex.

[Experimental reagents]

0.0025% heparin solution, 0.0125% protamine sulfate solution, physiological saline, picric acid.

[Experimental methods]

Capillary Tube Method

The experimental operation steps are as follows, as shown in Figure 5-1-1.

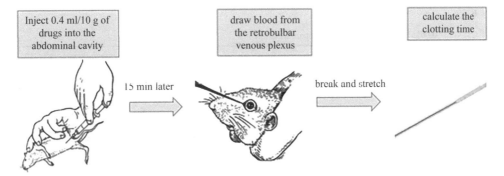

Figure 5-1-1   Schematic diagram of operational step

1. Injection of drug

Take 3 white mice, weigh and number them, and mark them with bitter acid. Inject 0.4 mL/10 g of each drug intraperitoneally, as follows: Rat A is injected with physiological saline, Rat B is injected with 0.0025% heparin solution, and Rat C is injected with 0.0025% heparin solution. After 15 minutes, inject 0.4 mL/10 g of 0.0125% protamine sulfate solution intraperitoneally into mouse C.

2. Blood sampling and calculation of clotting time

After 15 minutes from drug administration, use a capillary tube to puncture the medial canthus of each mouse and withdraw blood from the retrobulbar venous plexus on one side. Once the capillary tube is filled with blood, remove it and place it horizontally on the table, starting the stopwatch simultaneously. Every 30 seconds to 1 minute, snap off about 0.5 cm of the capillary tube and gently pull it apart in a left-right direction, observing for the appearance of fibrils at the broken end. Calculate the time from taking blood from the capillary tube to breaking the capillary tube and producing coagulation filaments. This is the clotting time of the capillary glass tube method in mice.

[Experimental records and results]

Collect the results from the entire laboratory, calculate the average clotting time for the three groups of mice, and fill in Table 5-1-1 below.

Table 5-1-1 Antagonistic Effect of Protamine Sulfate on Heparin Anticoagulant Activity

Group	Drug	Group						Average Clotting Time
		1	2	3	4	5	6	
A	Saline							
B	0.0025% Heparin							
C	0.0025% Heparin + 0.0125% Protamine sulfate							

[Precautions]

(1) Strictly control the injection speed of the drugs to avoid being too fast or too slow, aiming for consistency, especially when administering protamine sulfate, which should be injected slowly.

(2) Do not mix syringes used for injecting heparin and protamine sulfate to prevent precipitation.

(3) Ensure that the inner diameter of the capillary tubes is uniform, clean, and dry.

(4) Clotting time is affected by room temperature. A temperature of around 15°C is preferable during experiments. Avoid holding the capillary tubes filled with blood for extended periods to prevent influencing the experimental results.

(5) If no blood flows out after inserting the capillary tube into the medial canthus, gently rotate the capillary tube.

[Practice questions]

1. When treating bleeding caused by excessive heparin, which should be selected?

A. VitK.   B. Protamine Sulfate.

C. Aspirin.   D. Aminomethylbenzoic Acid.

2. The most commonly used route of administration for heparin anticoagulation *in vivo*

is _____.

    A. oral   B. intramuscular   C. subcutaneous   D. intravenous

3. Regarding heparin's anticoagulant mechanisms, which of the following statements is correct?

A. Directly inactivates coagulation factors II a, VII a, IX a, X a.

B. Directly binds to thrombin, inhibiting its activity.

C. Enhances the activity of antithrombin III .

D. Antagonizes VitK.

[Thinking questions]

How does protamine sulfate affect heparin's anticoagulant activity? What is the mechanism of their interaction? What are the clinical implications?

[Knowledye expansion]

The legendary discovery of heparin

The discovery of heparin is imbued with a legendary narrative. In 1916, Jay McLean, in his quest for a procoagulant substance, stumbled upon heparin, which possesses anticoagulant properties. This finding was initially dismissed as a "mistake" by his mentor, yet McLean persisted in his discovery and published his paper with his mentor's encouragement, thereby paving the way for heparin's widespread application in the medical field. This story underscores the importance of perseverance and courage as the keys to achieving breakthroughs in scientific exploration. In the face of unknowns and doubts, only by persisting and daring to explore can new scientific truths be discovered.

（房春燕）

Section 2　Reaction and rescue of insulin overdose

[Experimental objective]

(1) To observe hypoglycemic response caused by excessive insulin injection in mice, and rescue hypoglycemic mice.

(2) Be proficient in operating the experimental method of intraperitoneal injection of mice.

[Experimental principle]

Insulin is a protein hormone secreted by pancreatic islet β cells, which is stimulated by endogenous or exogenous substances such as glucose, lactose, ribose, arginine, glucagon, etc. The main physiological function of insulin is to regulate metabolism. Medicinal insulin is mostly extracted from the pancreas of domestic animals such as pigs and cattle. At present, insulin can also be synthesized artificially by DNA recombinant technology. Insulin is ineffective orally, and it is administered by injection, and subcutaneous injection is quickly absorbed. There are fast-acting, intermediate-acting, and long-acting insulin preparations. Insulin is the only hormone in the body that lowers blood sugar, and promotes the synthesis of glycogen, fat, and protein at the same time. After injecting excessive insulin into mice, the rapid decrease in blood sugar caused hypoglycemic shock, mental restlessness, convulsion and other phenomena.

[Experimental materials]

Ordinary balance or electronic scale, 1 mL syringe, large beaker, mouse cage.

[Experimental animals]

Mice, 18 ~ 22 g.

[Experimental reagents]

Acidic physiological saline, 50% glucose injection, insulin solution (2 U/mL).

[Experimental methods]

The schematic diagram of the experiment is shown in Figure 5-2-1.

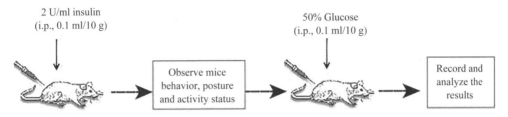

2 U/ml insulin
(i.p., 0.1 ml/10 g)

50% Glucose
(i.p., 0.1 ml/10 g)

Observe mice behavior, posture and activity status

Record and analyze the results

Figure 5-2-1   Schematic diagram of experimental steps

(1) Take three mice, labeled as , Ⅱ, Ⅲ, and weigh them. Ⅰ and Ⅱ are the experimental groups, and Ⅲ is the control group.

(2) Inject 0.1 mL/10 g of 2 U/mL insulin solution into the abdominal cavity of experimental group Ⅰ and Ⅱ mice, and 0.1 mL/10 g of acidic physiological saline into the control group mice Ⅲ.

(3) Place the mice in an environment of 30 ~ 37°C, record the time, observe and compare the expressions, postures, and activities of the two groups of mice. When the experimental group mice showed obvious reactions, mice Ⅰ were injected with 0.1 mL/10 g of 50% glucose injection for rescue, while mice Ⅱ were not treated for rescue.

(4) Compare the activities of mice Ⅰ, Ⅱ, and Ⅲ, record and analyze the results.

[Experiment Records and Results]

Record the above results in Table 5-2-1 and analyze them.

Table 5-2-1   Observation of response and rescue of insulin overdose

Number	Weight (g)	Drugs and doses	Reaction after admistration

[Precautions]

(1) Mice were fasted 18 ~ 24 hours before the experiment.

(2) Acidic saline configuration: 10 mL of 0.1 mol/L HCl was added to 300 mL of normal saline, and the pH value was adjusted to 2.5 ~ 3.5.

(3) 2 U/mL insulin solution configuration: it is advisable to use regular insulin, because the experimental phenomenon of ordinary insulin is obvious; It should be diluted to the desired concentration with acidic saline, as insulin is only effective in acidic environments.

(4) Experimental temperature: It can be room temperature in summer, and it is best to keep the insulin injected mice in an environment of $30 \sim 37°C$ in winter, because the temperature is too low, the reaction will be slow.

[Practice Questions]

1. The pancreas is mainly composed of _____ and blood vessels, which jointly regulate the balance of nutrients.

A. exocrine cells, endocrine cells, ductal cells

B. exocrine cells, endocrine cells, glandular cells

C. vesicle cells, β cells, ductal cells

D. alveolar cells, β cells, glandular cells

2. How should blood glucose be monitored during hospitalization for patients receiving intravenous insulin infusion or intensive care ICU?

A. Pre-meal + bedtime monitoring.

B. Monitoring every 4 hours.

C. Monitoring at 7 a.m. throughout the day.

D. Monitor every $1 \sim 2$ hours.

3. The correct sequence of intraperitoneal injections is _____.

① Grab the mouse so that its abdomen is facing up and its head is slightly drooping

② Grasp the skin on the back to tighten the skin of the abdomen, and pierce the skin under the skin about 1 cm on the side of the intersection of the root line of the two thighs and the midline of the abdomen

③ After the needle tip passes through the abdominal muscles, the resistance disappears, and there is no reflux in the retraction, and the drug is slowly pushed in

④ Advance the needle $3 \sim 5$ mm in the subcutaneous parallel midline of the abdomen, and then puncture it into the abdominal cavity at a 45° angle

A. ①②③④　　　B. ①②④③　　　C. ①③②④　　　D. ①④②③

[Thinking questions]

(1) What are the pharmacological effects and clinical uses of insulin?

(2) What adverse reactions can excessive insulin cause? How to rescue?

[Knowledye expansion]

China's synthetic insulin breakthrough

On September 17th, 1965, Chinese scientists synthesized crystalline bovine insulin with full biological activity, which was the first protein to be synthesized artificially in a laboratory. And later scientists from the United States and federal Germany completed similar work. At the beginning of 1956, the CPC Central Committee issued a call to "march towards science", and then the first medium and long-term science and technology development plan of New China, named the "1956—1967 Science and Technology Development Vision", was officially released. In June 1958, in the conference room of the Shanghai Institute of Biochemistry of the Chinese Academy of Sciences, under the chairmanship of Director Wang Yinglai, nine scientists discussed the next major topics to be studied by the institute. Someone has come up with a bold idea to "synthesize a protein". At the end of 1958, the synthetic insulin project was included in the 1959 national scientific research plan, and was codenamed "601", which was "the first major task in the 60s". However, prior to this, in addition to the manufacture of monosodium glutamate, China had never manufactured any form of amino acids, which are the basic materials for protein synthesis. In such extremely difficult conditions, everything had to start from scratch. In the era when the scientific research foundation was very weak and the equipment was extremely simple, after seven years of unremitting research, this project, which embodies the painstaking efforts of 100 scientific researchers from the Institute of Biochemistry of the Chinese Academy of Sciences, the Institute of Organic Chemistry and Peking University, has finally been successful. The successful synthesis of insulin by Chinese scientists marks a key step in the journey of human beings to explore the mysteries of life, which opens up the era of artificial protein synthesis, has had a significant impact on the history of life science development, and also lays the foundation for life science research in China.

（方　辉）

Section 3   The antagonistic effect of aspirin on thrombosis formation

[Experimental objective]

(1) Be proficient in experimental methods for arterial and venous bypass thrombosis.

(2) Analyze the causes of thrombosis and the mechanisms of aspirin's antithrombotic effect.

(3) Evaluate the antagonistic effect of aspirin on thrombosis.

[Experimental principle]

Arachidonic acid in cells exists in the form of phospholipids in the cell membrane. Multiple stimuli can activate phospholipase A, releasing arachidonic acid from membrane phospholipids. Free arachidonic acid is converted into prostaglandin G_2 (PGG_2) and prostaglandin H_2 (PGH_2) by the action of cyclooxygenase (COX). There are two isoenzymes in arachidonic acid cyclooxygenase: COX-1 and COX-2, both of which act on arachidonic acid to produce the same metabolites PGG_2 and PGH_2. Platelets contain thromboxane A_2 (TXA_2) synthase, which can convert the metabolic product PGH_2 of COX into TXA_2 and has a strong promoting effect on platelet aggregation. Vascular endothelial cells contain prostacyclin (PGI_2) synthase, which can convert the metabolite PGH_2 of COX into PGI_2. It is the most active endogenous platelet inhibitor discovered so far and can inhibit ADP, collagen induced platelet aggregation and release.

Aspirin acetylates the 530th serine residue of platelet cyclooxygenase, disrupting the enzyme's active center and preventing the synthesis of thromboxane (TXA_2). Due to the fact that platelets themselves do not have the function of synthesizing cyclooxygenase, the inhibitory effect of aspirin on platelet cyclooxygenase activity is irreversible. Aspirin inhibits cyclooxygenase on the endothelium of blood vessels, reducing the synthesis of prostacyclin (PGI_2). Under normal circumstances, the synthesis amount of TXA_2 far exceeds that of PGI_2. Low dose aspirin has a weak inhibitory effect on cyclooxygenase in endothelial cells and almost does not affect the synthesis of PGI_2. However, it can significantly inhibit platelet cyclooxygenase, resulting in a significant inhibition of TXA_2 synthesis. High dose aspirin has a strong inhibitory effect on the synthesis of PGI_2 and TXA_2. In addition, aspirin can also affect the release of platelet particulate matter, such as serotonin and PF_4, and inhibit platelet release.

This experiment used a polyethylene tube to connect the common carotid artery on one side and the external jugular vein on the opposite side of the rat to form a bypass blood flow. Place a section of silk thread in the middle of the polyethylene tube. When blood flows through, platelets come into contact with the rough surface of the silk thread or copper ring and adhere to it, causing a degranulation reaction and releasing active substances such as ADP, 5-HT, which promote platelet aggregation on the surface of the silk thread. First, small platelet thrombus is formed, followed by fibrin formation. When a large number of red blood cells are collected, a red thrombus is formed. By detecting the dry or wet weight of the thrombus, as well as the inhibition rate of thrombus formation, we can explore the mechanism of thrombus formation and evaluate the efficacy and mechanisms of antithrombotic and thrombolytic drugs.

The working principle is as shown in Figure 5-3-1.

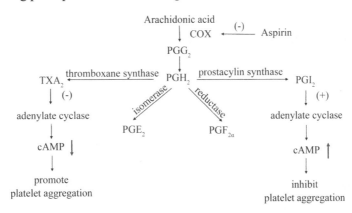

Figure 5-3-1　Schematic diagram of aspirin's antagonistic effect on thrombosis

[Experimental materials]

Rat operating table, 1 set of surgical instruments, arterial clip, polyethylene tube (with outer diameters of 1.6 mm and 1.3 mm), No. 4 surgical thread, 1mL syringe, 2 mL syringe.

[Experimental animals]

Rats, 250 ~ 300 g, male.

[Experimental reagents]

3% pentobarbital sodium solution, 2% aspirin solution, heparin physiological saline solution (50 IU/mL).

[Experimental methods]

(1) Take 2 rats from each group, weigh and number them according to A and B. Administer aspirin 5 mL/kg to mouse A by gavage every morning, and saline 5 mL/kg to mouse B for a total of 5 days.

(2) One hour after the last administration, rats A and B were anesthetized by intraperitoneal injection of 3% pentobarbital sodium (1.5 mL/kg), and then fixed in a supine position on the surgical table of the rats. The trachea was separated, and a plastic sleeve was inserted (which can be used to aspirate tracheal secretions) to separate the right common carotid artery and left external jugular vein.

(3) Cut a surgical thread with a length of about 6 cm, weigh it, and place it in a polyethylene tube. Fill the polyethylene tube with heparin normal saline solution. When one end of the polyethylene tube is inserted into the left external jugular vein, inject heparin normal saline (1 mL/kg) accurately into the polyethylene tube for anticoagulation, and then insert the other end of the polyethylene tube into the right common carotid artery.

(4) After opening the artery clamp, start timing and blood flows from the right common carotid artery into the polyethylene tube, returning to the left external jugular vein. After opening the blood flow for 15 minutes, interrupt the blood flow and quickly remove the silk thread for weighing. Subtract the weight of the silk thread from the total weight to obtain the wet weight of the thrombus.

[Experimental records and results]

Calculate the wet weight of thrombus measured by rat A and B and fill it in the Table 5-3-1.

Table 5-3-1　Anti-thrombotic effect of aspirin

Groups	Drugs	Dose (mL)	Thrombus wet weight/g
rat A	aspirin		
rat B	physiological saline		

[Precautions]

(1) The weight of animals in the control group and the treatment group should be strictly matched.

(2) Polyethylene pipes can only be inserted into blood vessels after being stretched thin, and the size of the pipe end diameter should be strictly controlled. Be careful not to twist the blood vessels after inserting the polyethylene tube into them.

(3) The surgical process requires speed, proficient technical operation, and appropriate dosage of heparin. The surgery should be completed within 15 minutes.

(4) Pay attention to timely suction of tracheal secretions and maintain smooth breathing.

[Practice questions]

1. The mechanism by which aspirin prevents thrombosis is to_____.

A. directly counteract platelet aggregation

B. reduce TXA2 generation

C. reduce thrombin activity

D. activate antithrombin E and enhance the effect of vitamin K

2. The typical gavage volume for rats is _____ mL.

A. 0.2 ~ 0.8　　　　B. 1 ~ 4　　　　　C. 5 ~ 6　　　　　D. 6 ~ 7

3. The dosage of that aspirin is commonly used for antithrombotic purposes is _____.

A. low dose　　　B. medium dose　　C. high dose　　　D. extreme dose

[Thinking questions]

(1) What is the effect of aspirin on the formation of blood clots in rats?

(2) What is the mechanism by which aspirin affects thrombosis? What is the clinical significance?

[Knowledye expansion]

"The universal elixir that comes out of the willow tree"—aspirin

In the 4th century BC, the "father of medicine" Hippocrate used willow leaves to make soup to treat headaches, allowing pregnant women to chew willow bark to relieve pain during childbirth and alleviate subsequent fever symptoms. In 1763, it was discovered that willow bark powder could treat fever caused by malaria. Until 1829, the active ingredient salidroside was successfully extracted and found to have strong pharmacological activity in vitro, laying the foundation for the development of aspirin in the future. Due to the complex process of extracting salicylic acid from willow trees, scientists synthesized salicylic acid for the first time in 1859 and once again verified its excellent antipyretic and analgesic effects. However, with its widespread clinical application, it has been found that salicylic acid can cause adverse side effects such as gastric ulcers and vomiting. In 1897, scientist Hoffmann from Bayer AG in Germany modified the structure of the compound and synthesized acetylsalicylic acid due to his father's rheumatism and the significant side effects of long-term use of salicylic acid. Through animal and clinical trials, it has been found that acetylsalicylic acid has better antipyretic and analgesic effects than salicylic acid, and has fewer side effects. In 1899, Bayer AG registered a patent for acetylsalicylic acid and named it aspirin. In the 1940s, American doctor Calvin found that patients with tonsillitis had excessive bleeding when using relatively high doses of aspirin, which led to the discovery of aspirin's anti thrombotic effect and its potential in preventing myocardial infarction.

The diligent and wise Chinese nation has a legend of Shennong tasting hundreds of herbs in ancient times. Our country's medical sages also recorded the medicinal value of willow trees in one of the four classic works of traditional Chinese medicine, *Shen Nong's Herbal Classic* and the oriental pharmaceutical giant *Compendium of Materia Medica*. Its active ingredient is salicylic acid. The *Shen Nong's Herbal Classic* records that "the roots, bark, branches, and leaves of willow can all be used as medicine, which has the effects of dispelling phlegm, improving vision, clearing heat and detoxifying, diuresis and wind prevention. External application can treat toothache." According to Li Shizhen's *Compendium of Materia Medica*, "Decoction of willow leaves can treat blood in the heart and abdomen, relieve pain, and treat scabies. Decoction of willow branches and root bark can be used to boil wine, rinse teeth, and relieve jaundice and turbidity. Willow catkins can stop bleeding, treat dampness and rheumatism, and relieve limb spasms."

（赵　超）

Section 4   The effect of oxytocin on uterine smooth muscle *in vitro* in guinea pigs

[Experimental objective]

(1) To observe the effects of different doses of oxytocin on uterus *in vitro*.

(2) Learn experimental methods for detached uterus.

[Experimental principle]

Oxytocin is a polypeptide hormone, and its chemical structure is shown in Figure 5-4-1. Different doses of oxytocin have different effects on the uterus. A small dose of oxytocin causes rhythmic contractions of the uterine fundus, which is beneficial for fetal delivery. High doses can cause tonic contractions, which are beneficial for postpartum hemostasis. Estrogen increases the sensitivity of the uterus to oxytocin, while progesterone reduces this sensitivity.

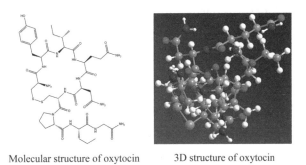

Molecular structure of oxytocin   3D structure of oxytocin

Figure 5-4-1   Chemical structure of oxytocin

There are specific oxytocin receptors on the plasma membrane of human uterine smooth muscle cells, and the density of oxytocin receptor expression varies at different stages of pregnancy. The basis for the uterine contraction effect of oxytocin is its binding to oxytocin receptors. Oxytocin acts on G protein coupled receptors in uterine smooth muscle cells, activating phospholipase C (PLC) and increasing the production of inositol triphosphate (IP_3). Subsequently, a large amount of Ca^{2+} is transferred into uterine smooth muscle cells, thereby enhancing the contractility of uterine smooth muscle and increasing its contraction frequency.

[Experimental materials]

BL-422 biological function experimental system, super constant temperature water bath, muscle strength transducer, bath tube, test tube, L-shaped hook, iron bracket, double concave clamp, spiral clamp, spring clamp, universal clamp, beaker, oxygen, needle, culture dish, suture, sewing needle, scissors, tweezers, 1mL syringe.

[Experimental animals]

Female non-pregnant rats weighing around 300 g.

[Experimental reagents]

0.005 U/mL oxytocin solution, 0.5 U/mL oxytocin solution, Le's solution, 0.5 mg/mL diethylstilbestrol.

[Experimental Methods]

1. Medication before experiment

24 ~ 36 hours before the experiment, 0.5 mg/mL of estradiol 0.5 mg was injected intraperitoneally to induce estrus.

2. Signal recording system connection

Turn on the BL-422 biological function experiment system, connect the transducer device, adjust the biological signal, adjust the temperature of the constant temperature water bath to (37.0 ± 0.5) °C, and add Le's solution to the bath to immerse the specimen.

3. Preparation of specimens

Take one guinea pig, strike the head to death. Quickly perform a caesarean section, find the uterus, cut off the lower end of the connection between the two corners of the uterus. Take out the uterus, place it in a culture dish containing Le's solution, carefully cut off the connective tissue and adipose tissue around the uterus, and cut the connection between the two corners of the uterus.

4. System debugging

Take one corner and tie both ends with threads. Fix one end on the L-shaped hook, place it in a bath containing 15 mL of Le's solution. Connect the other end to a muscle strength transducer, and adjust the resting tension by $1 \sim 2$ g. Administer oxygen and stabilize for 10 minutes. Draw a normal curve.

5. Medication

(1) Add 0.005 U/mL oxytocin solution 0.1 mL, observe smooth and rhythmic contractions of the uterine sarcomere, rinse after stabilizing the effect.

(2) Add 0.5 U/mL oxytocin solution 0.1 mL and observe the tonic contractions of uterine smooth muscle.

6. Observation and recording

Observe the changes in smooth muscle tension and record them after adding medication.

[Experimental records and results]

Fill in the experimental records and results in the table, as shown in Table 5-4-1.

Table 5-4-1   Effects of oxytocin on uterine smooth muscle

Drug	Concentration (U/mL)	Dose (mL)	Time	Smooth muscle tension (g)	Remarks
Oxytocin	0.005	0.1			
Oxytocin	0.5	0.1			

[Precautions]

(1) When making specimens, be gentle and avoid excessive pulling on the uterus. The shorter the operation time, the better.

(2) The amount of nutrient solution in the bath should be constant.

(3) When the working temperature is low ($32 \sim 35°C$), the specimen can maintain a longer working time. When the temperature is too high ($37 \sim 39°C$), the specimen is more sensitive, but the working time needs to be shortened.

[Practice questions]

1. The administration method of oxytocin does not include _____.

A. intramuscular injection   B. oral injection

C. intravenous injection   D. spray

2. The pharmacological effects of oxytocin do not include _____.

A. contraction of uterus   B. milk expulsion

C. contraction of vascular smooth muscle   D. oxygenation

3. What are the contraindications for oxytocin?

A. Abnormal birth canal.   B. Abnormal fetal position.

C. Placenta previa.   D. First-time parturient.

[Thinking questions]

(1) What are the precautions for medication during pregnancy?

(2) What are the types of medications that pregnant women can choose?

[Knowledge expansion]

Is oxytocin a "miracle drug"?

Oxytocin can be regarded as one of the "miracle drugs" in obstetrics, playing an important role in preventing and treating postpartum hemorrhage. In the 1990s, two British mothers died due to injections of oxytocin, and investigations found that the cardiovascular complications caused by oxytocin injections were related. South Africa has also reported two cases of maternal deaths caused by oxytocin, one of which was a sudden cardiac arrest resulting from intravenous injection of oxytocin during emergency cesarean section. Therefore, although oxytocin brings good news to mothers, there are still safety hazards if used improperly.

Oxytocin, also known as oxytocin, was originally extracted from the posterior pituitary gland of pigs, cows, and other animals. However, due to production process limitations and low purity, it can easily cause serious adverse reactions such as anaphylactic shock. In 1953, American scientist Vincent du Vigneaud brought about a significant change in the production process of oxytocin by artificially synthesizing it. The emergence of artificially synthesized oxytocin is a groundbreaking achievement in the history of pharmaceutical development, for which Vincent DiVinio was awarded the Nobel Prize. Its preparation process is simple, but the impurity content is still relatively high. In 1984, with the invention of solid-phase synthesis of peptide drugs, oxytocin with a purity of 99% emerged, and its inventor Robert also won the Nobel Prize for it.

（王　琳）

Section 5 The effect of diuretics on animal urine output

[Experimental objective]

(1) To observe the diuretic effect and characteristics of furosemide on anesthetized rabbits.

(2) To understand the acute diuretic experimental methods using bladder catheterization and ureteral catheterization.

[Experimental principle]

The generation of urine includes three processes: glomerular filtration, tubular secretion, and reabsorption. The process that affects tubular reabsorption can cause significant changes in urine volume.

Furosemide competitively inhibits the Na^+-K^+-$2Cl^-$- cotransporter by acting on the thick segment of the ascending branch of the renal tubular loop, suppressing the reabsorption of Na^+ and Cl^-, and further affecting the kidney's ability to dilute and concentrate urine, resulting in a strong diuretic effect. Under normal circumstances, continuous high-dose administration of furosemide can result in an adult's 24-hour urine output reaching $50 \sim 60$ L.

[Experimental materials]

BL422 functional experimental signal acquisition system, rabbit operating table, urinary catheter, bladder funnel (connected to rubber tube and droplet tube), intravenous infusion device, syringe, drip counter, baby scale, surgical knife, tissue scissors, ophthalmic scissors, vascular forceps, graduated cylinder, spring clip, etc.

[Experimental animals]

Rabbit, $2.0 \sim 2.5$ kg.

[Experimental reagents]

20% uratan, saline, 1% furosemide solution.

[Experimental methods]

1. Anesthesia

Take one rabbit, fast and avoid drinking water for 12 ~ 24 hours before the experiment. Weigh the rabbit and administer 30 mL/kg of saline by gavage 0.5 hours before the experiment to increase water load. Slowly inject 20% uratan solution (1.0 g/kg) through the ear vein, and fix the animal in a supine position on the rabbit operating table after anesthesia.

2. Operation

Trim the lower abdomen, make a midline incision of about 3 ~ 5 cm from the pubic symphysis upwards. Open the abdominal cavity along the white line of the abdomen, expose the bladder, and flip the bladder out of the abdomen. Carefully separate the two ureters, thread a line under the separated ureters, and ligate the bladder neck with a thread to block its passage to the urethra. Then make a 1 cm incision near the bladder tip on the ventral side of the bladder, avoiding blood vessels, and insert a water filled tube (with a droplet tube attached to the tube, and the bladder funnel should be aligned with the ureteral opening), ligate and fix it. Lower the tip of the dropper downwards below the bladder, release the spring clip clamped on the rubber tube of the sheath, and urine can be seen dripping out. The extracted urine should be dripped onto the contact point of the dropper, and recorded using the dropper device or directly recording the urine volume in milliliters. Finally, insert the bladder back into the abdominal cavity (without twisting) and cover the incision with saline gauze (Figure 5-5-1).

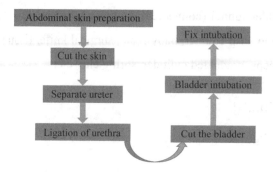

Figure 5-5-1　Abdominal surgery process diagram

3. Installation and adjustment of experimental equipment and recording

Turn on the computer and BL-422 functional experimental signal acquisition system according to the program, click on the experimental item bar in the menu, select the "Factors affecting urine production" item in the "Urinary System Experiment" under the "Experimental Items" menu, and test whether the recording of urine droplets, time recording, and stimulus symbols is good. Collect and record the normal number of drops per minute or total urine volume within 5 minutes after the urine is stable (Table 5-5-1).

4. Medication administration

Inject 1% furosemide 0.5 mL/kg (5 mg/kg) into the ear vein, continuously collect and record the number of urine drops per minute or urine volume each 5 minutes after administration, and continue for 20 minutes.

[Experimental records and results]

Table 5-5-1   Effects of Furosemide on urine volume in rabbits

Drug	Urination status (urine droplets/minute and urine volume mL/5 min)				
	Before administration	After administration			
		0 ~ 5 min	5 ~ 10 min	10 ~ 15 min	15 ~ 20 min
5 mg/kg Furosemide					

[Ureteral catheterization method]

After anesthesia, the rabbit is fixed supine on the operating table. A 3 ~ 5 cm incision is made along the midline from the pubic symphysis upwards, and the abdominal cavity is opened along the white line to expose the bladder. Two ureters are carefully separated on both sides of the bladder bottom, and two wires are threaded below them. One wire is ligated near the bladder end, and a small incision is made with an ophthalmic scissors towards the kidney direction above the ligature line to insert a polyethylene catheter. The other wire is ligated and fixed. Place the free ends of both catheters together into a measuring cylinder and collect and record the urine volume. Attention: The ureter of rabbits is delicate and fragile. When inserting the tube, the movements should be meticulous and light, and it is important to avoid inserting the ureter.

[Precautions]

(1) When separating the two ureters, be careful to avoid blunt separation of blood vessels.

(2) Before intubation, the bladder funnel and the connected rubber tube should be filled with water in advance.

[Practice questions]

1. The main adverse reactions of furosemide are _____.

A. arrhythmia   B. electrolyte disorders

C. elevated blood pressure   D. mental disorders

2. Which drug can treat both hypertension and diabetes insipidus?

A. Furosemide.   B. Etannic acid.

C. Hydrochlorothiazide.   D. Spironolactone.

3. Which drug is a high-performance diuretics that can be use in patients allergic to sulfonamide?

A. Furosemide.   B. Etannic acid.

C. Bumetanide.   D. Hydrochlorothiazide.

4. Spironolactone can be used for treating _____.

A. hyperkalemia   B. cirrhosis with edema

C. arrhythmia   D. angina pectoris

5. What diuretics can be used for hypertensive patients with hyperlipidemia?

A. Furosemide.   B. Indapamide.

C. Verapamil.   D. Hydrochlorothiazide.

[Thinking questions]

(1) What are the clinical applications and precautions of furosemide?

(2) Why is furosemide called a highly effective diuretic?

[Knowledye expansion]

Furosemide is listed as one of the banned drugs by the World Anti-doping Agency

In sports competitions such as weightlifting, taekwondo, martial arts, and combat that require weight classification, athletes use diuretics before weighing to quickly lose weight through heavy urination and participate in lower level competitions. Some athletes have also taken other stimulants. Before the doping test, they take furosemide to increase urine output, dilute the concentration of stimulants in urine, and avoid being detected as prohibited substances in urine. On December 18th, 2020, the China Anti-doping Center announced the results of a doping violation. Renowned mountain bike athlete Ma Hao was banned for two years for being tested for the banned substance furosemide outside the competition on December 1st, 2019. Amateur marathon runner Yang Qingchao won the men's bronze medal in the 2024 Hebei Marathon with a time of 2 hours, 31 minutes, and 38 seconds. Post match testing showed that the use of diuretic furosemide would face a comprehensive investigation. There are many cases like this. Although taking stimulants can improve athletic performance, it goes against the principle of fair and just competition, and can also cause harm to the human body. For example, furosemide can cause dehydration and reduce athletic ability, and can cause blood potassium deficiency and symptoms such as fatigue and spasms. Therefore, furosemide has been explicitly listed as one of the banned drugs by the World Anti-doping Agency (WADA), prohibiting athletes from using it both in and out of competition.

（王　琳）

Section 6   The effect of hydrocortisone on ear swelling induced by paraxylene in mice

[Experimental objective]

(1) To observe the effect of hydrocortisone on the capillary permeability of mouse

auricle and analyze its anti-inflammatory characteristics.

(2) To understand the mechanisms of experimental inflammation.

[Experimental principle]

The basic pathological changes of inflammation are degeneration, exudation, and proliferation. Corticosteroids have strong anti-inflammatory effects and can inhibit the occurrence of various inflammations. In the early stage of acute inflammation, it can increase the tension of blood vessels, reduce congestion, and decrease the permeability of capillaries, thereby reducing exudation and edema. Simultaneously it can inhibit leukocyte infiltration and phagocytic response, reduce the release of various inflammatory factors, thereby alleviating symptoms such as redness, swelling, heat, and pain. Corticosteroids exert anti-inflammatory and immunosuppressive effects through genomic and non-genomic effects. The classic genomic effect is mediated by the cytoplasmic receptors of glucocorticoids, which can upregulate the expression of anti-inflammatory proteins in the nucleus or inhibit the transfer of pro-inflammatory transcription factors from the cytoplasm to the nucleus (Figure 5-6-1). Non-genomic effects may be mediated by membrane receptors of glucocorticoids. Applying xylene to the ears of mouse can cause local cell damage, promote the release of inflammatory substances such as histamine and bradykinin, and cause acute inflammatory edema in the ears. The inflamed area is significantly swollen and the volume increases. In this experiment, the weight of mouse ears was measured to determine the degree of swelling and observe the anti-inflammatory effect of the drug.

The anti-inflammatory mechanism of glucocorticoids (genomic effects) is shown in Figure 5-6-1.

[Experimental materials]

Electronic balance, 1 mL syringe, squirrel cage, pipette, rough scissors, 8mm diameter punch, precision balance.

[Experimental animals]

White mouse, 25 ~ 30 g, male.

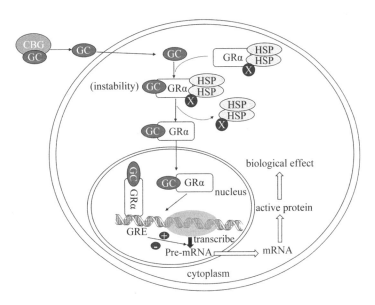

Figure 5-6-1　Gene regulation mechanism of glucocorticoids

[Experimental reagents]

0.5% hydrocortisone injection, xylene, normal saline, picric acid.

Note: CBG: corticosteroid-binding globulin; GC: glucocorticoid; GR: glucocorticoid receptor; HSPs: heat shock proteins; GRE: glucocorticoid receptor element.

[Experimental methods]

(1) Take 2 mice, weigh and label them with picric acid. Mouse A was intraperitoneally injected with 0.5% hydrocortisone injection at a dose of $0.05 \sim 0.1$ mL/10 g, while mouse B was intraperitoneally injected with an equal volume of normal saline. After 30 minutes, apply $0.05 \sim 0.1$ mL of xylene evenly to the front and back of the left ear of two mice using a pipette to induce inflammation, and do not apply the drug to the right ear as a blank control.

(2) After 2 hours, the mice were dislocated and euthanized. Both ears were cut along the ear canal, and 8 mm diameter punchers were used to make ear flaps in the same parts of the left and right ears. The mice were then weighed separately using a precision balance. The weight difference between the left and right ear pieces of each mouse is the degree of swelling, and the swelling degree and swelling rate are calculated according to the following formula.

$$\text{swelling degree} = \frac{\text{left ear piece weight - right ear piece weight}}{\text{swelling rate (\%)}} = \times 100\%$$

[Experimental records and results]

Summarize the experimental results of the entire laboratory, perform statistical analysis on the swelling degree of control mice and treated mice. The data is represented as $\bar{x} \pm s$, and perform inter group t test (Table 5-6-1).

Table 5-6-1   The effect of the drug on xylene induced ear inflammation in mice

Groups	Drugs	Number of mice	Average swelling degree(mg)	Average swelling rate(%)
mouse A	hydrocortisone			
mouse B	physiological saline			

[Precautions]

(1) This experiment should be conducted at room temperature, as too low a temperature can affect the experimental results.

(2) The application of xylene should be uniform, the dosage should be accurate, and the application area should match the removed ear piece.

(3) The mouse ear inflammation model can also be replaced with a 70% ethanol solution containing 2% croton oil.

(4) The puncher should be sharp, and the earpieces should be removed at once. The location of the earpieces for each group must be consistent.

[Practice questions]

1. Regarding intraperitoneal injection in mice, which one is incorrect?

A. When administering, the mice should have its abdomen facing upwards and its head positioned high.

B. During administration, the mice's abdomen is facing upwards and its head is tilted downwards.

C. The needle should not be inserted too high or too deep to avoid damaging the internal organs.

D. Insert the needle into the abdomen from one side of the lower abdomen towards the head at a 30° angle.

2. According to the classification of drugs based on its kinetic characteristics, hydrocortisone belongs to _____.

A. long acting glucocorticoids

B. long acting glucocorticoids

C. medium acting glucocorticoids

D. short acting glucocorticoids

3. Which one of the following are not pharmacological effects of glucocorticoids?

A. Anti-shock effect.

B. Immunosuppressive and anti-allergic effects.

C. Anti-inflammatory effect.

D. Anti rheumatic effect.

[Thinking questions]

(1) What is the mechanisms of action of glucocorticoids in combating acute inflammation?

(2) What is the difference in efficacy between local and systemic use of hydrocortisone? Why?

[Knowledye expansion]

"Half honey, half arsenic"—Glucocorticoids

The unity and struggle of both sides in the contradiction of things constantly promote the development of things from lower to higher levels. This theory is perfectly reflected in the duality of glucocorticoids. The glucocorticoids secreted by the human body can effectively resist harmful stimuli during stress responses. As a therapeutic drug, it has the effects of inhibiting immune response, anti-inflammatory, anti-toxic, and anti-shock, and is widely used in clinics. But at the same time, it has many adverse reactions, such as long-term non-standard use of glucocorticoids can cause iatrogenic Cushing's syndrome, manifested as central obesity, and can also cause high blood pressure, metabolic disorders of blood sugar, damage to gastrointestinal mucosa, osteoporosis, etc. Glucocorticoids have a negative feedback regulatory effect on the hypothalamus pituitary system. If glucocorticoids are used in large quantities for a long time, they can inhibit the pituitary gland, reduce the secretion of ACTH for a long time, and cause adrenal cortex dysfunction or even atrophy in patients. Sudden cessation of use at this time can cause serious consequences and endanger life. Therefore, the use of glucocorticoids must be regulated rather than abused. As students of medical schools, we should strive to lay a solid foundation, possess a solid theoretical foundation, establish good medical ethics and conduct in future work, always put patient safety firstly, and be a responsible and responsible medical worker who integrates medical skills and ethics.

（赵　超）

Section 7　Effects of magnesium sulfate and raw rhubarb on intestinal propulsion in mice

[Experimental objective]

(1) To observe the effects of magnesium sulfate and raw rhubarb on intestinal movement in mice.

(2) To master the anatomical method of mice and the measurement method of the total length of small intestine.

[Experimental principle]

Magnesium sulfate is a osmotic laxative, which dissociates into Mg^{2+} and SO_4^{2-} in the gastrointestinal tract after oral administration. Due to its low fat solubility, it is difficult to absorb in the gastrointestinal tract, forming hyperosmolar pressure in the intestine, absorbing water outside the intestine into the intestine and preventing water absorption, expanding the intestine, thus promoting intestinal peristalsis and diarrhea, and promoting bile secretion(Figure 5-7-1). Rhubarb is a traditional Chinese medicine with a strong purging effect. Its purging effect can be used for stagnation constipation caused by heat syndrome. Anthraquinone substances contained in it can stimulate the intestine, cause intestinal peristalsis to increase, inhibit intestinal water absorption and promote defecation. In this experiment, the effects of magnesium sulfate and raw rhubarb on intestinal tube propulsion in mice were observed by intragastric administration.

Charcoal propulsion method is a commonly used experimental method to evaluate the effect of drugs on gastrointestinal motility in mice. In this method, the effect of the drug is evaluated by observing the distance of the charcoal powder in the gastrointestinal tract of the mice.

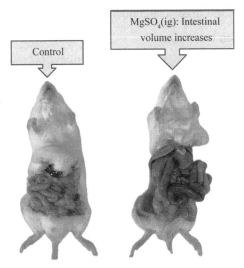

Figure 5-7-1   Schematic diagram of magnesium sulfate catharsis

[Experimental materials]

Surgical scissors, ophthalmic scissors, ophthalmic forceps, ruler, gavage needle, syringe (1mL), cotton ball, balance.

[Experimental animals]

Mice, weighing 23 ~ 25 g, either gender.

[Experimental reagents]

Magnesium sulfate (15%), activated carbon powder, raw rhubarb decoction (1 g/mL), sodium carboxymethyl cellulose.

[Experimental methods]

1. Experimental preparation

6 mice fasting for 24 hours were taken, weighed, labeled with picric acid, and divided into 3 groups for use.

2. Medication administration

Magnesium sulfate solution mixed with 5% carbon powder, raw rhubarb solution mixed with 5% carbon powder and normal saline solution mixed with 5% carbon powder were given to the three groups of mice by intragastric administration at a rate of 0.2 mL/10 g, and the completion time of intragastric administration was recorded.

3. Post administration treatment

20 minutes after administration, the mice were killed using cervical dislocation method. The abdominal cavity was opened to separate the mesentery, the gastrointestinal tract was stripped away, and the intestinal tube from the upper end to the pylorus and the lower end to the ileocecal part was cut out and placed in a tray to form a straight line. The length of the intestinal tube was measured as the "full length of small intestine", and the distance from the pylorus to the front edge of the carbon powder was measured as the "carbon powder propulsion distance".

4.Calculate the percentage of small intestine propulsion

The percentage of small intestine propulsion (%) = carbon powder propulsion distance/ full length of small intestine × 100%

[Experimental records and results]

The experimental results were recorded, the small intestine propulsion rate of mice in each group was calculated according to the formula, and recorded in the Table 5-7-1. The results of the whole class can also be collected and statistically analyzed.

Table 5-7-1　Effects of magnesium sulfate and raw rhubarb on intestinal propulsion in mice

Groups	Mouse number	Weight (g)	Dosage	Full length of small intestine (cm)	Charcoal dust advance distance (cm)	Propulsion rate (%)
Magnesium sulfate group						
Raw rhubarb group						
Saline group						

[Precautions]

(1) The time between the administration of the drug and the killing of the animal must be accurate to avoid experimental errors caused by different times.

(2) The more similar the weight of the experimental animals are, the better it is. The intestinal tube of the mice with the average weight of 23 ~ 25 g is relatively large and easy to operate.

(3) The change of intestinal volume can be observed by ligation of the upper and lower sections, weighing and quantifying.

(4) The colorant for the distance observation of intestinal propulsion can be administered orally with 10% activated carbon solution or other pigments (1% carmine solution), 0.2 mL/10 g body weight gavage.

(5) When opening the abdominal cavity of mice, tweezers should be used to lift and cut the belly fur to avoid damaging the intestine.

[Practice questions]

1. The clinical application of magnesium sulfate does not include _____.

A. constipation   B. food poisoning

C. eclampsia   D. routine medication for high blood pressure

2. Which type of laxative is similar to the laxative effect of raw rhubarb?

A. Volumetric laxatives.   B. Osmotic laxatives.

C. Irritant laxatives.   D. Lubricated laxatives.

3. Which one is the incorrect description about laxatives?

A. It is mainly used for functional constipation.

B. The elderly, pregnant women and menses should not use severe laxatives.

C. Magnesium sulfate catharsis is preferred when barbiturates are poisoned.

D. Salt laxatives should be used to eliminate poisons.

[Thinking questions]

(1) What kinds of laxatives are used clinically? What are the mechanisms of action and clinical indications?

(2) In addition to the anthracite method, what other methods can be used to observe the enteropropulsive effect in mice?

[Knowledye expansion]

Can laxatives also be abused?

Laxatives have a good effect on increasing gastrointestinal peristalsis and promoting defecation, and are clinically used for short-term relief of functional constipation. Constipation refers to the number of bowel movements less than three times a week, accompanied by difficulty in defecation and dry stool. But in recent years, many people have been taking laxatives for long periods of time to detoxify and lose weight, leading to a trend of laxative abuse. In fact, some laxatives have a very great impact on our health if taken for a long time, such as guide tablets, or the purging effect of rhubarb, senna, aloe vera in Chinese medicine, these stimulant laxatives may have very serious adverse reactions if taken for a long time. First of all, if you often use such laxatives to speed up defecation, it will lead to the function of intestinal automatic peristalsis becoming weaker and weaker, and finally may make constipation symptoms more and more serious. Even worse, there may be symptoms of being unable to defecate independently without taking laxatives. Secondly, eating such laxatives for a long time will also cause electrolyte disorders due to frequent diarrhea. If it is to lose weight and take such laxatives, food cannot be absorbed due to rapid intestinal peristalsis resulting in malnutrition. What's more, taking such laxatives for a long time may lead to melanosis in the intestine, which may induce intestinal tumors over time. Of course, if it is a dietary fiber type of volumetric laxatives or greasy laxatives, the adverse effects are relatively mild. So substance abuse is not just about psychotropic drugs. As students of medical college, it is of great significance to master the relevant pharmacology knowledge to improve our clinical rational drug use ability. When we use drugs clinically, we must choose them reasonably according to patients' conditions, take care of patients with a scientific, rigorous and realistic attitude, and contribute to the promotion of the Healthy China strategy.

（王雅娟）

Section 8　The effect of drugs on coagulation time in mice

[Experimental objective]

(1) To learn a simple method to determine the blood clotting time in mice.

(2) To observe the effect of procoagulant and anticoagulant drugs on the blood clotting time in mice.

[Experimental principle]

Blood coagulation refers to the process in which blood changes from a flowing liquid state to a jelly-like clot that cannot flow, which can be divided into endogenous and exogenous clotting pathways. The endogenous coagulation pathway refers to the fact that all factors involved in coagulation come from the blood system, usually activated by contact between blood and foreign object surface with negative charges (such as collagen fibers). The exogenous clotting pathway is a clotting process initiated by tissue factor (TF). The key process of blood clotting is the conversion of fibrinogen from plasma to insoluble fibrin. Clotting time refers to the time it takes for blood to leave the outside of a blood vessel to clot, generally the time it takes for blood to leave a blood vessel until fibrin filaments appear.

In this experiment, the mice were injected with etamsylate solution, heparin solution and normal saline to observe the effect of coagulant and anticoagulant drugs on the blood coagulation time in mice. Etamsylate can enhance platelet aggregation and adhesion, and can reduce capillary permeability, make blood vessels shrink, play a role in promoting coagulation. Heparin can promote the role of antithrombin III (AT III) in the blood, and play a powerful anticoagulant effect *in vivo* and *in vitro*.

[Experimental materials]

1mL syringe, glass capillary tube, slide, needle, stopwatch, cotton ball.

[Experimental animals]

Mice, weighing 18 ~ 22g, either gender.

[Experimental reagents]

2.5% etamsylate solution, 50 U/mL heparin solution, normal saline, picric acid solution.

[Experimental methods]

1. Experimental preparation

3 mice were weighed and labeled with picric acid.

2. Medication administration

Mice 1 were intraperitoneally injected with 2.5% etamsylate solution 0.2 mL/10g (5 mg/10 g). Mice 2 were intraperitoneally injected with 50 U/mL of heparin solution 0.2 mL/10 g (10 U/10 g). And mice 3 was intraperitoneally injected with normal saline 0.2 mL/10 g.

3. Blood collection

30 min after administration, the mice were given orbital canthus puncture with capillary tubes for blood sampling. When the blood filled the whole capillary tube, the stopwatch was activated immediately to start timing. Inner orbital canthus puncture is to extract blood from fundus venous plexus of mice. The specific method is shown in Figure 5-8-1.

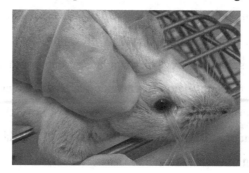

Figure 5-8-1   Schematic diagram of blood extraction from inner orbital canthus in mice

4. Determining clotting time

To measure the coagulation time, break a small section of capillary glass tube every 30 seconds (5 ~ 10 mm), and observe whether there is a fibrin filament. Until there is a fibrin filament connection between the two sections of glass tube, indicating that the blood has coagulated. Calculate the time from the beginning of the timing to the appearance of the fibrin filament, that is, the coagulation time.

5. Determining clotting time using glass slide method

Blood was taken quickly after puncture of inner orbital canthus with a small capillary tube. One drop of blood was dropped on each end of a clean and dry slide, and the stopwatch was immediately activated. The blood was stirred with a dry needle every 15 seconds until the needle could pick up fibrin filaments. Another drop of blood was provided for retesting. Record the clotting time as above.

6. Statistical analysis

Gather the experimental results of the whole class, and the average blood coagulation time of mice in the etamsylate group, heparin group and normal saline group was calculated, and the significance of the difference between the mean numbers was detected, so as to draw a conclusion about the influence of etamsylate and heparin on the blood coagulation time in mice.

[Experimental Records and results]

Record the experimental results of the whole class and make statistical analysis. See Table 5-8-1 for details.

Table 5-8-1　Effects of drugs on blood clotting time in mice

Groups	Number of mice	Dosing	Mean blood clotting time ± standard deviation		P value	
			Capillary method	Slide method	Capillary method	Slide method
Etamsylate Group						
Heparin group						
Saline group						

[Precautions]

(1) Coagulation time can be affected by temperature, the room temperature in this experiment is better around 15°C.

(2) The inside diameter of the capillary tube should be 1 mm and uniform.

(3) The action of breaking the capillary should be light. After breaking the capillary at both ends, slowly pull apart the capillary at both ends and check whether there are fibrin filaments (blood coagulation filaments) in the middle.

[Practice questions]

1. Clinical use of heparin is not included _____ .

A. DIC early stage　　　　　　　　　　B. myocardial infarction

C. in vitro anticoagulation　　　　　　　D. bleeding in preterm infants

2. The anticoagulant mechanism of coumarins is _____ .

A. inhibition of platelet aggregation

B. competitive inhibition of liver synthesis of coagulation factors II , VII , IX , X

C. antagonizing clotting factors in the blood

D. activating plasmin

3. For direct transfusions, add 2.5% sodium citrate _____ to each 100 mL of blood.

A. 5 mL   B. 10 mL   C. 15 mL   D. 20 mL

[Thinking questions]

(1) What are the main factors that affect clotting time?

(2) Which stages of blood coagulation are mainly affected by commonly used procoagulants and anticoagulants in clinics? What are the common uses in clinics?

[Knowledye expansion]

Thrombin and hemagglutinin

Thrombin and thrombin may look similar, but in reality they are completely different. Do not mistake the route of administration. Both thrombin and hemagglutinin have a hemostatic effect and are widely used in clinics. However, although they have similar names, they are used in completely different ways. Thrombin is a local hemostatic drug, which can be prepared into solution spray with normal saline or sprayed on the wound with dry powder, or oral or perfusion for digestive tract hemostasis. Intravascular, intramuscular or subcutaneous injection is strictly prohibited, otherwise it may lead to widespread thrombosis and endanger life. Hemagglutinin is a quick acting, long acting and safe hemostatic drug. It can be injected intravenously, intramuscularly, subcutaneously, or topically. Thrombin is one of the existing clotting factors in the body, while hemagglutinin is a non-clotting factor with a thrombin like effect, which is easy to degrade in the body without causing disseminated intravascular coagulation (DIC). The two have similar effects and different ways of administration. The slightest difference is a thousand miles away. As a medical worker, we directly serve human life and health. Each aspect and detail should be rigorous and meticulous, no room for any carelessness and fluke, because our 1% negligence may bring 100% harm to patients.

（王雅娟）

Section 9　Observation of antitussive effect of pentoverine

[Experimental objective]

(1) To learn the method of cough induced by ammonia water in mice.

(2) To observe the antitussive effect of pentoverine.

[Experimental principle]

Antitussive drugs can be divided into central antitussive drugs and peripheral antitussive drugs. Pentoverine is an amine ester derivative with central and peripheral antitussive effects. After absorption, it can slightly inhibit the bronchial receptors and afferent nerve endings, reduce cough reflex, relax spasmodic bronchial smooth muscle, reduce airway resistance, and have antitussive effects, which can relieve dry cough caused by various reasons.

Cough is one of the protective reflexes of the body. When the respiratory tract is stimulated by foreign bodies, it will induce the cough reflex. The cough induction methods commonly used in animal experiments include ammonia, citric acid and capsaicin. Concentrated ammonia is a strong chemical irritant that can stimulate respiratory receptors to trigger coughing. In this experiment, the cough inducing method of ammonia water was adopted. After inhaling ammonia aerosol, mice was stimulated respiratory receptors to induce cough reflex, and on this basis the antitussive effect of pentoverine on mice was observed (Figure 5-9-1).

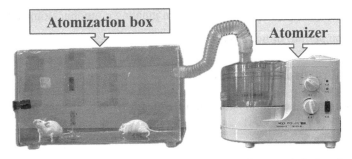

Figure 5-9-1　Schematic diagram of the experiment of ammonia induced cough

[Experimental materials]

Mouse intragastric needle, atomizer, atomization box, stopwatch, 1mL syringe.

[Experimental animals]

Mice, weighing $18 \sim 22$ g, either gender.

[Experimental reagents]

Concentrated ammonia (analytical pure), normal saline, pentoverine citrate tablet, platycodon grandiflorum decoction, picric acid.

[Experimental methods]

1. Experimental preparation

6 healthy qualified mice were prepared for the experiment, weighed and labeled, and randomly divided into 3 groups as follows: normal saline group, pentoverine group and platycodon grandiflorum group.

2. Medication administration

The mice in each group were given 0.2 mL/10 g by intragastric administration, and the administration time was recorded.

3. Observation of anticough effects

30min after gavage, the mice were put into a closed atomizing tank, 10mL of concentrated ammonia was put into the liquid storage cup of the atomizer to seal, and the atomizer was opened for 15s. The number of typical coughing movements (abdominal muscle contraction, mouth opening at the same time, sometimes coughing sound) of the mice in each group was observed. The time from inhaling ammonia atomization to coughing (cough incubation period) of mice was recorded.

[Experimental records and results]

The cough incubation period and cough frequency of mice in each group were recorded in Table 5-9-1.

Table 5-9-1　Observation of antitussive effects of antitussive drugs

Groups	Mouse Numbers	Weight (g)	Dosage (mg/kg)	Cough incubation period (s)	Cough frequency
Pentoverine group			21.0		
Platycodon Group			200.0		
Saline group			–		

[Precautions]

(1) The cough movements of mice must be observed carefully.

(2) Put 10 mL of concentrated ammonia water into the atomizer each time, and pour the residual liquid of the previous time before adding it again.

(3) It is best to cross the experimental group and control group animals when spraying.

[Practice questions]

1. Among the following cough suppressants, which are not central cough suppressants are _____.

A. codeine　　　　B. narcotine　　　　C. dextromethorphan　　D. pentoverine

2. Central cough suppressant are suitable for _____.

A. cold cough　　　　　　　　　B. cough with excessive phlegm

C. dry cough without phlegm　　　D. COPD cough

3. Which of the following is accurate about the strength of cough suppressants?

A. Pentoverine > Propiperine > Codeine

B. Codeine > Propiperine > Pentoverine

C. Propiperine > Pentoverine > Codeine

D. Propiperine > Codeine > Pentoverine

[Thinking questions]

(1) What steps can cough suppressants take to exert their cough suppressant effect?

(2) What are the advantages and disadvantages of central antitussive drugs? How to apply it reasonably in clinic?

[Knowledye expansion]

Dextromethorphan, an excellent cough suppressant, was controlled!

On May 7th, 2024, the State Drug Administration, the Ministry of Public Security and the National Health Commission issued a notice on the adjustment of the list of psychotropic drugs, which included dextromethorphan, compound preparation containing difenoxate, Nfurapine and lorcasserin in the second category of the list of psychotropic drugs, which came into effect on July 1st. Dextromethorphan, generally refers to dextromethorphan hydrobromide antitussive drugs, which antitussive effect is similar to codeine, but no analgesic effect, suitable for cough with little sputum caused by cold, acute and chronic bronchitis, pharyngitis, bronchial asthma and other upper respiratory tract infections. Although dextromethorphan has significant advantages in clinical treatment, with the widespread use of this drug, the phenomenon of abuse and dependence has gradually emerged in the population. Dextromethorphan can cause euphoria, hallucinations and other symptoms when taken in excess of doses, and over a long period of time, it is extremely easy to addiction, long-term abuse can cause brain damage and mental disorder. Therefore, there is a risk of abuse of dextromethorphan in life.

In recent years, the administration of dextromethorphan has been continuously strengthened. In December 2021, the State Food and Drug Administration issued an announcement to convert the oral monotherapy of dextromethorphan from over-the-counter to prescription. The announcement also revised the drug instructions. The newly revised instructions added the possible symptoms of excessive use of dextromethorphan, such as mental confusion, excitement, nervousness, etc., and deleted the statements of non-addiction and tolerance for long-term use. On December 1st, 2022, the "Prohibited List of Online Sales of Drugs (First version)" formulated by the State Food and Drug Administration came into effect, and dextromethorphan was banned online. In 2023, the NDA, the Ministry of Public Security and the State Post Bureau issued a notice on further strengthening the administration of drugs such as compound diphenoxylate tablets and dextromethorphan oral monodal preparations, requiring the relevant departments to be notified to strictly control drug production, strengthen supervision of drug production links, strengthen inspection of delivery channels, and severely crack down on violations of laws and regulations. A series of changes in the management of dextromethorphan reflect our country's emphasis to people's health. As medical students, we should be aware of the importance and particularity of medical work, improve our legal awareness while cultivating our own medical level, avoid drug abuse, and make full preparations for the future medical work.

（王雅娟）

Chapter 6   Pharmacology of chemotherapy drugs

Section 1   Toxic reactions of streptomycin and its relief

[Experimental objective]

To observe the toxic reactions of streptomycin sulfate in blocking neuromuscular junctions and the rescuing effect of calcium chloride.

[Experimental principle]

High-dose intramuscular injection of streptomycin or rapid administration can lead to neuromuscular junction blockade, causing myocardial depression, hypotension, limb weakness, and respiratory depression. The primary mechanism involves streptomycin binding to the calcium-binding sites on the presynaptic membrane, inhibiting the neutralization of negative charges by calcium ions, thereby preventing the release of acetylcholine mediated by calcium ions. This results in reduced acetylcholine release, manifesting as symptoms such as limb weakness and respiratory depression. Neostigmine or calcium supplements can counteract the muscle-relaxing effects induced by streptomycin.

[Experimental materials]

1 mL and 2 mL syringes, infant scales.

[Experimental animals]

Guinea pigs (approximately 300 g each).

[Experimental reagents]

25% Streptomycin sulfate, 5% calcium chloride solution, picric acid.

[Experimental methods]

1. Weighing and Marking

Take 2 guinea pigs, mark them with picric acid for identification, and weigh them. Observe their respiratory patterns, posture, gait, and limb muscle tone.

2. Administration and Observation

Group A: Administer 25% Streptomycin Sulfate intramuscularly at a dose of 0.24 mL/ 100 g. Observe the animal's responses (respiratory rate, posture, and limb muscle tone) 15 minutes after injection. If respiratory depression occurs, administer 5% calcium chloride solution intraperitoneally as a rescue measure at a dose of 1mL/100g and observe for recovery.

Group B: Administer 25% Streptomycin Sulfate intramuscularly at a dose of 0.24 mL/100 g. Observe the animal's responses (respiratory rate, posture, and limb muscle tone) 15 minutes after injection and record whether or not spontaneous recovery occurs (Figure 6-1-1).

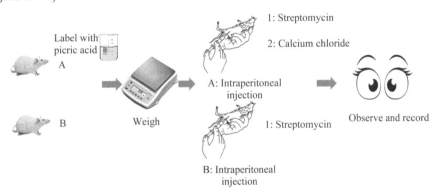

Figure 6-1-1   Schematic diagram of the experimental procedure

[Experimental records and results]

The detail are listed in Table 6-1-1.

[Precautions]

(1) The toxic reaction is slow after intramuscular injection of streptomycin, usually appearing 10 minutes after medication and gradually worsening.

(2) Pre-extract $CaCl_2$ for later use, rinse thoroughly with a syringe after use.

(3) If the first $CaCl_2$ rescue effect is not good, half the amount can be given again.

Table 6-1-1   Observation of streptomycin's toxic reactions and the rescuing effect of calcium chloride

Animal	Drug treatment	Respiration	Body position	Muscular tension
A	before using streptomycin			
	after using streptomycin			
	after using calcium chloride			
B	before using streptomycin			
	after using streptomycin			

[Practice questions]

1. Which class of antibiotics does streptomycin belong to?

A. Quinolones.

B. Macrolides.

C. Aminoglycosides.

D. Tetracyclines.

2. Which one of the following options are adverse drug reactions of streptomycin?

A. Superinfection.

B. Neuromuscular paralysis.

C. Liver damage.

D. Bone marrow suppression.

3. Which drug is used for the rescue of streptomycin toxicity?

A. Neostigmine.

B. Atropine hydrochloride.

C. Magnesium sulfate.

D. Normal saline.

[Thinking questions]

What toxic reactions of streptomycin were observed through this experiment? Why?

[Knowledye expansion]

The story of streptomycin

The discovery of penicillin was extremely miraculous and dramatic, ushering in a new era of antibiotics. The significance of the discovery of streptomycin is no less than that of penicillin, but its discovery is the result of careful design and long-term efforts. "Tuberculosis" is as famous as the Black Death. Because the patient has cough, hemoptysis and pale face, it is called the white plague, also known as "infectious cancer". Tuberculosis is a chronic infectious disease caused by a complex group of mycobacterium tuberculosis. Selman Waksman, a professor of soil science at Rutgers University in the United States, noticed that pulmonary tuberculosis bacteria would be killed quickly in the soil, and searched for microorganisms that could kill tuberculosis bacteria in the soil, isolated a substance that was fatal to tuberculosis bacteria-streptomycin, which stopped the rampant spread of tuberculosis. Waksman firstly used streptomycin in the treatment of tuberculosis patients, so he won the 1952 Nobel Prize in Physiology or Medicine.

（张朋飞）

Section 2　Determination of blood concentration of cefradine

[Experiment Objective]

(1) The blood concentration of ceftazidime was detected by HPLC to observe the change of blood concentration of cefradine.

(2) To master the calculation method and clinical significance of pharmacokinetics.

[Experimental principle]

Plasma half-life $(t_{1/2})$ is the time required for the plasma drug concentration to decrease by half, expressed as $t_{1/2}$. Most of the commonly used clinical drugs are eliminated in the body according to linear dynamics, that is the elimination rate is proportional to the instantaneous drug concentration. It means that the drug concentration is reduced according to a constant proportion, and the plasma drug concentration (logarithmic value) -time curve is a straight line. The plasma drug concentration (logarithmic value) -time curve of drugs is a parabolic curve belonging to a nonlinear dynamic elimination.Nonlinear elimination is caused by the saturation of the body's ability to eliminate drugs, and the blood drug concentration-time curve is a straight line. Determination of blood drug concentration can help us calculate important pharmacokinetic parameters such as $t_{1/2}$.

Cefradine is a first-generation semi-synthetic cephalosporin antimicrobial drug successfully researched in 1972. It is indicated for use in a variety of respiratory tract, genitourinary tract and soft tissue skin infections caused by sensitive bacteria. In addition to injection, Cefradin can be made into a variety of oral preparations, including Cefradin dry suspension, Cefradin tablets, Cefradin capsules and Cefradin granules.

[Experimental materials]

Centrifuge, centrifuge tube, capsule, syringe, a set of surgical instruments, High Performance Liquid Chromatograph.

[Experimental animals]

Rats, weighing 250 ~ 300 g, regardless of gender.

[Experimental reagents]

Cefradine for injection, cefradine control, methanol, acetonitrile, phosphoric acid, disodium hydrogen phosphate, and potassium dihydrogen phosphate, 0.9% sodium chloride injection, and ultrapure water.

[Experimental methods]

1. Animal handling

Take rats weighing 250 ~ 300 g, fast without water for 12 hours, and use a uniform standard meal during the trial period. 1 mL of blood was taken from the canthus. 5 min later, cefradine (0.2 g/kg) was injected intravenously. 1 mL of blood was taken from each canthus 5 min and 35 min after the administration of the drug, etc. All blood samples were placed in the blood collection tubes, left to stand for more than 15 min, and then centrifuged at 6000 r/min for 10 min to separate the serum.

2. Sample preparation

Take 300 μL of serum and add 450 μL of the methanol and 450 μL acetonitrile. Centrifuge the samples for 5 min, and then centrifuge at 4000 rpm and 4℃ for 10 min. Filter the supernatant to obtain the final product.

3. Chromatographic conditions setting

OSAKASODA CAPCELL PAK C_{18} (4.6 mm×250 mm, 5 μm) column was used. Mobile phase A was phosphate buffer (0.02 mol/L potassium dihydrogen phosphate solution adjusted the pH to 3.0 with phosphoric acid solution), and mobile phase B was methanol. The gradient elution was as follows: 0 ~ 2. 5 min (3% ~ 3%B)→2.5 ~ 11 min (3% ~ 25%B) →

11 ~ 13 min (25% ~ 40%B)→ 13 ~ 16 min (40%B) →16 ~ 19 min (40% ~ 80%B)→19 ~ 20 min (80% ~ 3%B)→20 ~ 30 min (3%B). Flow rate is 1.0 mL/min and detection wavelength is 220 nm with injection volume of 10 μL and column temperature of 30°C.

4. Preparation of control product

Weigh the appropriate amount of cephradine control product, add mobile phase A to dissolve, make a solution containing 60 μg/mL, as a control solution.

5. Data processing and analysis

Quantitative calculations were performed by the external standard method and blood concentration-time data were measured. Pharmacokinetic parameters were obtained by atrial fitting on a microcomputer using the 3p87 pharmacokinetic program (Figure 6-2-1).

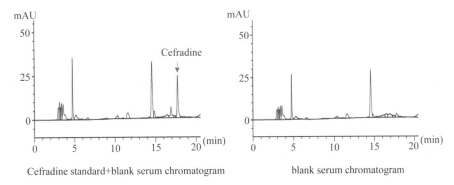

Figure 6-2-1   Chromatogram

[Experimental records and results]

The experimental results were recorded. The blood concentration and $t_{1/2}$ of cefradine at 5 min and 35 min after drug administration were calculated according to the formula. For details, seen in Table 6-2-1.

Table 6-2-1   Cefradine blood concentration and plasma half-life determination

Sampling time	Blood sample (mL)		serum (mL)	methanol (mL)	acetoni-trile (mL)		Supernat-ant (mL)	peak area	Concentr-ation (mg/mL)
Before dosing	1	Off-center	0.3	0.45	0.45	Off-center	0.9		
5 min after dosing	1		0.3	0.45	0.45		0.9		
35 min after dosing	1		0.3	0.45	0.45		0.9		

[Precautions]

(1) The rat beard should be subtracted to avoid hemolysis when blood was taken.

(2) Take care not to shake the blood collection tube violently to avoid hemolysis.

(3) Pay attention to balancing the placement of the centrifuge tubes during centrifugation.

(4) After configuring mobile phases A and B, they need to be filtered to remove insoluble impurities and prevent blocking of the chromatographic column.

(5) After mobile phases A and B was filtered, ultrasound is needed to remove bubbles to prevent affecting the results.

[Practice questions]

1. Which of the following drug belongs to the first generation cephalosporins?

A. Ceftazidime.　　　B. Cefradine.　　　C. Ceftriaxone.　　　D. Cefuroxime.

2. Which antibiotics require therapeutic drug monitoring during use?

A. Cefaclor　　　B. Amoxicillin　　　C. Vancomycin　　　D. Clarithromycin

3. The purpose of taking $NaHCO_3$ when taking sulfonamides is _____.

A. enhance antibacterial effect

B. promote drug absorption

C. inhibit drug excretion

D. alkalize urine and increase the solubility of sulfonamides in renal tubules

[Thinking questions]

(1) What is the significance of monitoring the blood concentration of antibiotics? Which antibiotics should be monitored clinically when they are used?

(2) What are the possible reasons for different blood concentrations of the same drug given to different patients?

[Knowledye expansion]

Gentamicin—Antibiotics independently developed in China

The discovery of penicillin opened an important chapter in the history of medicine, marking a new era in the synthesis of new drugs for humanity. As the first antibiotic independently developed by China, gentamicin is the pride of the Chinese people, and is also criticized for its serious adverse reactions such as deafness. Professor Wang Yue from the Fujian Institute of Vitamins, Chinese Academy of Sciences isolated a small single spore fungus from Fuzhou lake mud in 1965 and found that the antibiotic it produced was Gentamicin. It was produced for clinical use in 1969, during the 20th anniversary of the founding of the People's Republic of China and the 9th National Congress. Hence it was named "Gentamicin". Gentamicin made up for the shortcomings of penicillin and streptomycin, and had a low incidence of allergic reactions. It was widely used in the 1970s and 1980s. But with the widespread use of gentamicin, it has been found that it has significant ototoxicity and can cause permanent deafness. Many of the actors in the classic program "Thousand Armed Guanyin" on the 2005 Spring Festival Gala suffered from drug-induced hearing loss due to the use of such drugs (including gentamicin, streptomycin, kanamycin). Although gentamicin was once glorious and also criticized, it is still used in clinical practice for the treatment of diseases such as dysentery, enteritis, and severe infections such as sepsis. Antibiotics are the crystallization of technological innovation, and their discovery and application stem from the active exploration and bold attempts of outstanding scientists.

（王　蕾）

Section 3   Hemolysis test of injection

[Experimental objective]

(1) To observe the hemolytic reaction of injection and master the operation of the hemolysis test performed in a test tube.

(2) To master the method of rabbit heart blood collection and the preparation of red cell suspension.

[Experimental principle]

Hemolytic refers to the systemic toxicity of a drug preparation when it is administered through blood vessels, which is an integral part of preclinical safety evaluation. The original form of the drug and its metabolites, excipients, related substances and physicochemical properties (such as pH value, osmotic pressure, etc.) may cause hemolysis. Therefore, the local and/or systemic toxicity caused by injection should be studied before clinical application, so as to indicate the possible toxic reactions, toxic target organs and safe range during clinical application. Hemolytic reaction refers to the destruction of the red blood cell membrane or the appearance of many small holes, the reaction of hemoglobin flowing out of red blood cells due to extreme stretching. Agglutination is a serological reaction which a granular antigen binds to a corresponding antibody and small clumps of agglutination are visible to the naked eye in the presence of a dielectric medium.

In this experiment, a certain amount of caffeine citrate injection was added to 2% rabbit blood normal saline, and the hemolysis and agglutination reaction were observed within a certain time range to verify the safety of the injection.

[Experimental materials]

Rabbit fixator, scale, centrifuge, water bath, test tube, test tube brush, beaker, test tube holder, centrifuge tube, pipette gun, suction tip, 10 mL syringe.

[Experimental animals]

Rabbit, weighing 1.5 ~ 3.0 kg, regardless of gender.

[Experimental reagents]

Distilled water, normal saline, caffeine citrate injection.

[Experimental methods]

(1) Experimental preparation A rabbit was prepared for the experiment and weighed for use.

(2) Blood collection from rabbit heart Rabbit was dorsally fixed (or the assistant with left and right hands catching the rabbit hind limbs and forelimbs, the right side of the rabbit lying in the corner of the table). Cut a piece of hair in the left chest 2 ~ 4 ribs, disinfected with iodine and alcohol. Then, a 10 ~ 20 mL syringe equipped with a 7-gauge needle was used to puncture the most obvious place of the heartbeat. When the needle is inserted into

the heart cavity, blood flows into the syringe (or draw and puncture at the same time). After the blood is collected, the needle is quickly pulled out so that the hole in the heart muscle is easy to heal.

(3) Preparation of red blood cell suspension Take one rabbit and collect 10 mL of blood from the heart, and immediately placed into a beaker washed with normal saline in advance. The test tube brush was cleaned with normal saline, and the fibrin was removed with slight stirring. The blood was transferred into a centrifuge tube containing $5 \sim 10$ mL normal saline, mixed well and centrifuged at 2500 r/min for 5 min, then the supernatant was discarded. In this way, it was repeatedly washed $3 \sim 4$ times using the normal saline until the clear liquid was colorless and transparent. The washed red blood cells were prepared into 2% cell suspension with normal saline and set aside.

(4) Drug hemolysis test *in vitro.*

(5) Results judgement.

① Total hemolysis: the solution was clear red and no red blood cells remaining at the bottom of the tube (tube No. 7 in Figure 6-3-1);

② Partial hemolysis: the solution is clear or brown, with a small amount of red blood cells remaining at the bottom of the tube;

③ No hemolysis: all red blood cells sank, and the upper fluid was colorless and clear (tube $1 \sim 6$ in Figure 6-3-1);

④ Agglutination: no hemolysis, red blood cells agglutinated at the bottom of the test tube, and the cells cannot disperse after shaking.

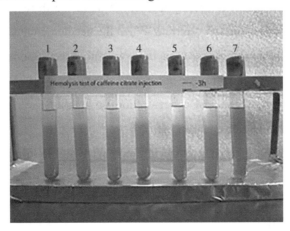

Figure 6-3-1   Schematic diagram of hemolysis test results for caffeine citrate injection

(6) Conclusion

① Preparations with partial hemolysis, total hemolysis, or agglutination reaction at 0.5 h should not be used intravenously;

② Preparations that do not show hemolysis and agglutination reaction at 3 h are judged to meet the requirements of the hemolysis test.

[Experimental records and results]

The hemolysis test results at 0 h, 0.25 h, 0.5 h, 0.75 h, 1 h, 2 h and 3 h were observed and recorded in Table 6-3-1.

Table 6-3-1   Design of hemolysis test

item	Test tube Number						
	1	2	3	4	5	6	7
Test solution (mL)	0.1	0.2	0.3	0.4	0.5		
Saline solution (mL)	2.4	2.3	2.2	2.1	2.0	2.5	
Distilled water (mL)							2.5
2% red blood cell suspension (mL)	2.5	2.5	2.5	2.5	2.5	2.5	2.5
result							

Note: Tube No. 6 was the blank control group, tube No. 7 was the positive control group; The results showed "+" for hemolysis and "−" for non-hemolysis.

[Precautions]

(1) The heart of a rabbit is usually located between the third and fourth ribs, and a needle needs to be inserted into the ventricle. When the needle tip enters the ventricle, blood will be sprayed into the needle tube. At this time, careful observation is needed. Once blood enters the needle tube, stop inserting the needle and slowly draw blood.

(2) The tested drug is the factory concentration, do not dilute.

(3) The test tube should be clean and dry.

(4) Beakers and test tubes that come into contact with blood must always be rinsed with normal saline.

[Practice questions]

1. When the patient has a hemolytic reaction, the excreted urine is strong brown or soy

sauce color. The main reason is that the urine contains _____.

A. bilirubin
B. red blood cells

C. hemoglobin
D. lymphatic fluid

2. Hemolysis refers to what changes occur in red blood cells in response to certain factors?

A. Red blood cell agglutination.
B. Red blood cell rupture.

C. Erythrocyte deformation.
D. Erythrocyte hyperplasia.

3. Where is the location of rabbit heart blood collection?

A. 1 ~ 2 intercostal.
B. 3 ~ 4 intercostal.

C. 5 ~ 6 intercostal.
D. 2 ~ 6 intercostal.

[Thinking questions]

(1) What factors of pharmaceutical preparations can cause hemolysis?

(2) What measures should be taken when hemolysis occurs clinically?

[Knowledye expansion]

Drug-induced immune hemolytic anemia

Drug-induced immune hemolytic anemia (DIIHA) is a rare complication in the clinical application of drugs (the incidence is about 1/1000000/ year), which is often missed diagnosis[1]. DIIHA often leads to serious adverse outcomes, including multiple organ failure and even death. Ceftriaxone is a broad-spectrum third-generation cephalosporin antibiotic, widely used in clinical treatment of various bacterial infections. There have been ceftriaxone DIIHA and multiple cases of hemolysis[1, 2] caused by ceftriaxone in clinical practice. It was reported that that ceftriaxone may[3] cause severe immune hemolysis in children, the elderly and patients with underlying diseases and poor immune function. The mechanism of ceftriaxone causing hemolysis is the formation of immune complex: after intravenous administration, ceftriaxone IgM antibody can appear in red blood cells, which then forms immune complex with ceftriaxone or its metabolites. It binds to the specific target protein on the erythrocyte membrane, activates the complement system, destroys red blood cells, leads to red blood cell rupture, and finally causes severe hemolysis reaction. The hemolysis caused by the activation of the complement system by this antibody is usually intravascular hemolysis. Therefore, ceftriaxone is recommended for clinical caution in children, the elderly and patients with underlying diseases, and clinical symptoms are closely observed.

（邹莹莹）

Section 4   Pyrogen examination of injection

[Experimental objective]

(1) To study the method and criterion of detecting pyrogen in injection by rabbits.

(2) To master the methods of detecting the anal temperature of rabbits.

[Experimental principle]

Pyrogen mainly derives from the metabolic products of bacteria. Chinese herbs contain starch, sugar, protein and other components that are conducive to the growth and reproduction of bacteria. If they are exposed to the air for too long time during the extraction process, they are easy to be contaminated by bacteria to produce pyrogen. About half an hour after the infusion containing pyrogen is injected into the human body, the patient will appear chills, high fever, sweating, nausea and vomiting. Severe cases may experience coma, shock, and even life-threatening situations. The rabbit method is an *in vivo* pyrogen test based on the principle that the rabbit's response to pyrogen is similar to that of humans. The method is to inject the test product into the rabbit ear border vein, and measured the animal body temperature several times in the specified time And observe the temperature changes so as to evaluate whether the test product induces the body fever reaction potential possibility. This method is also the pyrogen test method stipulated in our pharmacopoeia.

In this experiment, 25% or 50% glucose injection solution (other injections also available) commonly used in clinics as test drugs to observe whether it will affect the body temperature of rabbits after intravenous injection.

[Experimental materials]

Rabbit fixed box, weighing scale, anal thermometer, 10 mL syringe and needle, tweezers, alcohol cotton ball and dry cotton ball.

[Experimental animals]

Rabbit, weight 1.7 ~ 3.0 kg, male or female (female rabbits excluded pregnancy).

[Experimental reagents]

Experimental product (25% or 50% glucose injection or other injection), liquid paraffin wax.

[Experimental methods]

The experimental procedure is as follows, shown in Figure 6-4-1.

(1) Preparation before the experiment 1 to 2 days before the pyrogen test, rabbits should be exposed to the same temperature as possible. Rabbits that have not been tested for pyrogen should have their body temperature predicted within 7 days before the test and be selected. After fasting for 2 to 3 hours, the temperature of the rabbit should be measured once every 1 hour with the anal thermometer (the stimulation of the rabbit should be avoided as much as possible during the temperature measurement, and the depth of the thermometer should be the same for each rabbit, generally about 5 cm), 4 times in all. If the body temperature of the 4 times is in the range of 38.0 ~ 39.6°C, and the difference between the highest and lowest body temperature is not more than 0.4°C, the rabbit can be used for test.

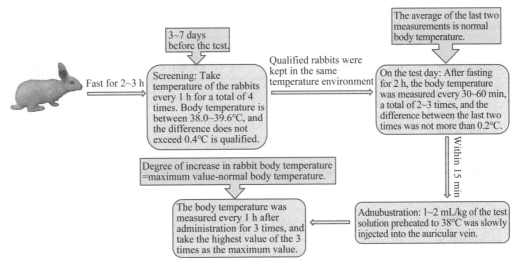

Figure 6-4-1   Schematic diagram of the operating procedure of pyrogen test in rabbits

(2) Determination method On the day of the test, after fasting for 2h, the rabbit's body temperature was measured once every 30 ~ 60 min with an anal thermometer, a total of 2 ~ 3 times. The difference between the last two body temperatures should not exceed 0.2°C. meaning that the average of the two body temperatures was taken as the normal body temperature of the rabbit. The normal body temperature should be within 38.0 ~ 39.6°C, and the temperature difference between the rabbits should not exceed 1°C. Three applicable rabbits were selected, 1 ~ 2 mL/kg of the test product solution preheated to 38°C was slowly injected into the ear limbo vein within 15 min after the normal temperature was determined. And then the temperature was measured once every 1h according to the previous method, a total of three times. Subtract the normal body temperature from the highest body temperature among the three times, that is the increased degree in the rabbit's body temperature.

[Experimental records and results]

The anal temperature measurements of rabbits were recorded and filled in Table 6-4-1.

[Result judgment]

(1) In 3 rabbits, if the temperature increase is below 0.6°C, and the total temperature increase of 3 rabbits is below 1.4°C, the test product should be considered to meet the requirements.

Table 6-4-1   Pyrogen test of injection

Date of examination			Room temperature		Checker	
Check name	Physicochemical properties and content				Lot number	
Rabbit number		1	2	3	4	5
Weight						
1st measurement						
2nd measurement						
Normal body temperature						
Time to inject the test product						
1st measurement						
2nd measurement						
3rd measurement						
Degree of increase in rabbit body temperature						
Examination conclusion						

(2) If only 1 rabbit in the 3 rabbits had a temperature increase of 0.6°C or more, or if the temperature increase of the 3 rabbits are all below 0.6°C, but the total temperature increase reaches 1.4°C or more, 5 rabbits should be selected for retest. In the retest, when the number of rabbits with a temperature increase of 0.6°C or above is not more than 1 among the 5 rabbits, and the total number of elevated body temperature of 8 rabbits (3 rabbits in initial test and 5 rabbits in retest) is not more than 3.5°C, the tested product should be considered to meet the requirements.

(3) When the number of rabbits with temperature increase of 0.6°C or above was more than 1 among the 3 rabbits in the initial test. Or more than 1 rabbit in the 5 rabbits in the retest had a temperature increase of 0.6°C or above. Or when the total body temperature increase of 8 rabbits exceeds 3.5°C, the tested product should be considered as not meeting the regulations.

[Precautions]

(1) Pyrogen test method is an absolute method, there is no standard product for test comparison at the same time, and it is judged by the degree of fever reaction of the specified animal. There are many factors affecting the change of animal body temperature, so the test must be carried out in strict accordance with the required conditions.

(2) The test syringes, needles and all utensils in contact with the test product should be heated in the oven for 250°C, 30 min or in the oven for 180°C, 2 hours to remove the pyrogens.

(3) Measuring the temperature of the rabbit or injection should be gentle, so as not to cause the animal to struggle and make the temperature fluctuate. When measuring the temperature, the mercury head of the anus thermometer is coated with liquid paraffin. Gently insert 5 cm deep into the anus and measure the temperature for at least 1.5 minutes. It is best to use the same thermometer for each rabbit's temperature measurement, and the temperature measurement time should be the same to reduce errors.

(4) The methods described in this experiment are mainly used for teaching experiments. Other matters can be referred to pharmacopoeia.

(5) It is also possible to add an appropriate amount of typhoid-paratyphoid vaccine or self-made non-sterile glucose solution into the test product, so that students can observe positive results.

[Practice questions]

1. Pyrogen test for injection is performed by _____.

A. limulus method   B. rabbit method

C. gel adsorption method   D. ultrafiltration

2. which following statement regarding the quality requirements for injections is incorrect?

A. Sterile   B. Colorless   C. Pyrogen free

D. pH should be equal to or close to the pH of the blood

3. The main components of pyrogen are _____.

A. heterologous proteins   B. lipopolysaccharides

C. cholesterol   D. Phospholipids

[Thinking questions]

(1) What are the requirements of pyrogen test for rabbits? What should be noted in the test?

(2) What means is pyrogen produced by in injection? How to remove?

[Knowledye expansion]

Be cautious of injection thermogenic reactions！

The generation of pyrogens in injections is multifaceted, such as from raw materials, from the utensils or containers used to prepare injections, from the solvents used in injections, and from contamination during the preparation process. Strict control and management are required at multiple stages, including packaging materials, injection water, raw materials, production equipment, and preparation processes, to reduce the generation and contamination of heat sources. In clinical practice, when administering large amounts of intravenous infusion, if the medication contains pyrogen, patients may experience symptoms such as chills, high fever, sweating, dizziness, vomiting, etc. within $0.5 \sim 1$ hour. During high fever, the body temperature can reach 40 ℃, and in severe cases, shock may occur. This phenomenon is called pyrogen reaction. According to incomplete statistics, there are currently over a hundred types of traditional Chinese medicine injections on the market in China. Among these injections, there are also some cases of adverse reactions, and regulatory authorities have tightened and restricted the use of related traditional Chinese medicine injections. For example, on January 11, 2022, the National Medical Products Administration announced that it would cease the production, sale, and use of Lianbizhi injection in China and cancel its drug registration certificate from that day on. Products that have already been put on the market for sale are recalled by the holder of the drug marketing authorization. Therefore, pharmaceutical manufacturers need to strictly control the quality of drugs to ensure their safety and effectiveness. Regulatory authorities should also strengthen the supervision of drugs, timely discover and handle drugs with quality problems, and ensure the safety of public medication. As a student majoring in medicine, whether engaged in drug production or clinical use in the future, it is necessary to be vigilant about the thermogenic reactions of injections and ensure the safety of medication for the public.

（邹莹莹）

Section 5　The inhibitory effect of doxorubicin on tumor cell growth *in vitro*

[Experiment objective]

(1) To observe the inhibitory effect of tumor cell growth of doxorubicin *in vitro* detectedby MTT assay.

(2) Master the experimental method of cell growth detection by MTT assay.

[Experimental principle]

Doxorubicin (The structural formula is shown in Figure 6-5-1), also known as Adriamycin, is an anticancer antibiotic. Its mechanism of action is to embed into tumor cell DNA, interfere with transcription and replication processes, cause DNA damage and cell cycle arrest, and ultimately induce cell death. It has a broad spectrum of antitumor activity, effective against a variety of cancers, and is lethal to tumor cells in all phases of the cell cycle, making it a non-specific phase drug. Clinically, it is used to treat malignant tumors such as acute leukemia, lymphoma, breast cancer, lung cancer, and bladder cancer.

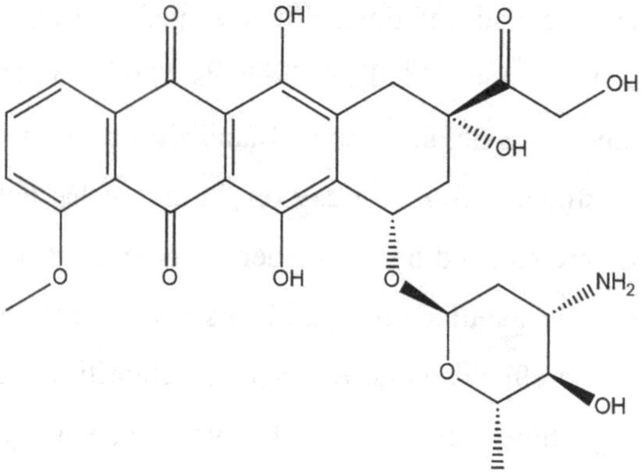

Figure 6-5-1　Chemical structure of doxorubicin

MTT〔3-(4,5-dimethylthiazol-2-yl)-2,5-diphenyltetrazolium bromide〕is a yellow tetrazolium salt that can be reduced to purple formazan by the mitochondrial dehydrogenase enzymes in living cells. The degree of reduction of MTT can reflect the activity of the cells, thereby being used to assess the inhibitory effect of drugs on cell growth.

[Experiment materials]

Medical purification workstation, benchtop centrifuge, enzyme-linked analyzer, CO_2 incubator, experimental pipettes, pipette tips, centrifuge tubes, and other glassware are all high-pressure sterilized and sterile, 96-well culture plates, etc.

[Experimental cell strain]

Human non-small cell lung cancer A549 cell strain.

[Experimental reagents]

Doxorubicin (stored at a concentration of 5 mg/mL), RPMI-1640 cell culture medium, fetal bovine serum, MTT (stored at a concentration of 5 mg/mL), DMSO, 0.25% trypsin, and Trypan blue dye.

[Experimental methods]

1. Cell culture and passaging

After resuscitation, cells are cultured using RPMI-1640 medium containing 10% fetal bovine serum, 100U/ml penicillin, and streptomycin. The culture conditions are at 37°C in a humidified atmosphere with 5% CO_2. When the cell confluence reaches 70% to 80%, passaging is performed. First, gently decant the culture medium and wash the cells with neutral PBS 1 to 2 times. Then, add an appropriate amount of trypsin pre-warmed to 37°C and gently rotate the culture flask to ensure full contact between the trypsin and the cell layer. Digest for 2 to 5 minutes at room temperature or incubate for 1 minute at 37°C until the cells detach. After aspirating the trypsin, add fresh medium containing serum to terminate the digestion process, and form a single-cell suspension by gently pipetting. Centrifuge at 800 rpm for 5 to 10 minutes, collect the cells, and passage at a ratio of 1 : 2 or 1 : 4.

2. Drug treatment

Select cells in the logarithmic growth phase, stain with trypan blue, and count them, adjusting the cell concentration to 2.5×10^4 cells/mL. Seed the cells into a 96-well culture plate with 200 μL per well. After the cells adhere overnight, add different final concentrations of doxorubicin (0.5, 1, 2, 4, 8, 16 μg/mL) to each drug treatment group, while the negative control group receives complete culture medium, and continue to culture for 48 hours with 4 replicates per group. Color development step: After 48 hours of culture, add 20 μL of 5 mg/mL MTT solution to each well and continue to incubate for 4 hours.

3. Termination of culture and absorbance measurement

After aspirating the supernatant from each well, add 150 μL of DMSO and gently agitate for 10 minutes to dissolve the formed crystals. Use an enzyme-linked analyzer to measure the absorbance of each well at a wavelength of 570 nm and record the data.

[Experimental records and results]

Record the absorbance values of each experimental group and analyze the results. Result analysis method:

Calculate the growth inhibition rate (GI) using the formula: GI (Growth Inhibition Rate) = 1− (OD value of the drug group / OD value of the negative control group) × 100%.

Use the NDST software to calculate the IC_{50} value of the drug after 48 hours of action according to the Bliss method.

[Precautions]

(1) The cell inoculation concentration should be appropriate, with 10^3 to 10^4 cells per well being ideal, and the OD values measured in the range of 0.4 to 0.8 are optimal for a linear relationship.

(2) The values from the outermost wells of a 96-well culture plate are biased when reading, and are generally not used. Set up a blank control without cells but with culture medium parallel to the experiment. Keep other experimental steps consistent, and finally adjust the zero with the blank in the colorimetric assay.

[Practice questions]

1. The mechanism by which doxorubicin produces anti-tumor activity is _____.

A. inhibition of DNA replication   B. methylation with DNA

C. inhibition of dihydrofolate reductase   D. interference with cell mitosis

2. When measuring cell activity using the MTT method, the absorbance is measured using an enzyme-linked immunosorbent assay at a wavelength of _____ nm.

A. 570   B. 480   C. 400   D. 440

[Thinking questions]

(1) The basic principle of the MTT method for detecting the inhibitory effect of drugs on the growth of tumor cells.

(2) The specific molecular mechanism by which doxorubicin inhibits the growth of tumor cells.

(3) Apart from MTT assay, what other experimental methods can be used to evaluate cell proliferation?

[Knowledye expansion]

The discovery of doxorubicin

Doxorubicin was initially extracted and isolated from the genus Actinobacteria in the mid-1960s, which is known for its natural presence in soil. It has become a "star" drug in the scientific research field of cancer treatment because it has been widely used in breast cancer, lung cancer, lymphatic cancer, ovarian cancer and other cancers in clinical treatment. Erythromycin is considered the prototype of anthracycline antibiotics, and researchers have discovered multiple anthracycline antibiotics or analogues. According to statistics, there are currently over 2000 doxorubicin analogues. The independently developed anti-tumor drug doxorubicin hydrochloride liposome injection in China was successfully launched in 2012, providing a powerful "weapon" for doctors and patients to face diseases.

（史立宏）

Section 6   The *in vitro* antibacterial effect of penicillin G

[Experimental objective]

(1) Master in experimental methods for *in vitro* determination of antibiotic antibacterial activity, including data recording and analysis.

(2) Understand and master the experimental techniques and scientific principles of the tube method and the paper disc method for determining the minimum inhibitory concentration (MIC) of antibiotics.

[Experimental principle]

Penicillin G is a bactericidal agent that exerts its effects during the rapid growth phase of bacteria, demonstrating significant antibacterial activity against Gram-positive bacteria and Gram-negative cocci. However, its bactericidal action against Gram-negative bacilli is relatively weaker. The primary mechanism of bactericidal action of penicillin G lies in its ability to interfere with the synthesis of bacterial cell wall peptidoglycan, leading to structural damage of the cell wall. This damage causes the bacteria to lose their natural protective barrier, resulting in cellular expansion and eventual lysis and death.

When assessing the *in vitro* antimicrobial activity of a drug, we typically use two key indicators: the Minimum Inhibitory Concentration (MIC) and the Minimum Bactericidal

Concentration (MBC). The MIC refers to the lowest concentration of a drug that can inhibit the growth of a pathogen under in vitro culture conditions, which is usually determined after 18 to 24 hours. The MBC, on the other hand, is the lowest concentration of a drug that can completely kill the bacteria present in the culture medium. If a drug can effectively inhibit or kill the pathogen at a low concentration, the pathogen is said to be "sensitive" to the drug. Conversely, if the drug cannot inhibit or kill the bacteria even at high concentrations, it is referred to as "resistant" or "non-sensitive."

To detect the sensitivity or resistance of bacteria to various drugs, we usually conduct susceptibility testing. Under *in vitro* culture conditions, the commonly used methods are the tube method and the disc method.

The tube method, also known as the dilution method, involves carrying out serial dilutions of the drug in a series of containers with bacterial culture medium, then adding the test bacteria. After a period of cultivation, the reaction of the bacteria to the drug is observed. Since there are differences in the growth rate and quantity of the test bacteria at different drug concentrations, this will lead to different degrees of turbidity in the culture medium, thereby reflecting the antimicrobial effect of the drug.

The disc method is a form of diffusion technique, where a disc impregnated with a drug is placed on a solid culture medium that has been inoculated with the test bacteria. The diffusion of the drug through the medium and the formation of an inhibition zone are observed. The presence and size of the inhibition zone can infer the inhibitory effect of the drug on bacterial growth. The greater the distance the drug diffuses, the stronger its bacteriostatic ability is indicated to be. Based on the size of the inhibition zone, we can assess the antimicrobial efficacy of the drug: an inhibition zone less than 10 millimeters indicates insensitivity, 10 millimeters indicates slight sensitivity, 11 to 15 millimeters indicates moderate sensitivity, and 16 to 20 millimeters indicates high sensitivity.

Staphylococcus aureus is a gram-positive coccus, while Escherichia coli is a gram-negative bacillus. By employing the tube method and the disc method, we can observe the differences in the antimicrobial activity of penicillin G against these two common clinical pathogens, thereby gaining a preliminary understanding of the characteristics of penicillin G's antimicrobial action.

[Experimental materials]

Sterilized small test tubes, test tube racks, pipettes (0.5mL, 2mL), sterilized cotton swabs, small forceps, circular filter paper (diameter 6 mm), culture dishes, and broth agar plates.

[Experimental strains]

Staphylococcus aureus standard strain (ATCC29213), Escherichia coli standard strain (ATCC35218).

[Experimental reagents]

Sterilized beef broth, MH medium, penicillin G.

[Experimental methods]

1. Tube Method (Dilution Method) Procedure:

(1) Tube Preparation: Select 10 clean, transparent, crack-free sterile test tubes and label them from 1 to 10.

(2) Culture Medium Addition: Accurately add 0.5 mL of pre-prepared beef broth culture medium to each test tube.

(3) Drug Dilution Preparation: Prepare a stock solution of penicillin G at 40 U/mL and allow it to equilibrate to room temperature.

(4) Serial Dilution Process: Add 0.5 mL of the stock solution to tube 1 as the initial concentration. Mix the solution in tube 1 thoroughly using a pipette, then transfer 0.5 mL to tube 2. Repeat this process up to tube 9, ensuring thorough mixing before each transfer; discard 0.5 mL of the solution from tube 9 to reduce error.

(5) Control Group Setup: Tube 10 serves as the control group, with no drug added, only culture medium and bacterial suspension.

(6) Bacterial Inoculation: Prepare bacterial suspensions of Staphylococcus aureus and Escherichia coli adjusted to approximately 10^8 CFU/Ml. Add 0.5 mL of the bacterial suspension to each test tube and gently shake to mix evenly.

(7) Incubation Condition: Place all test tubes in an incubator at 37°C and incubate for 18 to 24 hours.

(8) Observation and Recording: After incubation, observe for signs of bacterial growth in each test tube, such as turbidity or precipitation. Record the highest drug concentration at which bacterial growth is not observed, which will be the MIC for penicillin G.

2. Disc Method (Diffusion Method) Procedure:

(1) Culture Medium Preparation: Melt MH agar and adjust to $45 \sim 50°C$, pour into sterile petri dishes and allow to solidify.

(2) Bacterial Suspension Adjustment and Inoculation: Adjust the bacterial suspension to 0.5 McFarland standard using a McFarland turbidity standard. Use a sterile cotton swab to evenly inoculate the surface of the culture medium. Take care not to apply too much pressure to avoid damaging the agar surface.

(3) Drug Concentration Preparation: Dilute penicillin G to different concentrations ranging from $62.5 \sim 2000$ U/mL as required.

(4) Disc Treatment: Select appropriately sized sterile round filter paper discs, immerse two discs in the same concentration of drug solution to ensure complete saturation. Remove the discs and use a sterile forceps to gently remove excess solution, avoiding accumulation at the edges of the discs.

(5) Application of Discs: Place the drug-soaked discs on the inoculated culture medium surface, ensuring accurate spacing and positioning of the discs. Once placed, do not move or adjust the discs to avoid affecting drug diffusion.

(6) Incubation Conditions: Invert the petri dishes to prevent disc drying or movement, then place in an incubator at $37°C$ and incubate for 18 to 24 hours.

(7) Observation and Measurement: After incubation, observe from the back of the petri dish whether a clear inhibition zone has formed around each disc. Measure the diameter of the inhibition zone with a caliper and record the data.

(8) Data Analysis: Evaluate the antimicrobial effect of penicillin G against Staphylococcus aureus and Escherichia coli based on the size of the inhibition zones and compare the results.

[Experimental records and results]

Record the results of the experiment as shown in the Table 6-6-1 and Table 6-6-2.

Table 6-6-1 Penicillin G tube method results record for Staphylococcus aureus

Tube Number	1	2	3	4	5	6	7	8	9	10
Dilution Factor	1	2	4	8	16	32	64	128	256	0
Final Concentration (U/mL)	10	5	2.5	1.25	0.625	0.313	0.16	0.08	0.04	–
Turbidity (Presence/Absence)										

Table 6-6-2 The inhibitory zone diameter of penicillin G for Staphylococcus aureus
and Escherichia coli (mm)

Bacteria type	Penicillin G Concentration (U/mL)					
	2000	1000	500	250	125	62.5
Staphylococcus aureus						
Escherichia coli						

[Precautions]

(1) Staphylococcus aureus and Escherichia coli are both potential pathogens, so personal protective measures should be strictly followed during the experiment, and care should be taken to prevent bacterial contamination of other items or the environment.

(2) Ensure accurate measurement of liquids during the operation. When using the tube method, observations should be meticulous. When performing the disc method, the placement of the discs should be carefully planned in advance.

(3) Sterile operation is required. The experimental bench should be thoroughly cleaned before the experiment, and disinfected with ultraviolet lamps or disinfectants.

(4) Preparation and sterilization of the culture medium.Ensure the components of the culture medium are accurate and error-free, and avoid overheating during the sterilization process to prevent damage to the nutritional components in the culture medium.

(5) Preparation of experimental materials. All materials should be checked for completeness before the experiment to avoid affecting the results due to equipment issues during the process.

(6) Recording and organizing experimental results. Each step's conditions and observations should be recorded in detail during the experiment, and data should be organized promptly after the experiment is concluded.

(7) Cleaning and disinfection after the experiment. All used equipment should be thoroughly cleaned and disinfected after the experiment to prevent cross-contamination.

(8) Experimental safety. when handling potential pathogens, appropriate personal protective equipment should be worn, such as laboratory coats, gloves, and masks.

[Thinking questions]

(1) What could account for the differences in the antimicrobial activity of penicillin G against Staphylococcus aureus and Escherichia coli?

(2) In the disc diffusion test, how can one interpret the observation that the zone of inhibition diameter at a certain concentration of penicillin G is significantly smaller than at other concentrations?

[Knowledye expansion]

The discovery of penicillin

The discovery of penicillin is a story filled with serendipity and scientific insight. In 1928, the British bacteriologist Alexander Fleming accidentally discovered this revolutionary antibiotic in the laboratory at St. Mary's Hospital Medical School, London. At that time, he was about to go on vacation but left behind some unwashed petri dishes. Upon his return, he found that one of the dishes had been contaminated by a greenish mold. A zone devoid of bacterial growth around this mold piqued Fleming's great interest.

Fleming found that this mold, later identified as Penicillium, could kill a variety of bacteria, including Staphylococcus aureus, a common pathogen. He realized that this might be a substance with powerful bactericidal properties, so he began to research and ultimately isolated penicillin. However, Fleming encountered difficulties in extracting and purifying penicillin, and his research was not widely recognized or applied for a period of time.

It was not until 1939 that Howard W. Florey and Ernst B. Chain at the University of Oxford repeated Fleming's work and successfully purified penicillin, making it available for clinical treatment. During World War II, the large-scale production and application of penicillin saved countless lives, marking the beginning of the antibiotic era. Fleming, Florey, and Chain were jointly awarded the Nobel Prize in Physiology or Medicine in 1945 for their contributions to the discovery and application of penicillin.

The discovery of penicillin not only ushered in a new era of antibiotic therapy but also promoted the search for and research of other antimicrobial substances, greatly improving human health conditions and life expectancy. Although resistance to penicillin and allergic reactions to it have emerged subsequently, the discovery of penicillin is undoubtedly a milestone in the history of medicine.

（史立宏）

Chapter 7　Experimental design

Section 1　The objective and significance of experimental design

Experiment design is a kind of planned research, which is the core of scientific research work. The scientificity, rationality and feasibility of experiment design will determine the reliability of experimental conclusions directly. In general, experiment design is a general procedure of scientific research, including the process of question raising, hypothesis formation, variable selection, experimental method, result analysis, paper writing and other scientific research. While in the narrow sense, experiment design refers to the design of a reliable experimental scheme, and the implementation of the experiment and its related statistical analysis process according to the scheme, focusing on the process from the establishment of hypotheses to the conclusion. In this chapter, the design of pharmacological experiments falls into the latter category.

The objective of the experiment design is to obtain a deep understanding of the research object through reasonable variables, condition setting and data analysis, so as to explore the essential characteristics, regularity and function of things, provide real and reliable data basis for researchers, and promote the continuous update and development of scientific knowledge. For pharmacological experiments, due to experimental errors and differences between experimental subjects (such as experimental animals, isolated organs, etc.), experimental conditions must be strictly controlled to eliminate factors that may interfere with the results to obtain accurate and reliable experimental conclusions, so as to further understand the law of interaction between drugs and the body.

The significance of experiment design lies in the strict control of experimental errors through the purposeful, planned and step-by-step arrangement of various experimental factors, thus the experimenter will obtain abundant and reliable data to the maximum extent with less manpower, material resources and time. A thorough and perfect experimental design can correctly reflect the inherent laws of the development of things, provide useful guidance and reference for scientific research and technological application, and promote the development and technological innovation in the field of science.

In general, experiment design is the basis of experimental process, the premise of experimental data processing, and an important guarantee for improving scientific research results. In the medical scientific research work, whether laboratory research, clinical efficacy observation or field investigation, the research plan should be carefully considered according to the purpose and conditions of the experiment, combined with the requirements of statistics, and the whole process of the experiment.

（王姿颖）

Section 2　The basic elements and principles of experimental design

| The basic elements of experimental design

Experiment design includes three basic elements: experimental object, treatment factor and observation index.

1. Experimental object

The experimental object refers to the object being tested, which can be normal or pathological. The experimental objects of pharmacological experiments are mainly human and animal, including tissues and organs both in vivo and *in vitro*.

Human being are the subjects of clinical pharmacology studies, including healthy volunteers and patients. Human experiments must follow the Declaration of Helsinki, that is, in the process of human experiments, the consideration of the health of the subjects must take precedence over the interests of science and society, scientific research in line with medical purposes must be adhered to, the rights and interests of the subjects must be protected, and the subjects' personality and right to informed consent must be respected.

For animals, generally speaking, different experimental animals may have similar responses to the some same drug, but various experimental animals will have quantitative and qualitative responses to the drug due to species differences. Therefore, different experimental animals should be selected according to the experimental purpose, method and the characteristics of the animals themselves.

Commonly used experimental animals in pharmacological experiments include rats, mice, guinea pigs, frogs (or toads), rabbits, cats, dogs, sheep, etc., and sometimes primates may be selected in special cases.

2. Treatment factors

Treatment factors refer to the external intervention applied to the experimental subjects, including physical factors (such as sound, light, heat, rays, etc.), chemical factors (such as toxins, nutrient solutions, etc.), biological factors (such as bacteria, viruses, etc.), drug factors, trauma, surgery and other factors. The first purpose of applying the processing factors is to replicate the human disease models, observe the manifestations of the diseases, and analyze the etiology and pathogenesis of the diseases. The second is to observe the intervention effect of drugs or other therapeutic means.

In the process of experiment design, treatment factors may be single or multiple. Single-factor design means that only one treatment factor is involved and the effect on the experimental object is observed. Multi-factor design refers to giving multiple treatment factors and observing the effects on the experimental subjects. Multi-factor analysis, also known as multivariate analysis or multivariate analysis, is a kind of analysis method to study the relationship between multiple related factors and the relationship between samples with these factors. The main objective of this method is to simplify complex problems, grasp the main contradiction of things, and reduce the workload. Orthogonal test, regression analysis, cluster analysis and so on all belong to multi-factor analysis methods.

3. Observation index

Observation index is a marker that reflects the change of physiological or pathological state of experimental subjects after treatment by various factors. The selection of observation index should be based on the premise of repeatability, feasibility and acceptance as far as possible. Advanced instruments, stable techniques and quantitative indicators should be used to reduce the influence of subjectivity on the judgment of experimental results.

‖ Basic principles of experiment design

Experiment design is a subject based on logical reasoning and statistical analysis, which should follow the three basic principles which are repetition, control and randomization.

1. Principle of replication

Replication is also known as reproducibility. Due to individual differences or experimental errors, it is often difficult to obtain reliable conclusions based on the results obtained from only one experiment or one sample. The more repetitions within a certain range, the results will be more reliable. In addition to increasing accuracy and reliability, replication also allows the experimenters to understand the variation. But if the sample size is too large, the consumption of manpower, material resources and time is not in line with economic principles. Therefore, in the design of pharmacological experiments, the researchers should consider how to conduct experiments with appropriate samples to ensure the accuracy of results.

The following factors will be considered in the estimation of sample size:

(1) Coefficient of variation (CV)

The larger the coefficient of variation is, the larger the sample should be. If the coefficient of variation is small, only a small sample is needed to obtain a significant difference.

(2) Confidence limit

If the confidence limit is small, the sample needs to be increased. On the contrary, if the confidence limit is large, the sample can be small.

(3) Probability (P-value)

If the P-value is required to be small, the sample must be increased. Conversely, if the P-value is set large, the sample can be small.

In animal studies, for small animals (mice, frogs, etc.), the sample size should be no less than 10 cases per group in measurement data, and no less than 30 cases in count data. For medium animals (rabbits, guinea pigs, etc.), the sample size should be no less than 6 cases per group in measurement data, and no less than 20 cases in count data. For large animals (dogs, cats, sheep, etc.), the sample size should be no less than 5 cases per group in measurement data, and no less than 15 cases in count data.

In clinical studies, the sample size should be $5 \sim 10$ cases of refractory diseases (cancer, rabies, etc.), $30 \sim 50$ cases of severe disease (shock, heart failure, meningitis, etc.); while in general or chronic diseases should be $100 \sim 500$ cases.

2. The principle of comparison

In order to observe the effects of treatment factors on experimental subjects, comparison before and after treatment or between different groups should be carried out during the experiments. An appropriate control group must be raised in the experiment design. On the course of comparison, the experimentors should follow the principle of "homogeneity comparison", that is, any other condition except the factors studied should be identical so as to eliminate the interference of non-treatment factors on the experiment results. The control can be divided into negative control and positive control due to the treatment factors. And the control can also be divided into self-control and inter-group control based on the experimental object.

(1) Negative control

Negative control includes the following items: ① Blank control, also known as normal control, which are normal subjects without any treatment factors. ② Sham-treatment control, which is commonly used in pharmacological experiments. That is, apart from the appointed treatment factors (such as drugs), the subjects are treated with the same procedures such as anesthesia, surgery or given drug-free solvents, etc. This control method is commonly used. ③ Placebo control is a negative control commonly used in clinical trials. Placebo is a drug-like preparation made of a substance without special pharmacological activity.

(2) Positive control

Positive control also known as the standard control, that is, the experimental results are compared with the standard value. Positive control includes the following items: ① Standard control, which is using the typical drug or standard drug as the control in order to assess the strength of the drug. ② Positive control also refers to use the effective drug with the national approval number as the control. If a new drug is significantly superior to the old one, the value of the new drug might be affirmed.

(3) Self control

Self control refers to the same subject itself compared before and after treatment.

(4) Intergroup control

Intergroup control refers to several parallel design in the experiment group compared among groups.

3. The principle of random

Considering there are individual differences in the responses of experimental subjects to treatment factors, the grouping should be based on the principle of randomization. Each individual has an equal opportunity to receive treatment in the experiment so as to avoid or reduce intentional or unintentional biases. The commonly used random grouping methods include complete random grouping method, random block method, Latin square stochastic method and paired stochastic method. The most commonly used method in pharmacological experiments is the random block method. The grouping process is as follows: ① Queuing: all animals are ranked according to a certain condition. ② Blocking: all animals are divided into several areas with the number of animals in each area which is equal to the number of groups. ③ Take random numbers refer to affiliated Table X random number table, note that the numbers in the table must be used continuously, while the choice of direction is more flexible (horizontal or vertical). ④ Determine the divisor: the divisor reprensents the possibility of each animal in each block being divided into each group. ⑤ Calculate the remainder: divide the random number by the corresponding divisor to get the remainder. Note that there may be two special cases as the dividend is less than the divisor or exact division. In those cases, the divisor is used instead of the remainder. ⑥ Determine the groups: the animals in each group are assigned according to the numbers of the remainder.

Take "14 mice divided into four groups" as an example. The detailed grouping procedures and results are shown in Table 7-2-1 and Table 7-2-2.

Table 7-2-1　An example of random block grouping

Number	1	2	3	4	5	6	7	8	9	10	11	12	13	14
Weight (g)	18	18	18	19	19	19	19	19	19	20	20	21	21	21
Random number	68	65	84	68	95	23	92	35	87	02	22	57	51	61
Divisor	4	3	2	1	4	3	2	1	4	3	2	1	4	3
Remainder	4	2	2	1	3	2	2	1	3	3	2	1	3	1
Group	4	2	3	1	3	2	4	1	3	4	2	1	3	1

Table 7-2-2　The results of grouping

Group	Animal number(weight)			
1	4(19)	8(19)	12(21)	14(21)
2	2(18)	6(19)	11(20)	
3	3(18)	5(19)	9(19)	13(21)
4	1(18)	7(19)	10(20)	

（王姿颖）

Section 3   The main content and method of experimental design

The main content of experimental design includes the following items:

Ⅰ To establish clear aims and tasks

Before the experiment design, the first thing for the researcher is to establish clear experimental targets, which is the core of the problem. The aims of experiment must be prominent, avoiding to be too much.

Ⅱ To ensure the main elements of the experimental design

1. Select the appropriate experimental subjects

In the experiment design, it is necessary to specify what kind of experimental objects should be used according to the purpose and content of experimental observation, combined with the physiological characteristics of experimental objects and their sensitivity to treatment factors and actual conditions. The consistency and representativeness of experimental objects must be ensured in the experiment design. (For detail, please see section)

2. Set up stable and reliable processing factors

Treatment factors refer to certain factors that are planned to be applied to experimental subjects in an experimental study, such as nutrient solution, feed, etc. For example, several therapies or drugs to treat a disease in nutritional experiments and different doses of a drug in pharmacological studies all belong to treatment factors. Accepted and reliable treatment methods should be used in experimental design. Take an example, to study the effect of lipid-regulating drugs, experimental hyperlipidemia models is commonly used by feeding experimental animals with a certain proportion of high-fat diet. If someone wants to improve or innovate the typical method, besides a scientific basis, it is still necessary for him to test the stability and sensitivity of the method, and compare it with the standard method to ensure that it is reliable before application.

In the whole process of the experiment, the treatment factors should always remain constant. If the treatment factor is a drug, the composition, content, batch number of the drug must remain unchanged. If the treatment factor of the experiment is surgery, the proficiency level of the operator should be consistent before the experiment.

3. Select reliable observation indexes

Observation index may reflect the effects of experimental factors on experimental subjects, which need to meet with the following requirements. ① can reflect the nature of the problem being studied and have specific reliability, ② as objective as possible to avoid or reduce the interference of subjective factors, ③ better to be quantitative reaction, which can be measured quantitatively to obtain accurate data.

III Highlight the three principles of experimental design

The principle of replication, comparison and randomness should be reflected by determining the sample size in the experimental design, setting up appropriate control group and randomly grouping experimental objects respectively. The specific scheme is described in Section 2 of this chapter.

IV Organization and implementation of experiments

Detailed experimental steps, technical means, manners of control and implementation methods may ensure the progress of the experiment.

V Map out the record format of experiment

The original record is not only the important document of the experiment but also the basis for judging the experimental results. In the experiment design, the format of the experimental record should be prepared to ensure the orderly conduct of the experiment. In general, experimental records should include: ① conditions of experimental subjects: such as the species, gender, weight of experimental animals, ② setting of treatment factors: such as drug source, batch number, dosage form, concentration, dose, route of administration, etc., ③ experimental environmental conditions: such as laboratory temperature, humidity, etc., ④ experimental schedule, methods and procedures, ⑤ data or graphs to observe the change of indicators, ⑥ information of experimenter, etc.

VI Statistics

The experimental data were divided into measurement data and counting data, corresponding to quantitative response and qualitative response in pharmacological effects.

The former refers to data with continuous quantitative changes that can be measured with specific tools, such as weight, blood pressure, blood glucose, etc. The latter refers to whether the effect occurs (all or none, positive or negative), such as death or survival, effective or ineffective. In the experimental design, the statistical treatment method of experimental results should be prepared. Generally speaking, the measurement data can be used student's t test or ANOVA, and the counting data can be used x^2 test or Fisher direct probability method.

In conclusion, when doing experiment design, the researchers must clarify their mind. Hypothesis is proposed according to the experimental purpose. Subjects and variables are determined based on the hypothesis. Corresponding methods and measures are adopted according to the experimental variables. Experimental procedures are arranged according to the variable control. Suitable equipment and reaction conditions are selected. In the process of implementation, comparison and control should be emphasized so as to ensure that the experiment to be as scientific and effective as possible.

（王姿颖）

Section 4　Types of experimental design

Experimental design covers a variety of types from basic scientific research to practical application fields. Researchers can choose suitable experiment design types according to different research purposes and conditions. Commonly used experiment designs include the following types：

1. Factor design

According to the number of independent variables in the experiment, the design can be divided into single-factor design and multi-factor design. The former is simple and easy to be carried out, which is suitable for the relatively simple situations. The latter might take multiple influencing factors into account and is suitable for complex situations.

2. Quasi-experiment design

Considering that some irrelevant variables may affect the experimental results which is difficult to properly be controlled in practice, quasi-experimental design can be adopted. The characteristic of quasi-experimental design is that no randomization procedure is adopted.

The choice, grouping, processing and allocation of subjects are not randomly arranged.

3. Non-experiment design

Non-experiment design is used to determine naturally occurring critical variables and their interrelationships. There are several research methods for non-experiment design, such as natural observation method, correlation method, interview method and so on.

4. Pre-experiment design

Pre-experimental design refers to that a small-scale experiment is conducted to test the feasibility and effect of the experiment before the formal experiment.

5. True experiment design

True experimental design means that experiments conducted under strictly controlled conditions, usually involving random assignment and the setting of a control group.

6. Market testing

Market testing is a type of specific experiment design for the field of market research that is used to evaluate the market response and effectiveness of a product or service.

7. Parallel group design

Parallel group design is also known as group design, which means that the eligible subjects were randomly assigned to the experimental group and the control group to receive different treatments respectively. The effectiveness and safety information were collected to illustrate the effect of the intervention by comparison. The advantage of this design is that it can effectively avoid selection bias and increase the equilibrium comparability of treatment groups.

8. Factorial design

Factorial design is a method by combining the levels of two or more treatment factors to evaluate various possible combinations. Factorial design is suitable for analyzing the main effects and interactions of multiple factors.

9. Matching design

Matching design refers to conduct experimental research by matching the research subjects into pairs according to certain conditions.

10. Random block design

The process of random block design is as follows. First, research objects with similar conditions are matched into groups, and then assigned to different processing groups according to randomization method to enhance the balance among the processing groups.

11. Repeated measurement design

The efficiency indexes of the same subject are repeatedly observed at multiple time points to explore the changes of the same subject at different time points.

12. Single-blind and double-blind design

Single-blind and double-blind design are related to the state of knowing the grouping information. Participant in the design of single-blind design doesn't know whether he (or she) belongs to the experimental group or control group, while in the design of double-blind, both the participants and researchers don't know the grouping information.

Section 5　The procedure and requirement of experimental design

| The procedure of experimental design

The steps of experimental design refer to the experimental design carried out by the experimenter according to certain procedures and methods in specific practice. As follows:

1. Raise the proposal

Before the experimental design, it is necessary to clarify the research problem, which is the starting point and basis of the experiment. By referring to the literature related to the subject, the researchers may understand the current developments and advanced methods worldwide, so as to set up a scientific, innovative and feasible proposal.

2. Set up the experimental objectives

The researchers should clarify the objectives and expected results of the experiment according to the research questions. Experimental objectives should be closely related to the research problems and have specific measurable criteria.

3. Determine the experimental variables

Experimental variables are the subjects that may affect the results of the experiment and should be controlled and adjusted. Both independent and dependent variables should be clearly defined during experimental design.

4. Design the experimental procedure

The researchers should determine the experimental steps and the operation process based on the research target. The experimental procedure should be systematic and logical to ensure the reliability and effectiveness of the experiment.

5. Determine the research object and sample size

The researchers should determine the representative types of research subjects and sample size for the experiment according to the research question and experimental objectives.

6. Set out methods for data collection and processing

The researchers should set out methods for experimental data collection and processing. The data collection method should be accurate and repeatable, and the data processing method should match the research problem and the experimental goal.

7. Conduct pre-experiment

Before the formal experiment, pre-experiment might be helpful for the researchers to check the feasibility of experimental steps and operating methods, so as to find and solve potential problems in time.

8. Conduct formal experiments

Conduct formal experiments according to the requirements of the experimental design and plan is the main content of the research work. In the process of experiment, it is necessary to carefully record the original experimental data and experimental operation to ensure the reliability and reproducibility of the experiment.

9. Data analysis and result interpretation

Conduct data analysis and result interpretation based on experimental data is also very important. Data analysis should follow scientific statistical methods and data processing principles. The discussion of the results should be consistent with the experimental objectives and research questions.

10. Get the conclusion

By objectively analyzing and evaluating experimental data and results, the researchers may draw the conclusion which can provide answers to research questions and suggestions for further research.

‖ The requirements of experimental design for students

Students' experiment design is a kind of independent learning activity, which is based on the study of the subject, designed and carried out by the students themselves. Through experiment design, students are trained to search and consult literature, think independently, analyze and solve problems. This kind of learning experience will offer a solid foundation for their scientific research career in the future.

The main requirements for students' experiment design report include the following items: ① title, ② background (including main references), ③ objective, ④ materials, ⑤ methods, ⑥ expected results and ⑦ expected conclusions.

（王姿颖）

Chapter 8　Case analysis

Case 1

[Case]

Patient Zhang, female, 42 years old. Admitted due to severe abdominal pain. Before admission, the patient had intermittent upper abdominal colic attacks for several years, accompanied by symptoms such as nausea, vomiting, and diarrhea, diagnosed as gallstones and chronic cholecystitis. Before admission, the patient had been injected with morphine due to pain. After taking the medication, the patient experienced severe vomiting, slowed breathing, and controlled diarrhea. After admission, intravenous infusion of cefradine and intramuscular injection of 50 mg of pethidine and 0.5 mg of atropine were administered every 3 ~ 4 hours, while surgical treatment was performed simultaneously. The postoperative patient experienced pain in the wound and continued to use pethidine. The patient really wants to be injected with pethidine. If not used for a day, the limbs will feel cold, the emotions will be uneasy, the hands and feet will become numb, the anger will be urgent, the speech will be vague, and even the temper will be angry. She needs to inject pethidine 4 times a day, 300 ~ 400 mg per day, and add sedative hypnotic drugs at night to help her fall asleep peacefully. Afterwards, the patient was transferred to a psychiatric hospital.

[Discussion]

(1) Try to analyze whether the patient's use of morphine and pethidine before and after admission is appropriate?

(2) What are the possible reasons for patients to continue using pethidine after discharge?

(3) What is the basis for using pethidine in combination with atropine?

(4) What is the reason for the patient's slow breathing and controlled diarrhea after using morphine before admission?

（高　伟）

Case 2

[Case]

Patient Yang, male, 66 years old. Admitted due to pneumothorax. The patient has a history of rheumatoid arthritis for 17 years. He has been taking prednisone irregularly for a long time, and has been suffering from chronic cough for more than 30 years. He was admitted to the hospital with chronic bronchitis, pulmonary tuberculosis accompanied with pneumothorax this time. After admission, the patient underwent vacuum aspiration and closed chest drainage, and was given anti-infection and anti-tuberculosis treatment. During hospitalization, the patient experienced repeated episodes of fever, cough, sputum, pneumothorax, and presented with psychiatric symptoms, suggesting pulmonary encephalopathy. Intravenous infusion of lung brain mixture (containing dexamethasone) and prednisone resulted in significant upper abdominal pain and black stool after 4 days, as well as a decrease in blood pressure. The patient died on the fourth day after the onset of bleeding.

[Discussion]

(1) What complications did the patient experience after using hormones? What is the mechanism of occurrence?

(2) Please discuss how to use glucocorticoids correctly? What insights can be gained from this case?

（高　伟）

Case 3

[Case]

Patient Wu, female, 55 years old. Ms. Wu has a history of hypertension and coronary heart disease for 10 years. The doctor recommended that she take aspirin 100 mg orally every day, and she strictly followed the prescribed regimen to take the medication. At first everything was normal, but after taking aspirin for three months, she began to experience digestive symptoms such as upper abdominal pain and nausea. At first, the patient thought it was a diet issue, but her symptoms continued to worsen and she began to experience black stool. She realized the seriousness of the situation and immediately went to the hospital for treatment. After examination, the doctor diagnosed her with gastric ulcer bleeding caused by aspirin. The patient was urgently arranged to be hospitalized for treatment, receiving medication for hemostasis and gastric mucosal protection, and discontinuing aspirin. After communicating with the patient and her family, the doctor suggested switching to alternative medications such as clopidogrel and administering proton pump inhibitors to protect the gastric mucosa. In the subsequent follow-up examination, the patient's symptoms gradually improved and her stomach ulcer healed well.

[Discussion]

(1) What is the basis for the use of aspirin in this case?

(2) Try to analyze the mechanisms of adverse reactions that occurred after the use of aspirin in this case. Besides, what other adverse reactions may occur?

（高　伟）

Case 4

[Case]

Patient Wang, male, 45 years old. He took cefixime for 3 days due to acute respiratory infection. After treatment, his condition quickly improved. On the fourth day, he drank 4 bottles of beer while gathering with friends. A few hours later, the patient began to experience symptoms such as facial flushing, headache, nausea, palpitations, and felt unwell. He was immediately taken to the hospital and diagnosed with suspected "withdrawal symptoms", namely disulfiram-like reactions (similar to those caused by disulfiram for alcohol abstinence). Symptomatic treatment was provided, including fluid replacement, antiemetics, and monitoring vital signs. The condition improved and the body gradually recovered. During this process, the patient was informed of the serious risk of developing a disulfiram reaction.

[Discussion]

(1) Please analyze the mechanism of the disulfiram reaction?

(2) What are the dangers of taking cephalosporin drugs while drinking alcohol?

（高　伟）

Chapter 9　Common experimental instruments

Section 1　Information integrated signal acquisition and processing system

[Experimental objective]

    (1) Learn how to use information integrated signal acquisition and processing system.

    (2) Master the operation method of signal acquisition and processing system.

[Experimental principle]

    Along with the advances of science and technology and society, the electronic computer is widely used in management, finance, information networks, scientific research, and other fields. In pharmacological experiments, most of the experimental operations can be achieved by combining the biological signal acquisition system with the computer. Although there may be differences in signal acquisition equipment and analysis software produced by different manufacturers, the core components and basic principles are generally similar. There are a variety of signals emitted by living organisms, among which only electrical signals can be directly input into the amplifier, while non-electrical signals (such as blood pressure and tension) need to be converted into electrical signals by the corresponding sensors before they can be input into the amplifier. Electrical signals are amplified and filtering processed (to remove the interference signal of the biological signals, for example, 50 Hz AC power interference, the interference signal intensity is often greater than the biological electrical signals themselves. If they do not be filtered, it will hide the actual signal), and then converted to digital signals for computer processing, so as to get a clear signal of the image.

    The biological signal acquisition and processing system is an integrated signal acquisition, processing, and displaying system. It can replace traditional laboratory equipment, such as amplifier, recorders, stimulators, oscilloscopes, and electrocardiogram machines. And it has the capability of data processing, which is widely used in domestic colleges and universities. The application of this system significantly improved the experimental teaching method and realized the networking, digitalization and integration of educational means. The system consists of a host computer, system, sensor, software and printers, mainly used for the observation and test of organisms or *in vitro* tissue of the biological electrical signal and the signal such as tension, pressure and temperature, etc. And it can record and analyze the changes of the organism in different experimental conditions. This chapter focuses on the application and precautions of the biological signal acquisition and processing system.

[Experimental apparatus]

BL-422I information integrated intelligent signal acquisition and processing system

[Experimental animals]

It can detect and record functional signals of rabbits, toads, rats and other experimental animals.

[Experimental reagents]

Based on the pharmacological experiment projects.

[Experimental method]

This part mainly introduces the composition and basic application of BL-422I biological function experiment system.

1. Composition of the system

BL-422I informatization integrated signal acquisition and processing system adopts the integrated design principles and integrates the mobile experiment platform, biological acquisition system, respiratory system, temperature measuring system, lighting system and synchronization demonstration system. Experimental data, report processing paperless, assist the teacher in the experiment information management. Help researchers obtain more objective and comprehensive experimental data, which can be used in various physiological, pharmacological, and pathophysiological experiments.

BL-422I biological function experiment system is a multi-channel biological signal acquisition, amplification, displaying, recording, and processing system configured on a microcomputer. It consists of four parts: computer, system hardware, biological signal display and processing software and control unit. The system detects biological electrical signals in biological organs in vivo or in vitro or tension, pressure and other non-electrical signals, and can be carried out on the experimental data storage, analysis and processing.

2. Operation of switching machine

1) Boot the operating

(1) Please press the main power button on the right side of the machine, as shown in Figure 9-1-1.

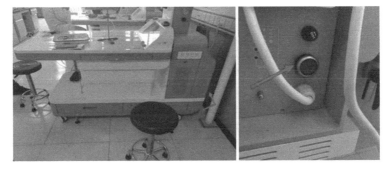

Figure 9-1-1　Schematic diagram of BL-422I biological function experiment system start-up

(2) After pressing the total power, wait for Windows to enter the desktop;

(3) Normal experiments can be performed after the BL-422I system is connected with the plate.

2) Shutdown operation

(1) Be sure to use the tablet to turn off Windows system (please follow Figure 9-1-2);

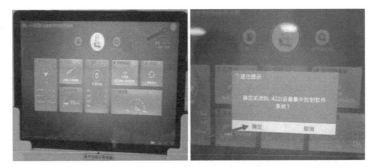

Figure 9-1-2　BL-422I biological function experimental system shutdown

(2) Be sure to wait for 1 minute (after being integrated systems all stop running) to close the machine's total power supply.

3. Brief steps for the operation of the main interface

Software panel interface: BL-422I supporting software is the software shared by the 420N biological acquisition equipment, which is the main hardware of the system. It uses Windows system as the software platform, applies both Chinese and English bilingual and graphical operation interface, and presets 55 experimental modules in ten categories. Determine the specific operational steps based on the experimental project . The main interface of the software is seen in Figure 9-1-3. Enable software, insert the corresponding transducer or accessory according to the instructions, and then follow the instructions to operate (Figure 9-1-4).

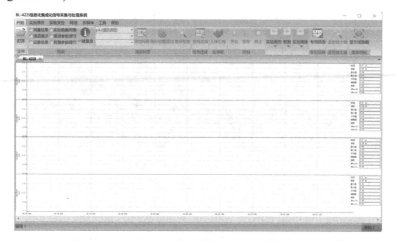

Figure 9-1-3   Main interface of BL-422I biological function experiment system

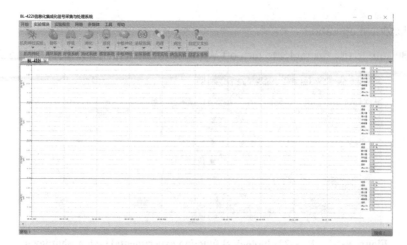

Figure 9-1-4   Alternative experimental items for the BL-422I biological function experimental system

[Precautions]

(1) Be sure to follow the operating instructions, especially do not use the Windows interface to shut down the machine.

(2) Take care of the equipment and prevent violent insertion and disassembly of the transducer.

[Practice questions]

1. The main advantage of BL-422I information-based integrated intelligent signal acquisition and processing system is _____.

A. highlight intelligence

B. integration of biological information acquisition function

C. highlight the information

D. none of the above is true

2. The working principle of BL-422I information integrated intelligent signal acquisition and processing system is _____.

A. artificial intelligent

B. biological signals into electrical signals and digital signals

C. the digital signal was entered manually

D. according to the experimental animals

[Thinking questions]

(1) What is the working principle of biological information acquisition system?

(2) How to use an information-based integrated signal acquisition and processing system to design an experiment on the effects of sulfamethoxazole drugs on rabbit kidney function?

[Knowledye expansion]

Continuous innovation in the field of medical technology in China

In the fields of the people's livelihood and technology, significant progress has been made in China. Medical heavy ion accelerators, magnetic resonance, color ultrasound, and CT localization of high-end medical equipment replacement made significant breakthroughs. As important tools of modern medical diagnosis, high-end medical equipment such as CT, color ultrasound and magnetic resonance imaging provide strong support for the Healthy China strategy. Especially in the fight against the new crown in the process of the outbreak, CT as a key equipment of diagnosis and treatment has played a vital role. According to the research report on China's Medical Imaging Industry Chain in 2020, CT has become one of the fields with a high degree of localization in China's medical imaging industry, and many domestic high-end CT equipment has reached the international advanced level. However, 20 years ago, whether it was a tertiary hospital or county-level medical institution, CT equipment was not only limited in quantity but also relied on imports. The high price made it difficult for primary medical institutions to afford, and it was difficult for ordinary people to afford the examination cost.

In the face of this challenge, several local medical imaging equipment enterprises insist on independent research and development and gradually break the monopoly of foreign brands. Nowadays, several Chinese enterprises have successfully developed and produced high-end CT equipment, realizing the transition from relying on imports to independent production. This transformation not only reduces medical costs, and improves the accessibility of medical services, but also enhances China's independent innovation ability and international competitiveness in the field of medical science and technology.

（崔晓栋）

Section 2　Spectrophotometer

[Experimental objective]

(1) Learn how to use a spectrophotometer.

(2) Master the operation method of spectrophotometer.

[Experimental principle]

The working principle of a spectrophotometer is based on the selective absorption of light (wavelength of light) by substances. Different substances have their own absorption wavelengths. So when monochromatic light after light dispersion passes through a solution, certain wavelengths of light will be absorbed by the solution (reducing light energy). Therefore, at a certain wavelength, there is a certain proportional relationship between the concentration of substances in a solution and the degree of reduction in light energy, which conforms to Beer's Law.

The 721 spectrophotometer is a simple and easy-to-use universal instrument for spectrophotometry (Figure 9-2-1), capable of measuring transmittance, absorbance, and concentration within the allowable measurement range of 360 ~ 800 mm. Due to its relatively simple structure and high sensitivity and precision in measurement, it is widely used for qualitative and quantitative analysis in medical and health, clinical laboratory, biochemistry, petrochemicals, environmental testing and quality monitoring departments.

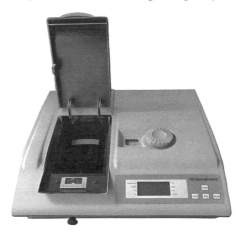

Figure 9-2-1   Spectrophotometer

[Usage method]

A spectrophotometer can use a series of spectroscopic devices to decompose complex light components into monochromatic light of specific wavelengths. When the sample is irradiated with monochromatic light for testing, some of the light is absorbed. By measuring the energy of the incident and transmitted light before and after passing through the sample, the absorbance of the tested substance at a specific wavelength or within a certain wavelength range can be detected. And then the substance can be qualitatively and quantitatively analyzed. The commonly used wavelength ranges are: UV range of 200 ~ 400 nm, visible range of 400 ~ 760 nm, and infrared range of 2.5 ~ 25 μm. The instruments used can be divided into ultraviolet spectrophotometer, visible spectrophotometer, infrared spectrophotometer or atomic absorption spectrophotometer.

1. Preparation before using the instrument

① First, connect the power supply, turn on the power switch, the indicator light will turn on. Open the colorimetric chamber and preheat for 20 minutes. ② Rotate the wavelength selection button to choose the desired monochromatic light wavelength. ③ Press the MODE button, select the transmittance (T), open the dark box cover of the colorimetric dish, place the colorimetric dish, press the zero adjustment button (0%T), and make the screen display 0.00. Close the dark box cover of the colorimetric dish, push the colorimetric dish lever to the blank correction position, press the OA button to adjust (100%T), so that the screen displays 100. After stabilization, press the MODE button to select the absorbance (A), and then proceed with the measurement work.

2. Sample testing

Place the colorimetric dish containing the solution in the colorimetric dish rack, cover the colorimetric dish dark box cover, pull the colorimetric dish rod to place the sample solution on the optical path, read the absorbance value, and immediately open the colorimetric dish dark box cover after reading. Measure three times and take the average. After the measurement is completed, take out the colorimetric dish, wash it, and invert it on filter paper to dry. Turn off the power switch and unplug the power plug.

[Precautions]

(1) Be careful, cautious, and strictly follow the operating requirements when using instruments.

(2) The instrument should be placed on a fixed and non-vibrating instrument to prevent vibration, moisture, magnetic fields, and direct sunlight.

(3) The tested sample should ensure that the solvent and solute are fully dissolved and stable, without suspended solids or volatility, to avoid unstable instrument detection.

(4) It is strictly prohibited to hold the optical surface of the colorimetric cup by hand.

After using the colorimetric cup, it should be immediately rinsed with tap water and then washed with distilled water. After washing, the colorimetric cup should be inverted and dried, or the water should be sucked off with filter paper, and then gently wiped dry with lens wiping paper.

(5) The colorimetric dishes for different testing items cannot be mixed. Quartz colorimetric dishes are used for UV region colorimetry, and glass colorimetric dishes are used for visible region colorimetry.

[Practice questions]

1. A spectrophotometer is based on the selectivity of substances towards _____.

A. electricity　　　　B. light　　　　　　C. water　　　　　　D. atoms

2. Hold _____ of the colorimetric cup with your hands.

A. optical surface　　　　　　　　　　B. frosted glass surface

C. top surface　　　　　　　　　　　　D. side surface

[Thinking questions]

(1) What is the working principle of the 721 spectrophotometer?

(2) What should be noted when operating a 721 spectrophotometer?

（李文涛）

Section 3　Physiological and pharmacological electronic stimulators

[Experimental objective]

Learn the operating principles and usage methods of physiological and pharmacological electronic stimulators.

[Working principle]

Electrical (square wave) stimulation is one of the most commonly used experimental methods in physiology and pharmacology. There are hundreds of pharmacological experimental methods that use electrical stimulation, but the strength of the stimulator function, the width of the square wave setting range, the quality of the waveform, and the ease of use often become the key to the success or failure of the experiment.

The YLS-9A stimulator is a multi-purpose square wave stimulator, as shown in Figure 9-3-1. The output voltage range is wide, up to 200 V, with current limiting protection function and adjustable current limiting. The maximum output current is 2 mA, and the stimulation output is completely isolated from the control circuit. Multiple types of output square waves can be customized through parameter settings. The output can be triggered by a switch or an external input signal. When triggered by an external input signal, it can be set as a delayed output with adjustable delay time. The output square wave includes three waveforms: positive pulse, positive pulse + gap + negative pulse, and positive pulse + negative pulse. The number of output pulses can be adjusted, and the voltage and current during output process can be adjusted, which can meet the needs of various experiments such as physiology and pharmacology. The instrument adopts a liquid crystal panel to display the current output parameters in Chinese, which is very intuitive and can store 8 set waveform parameters, making it convenient for experimental personnel to operate.

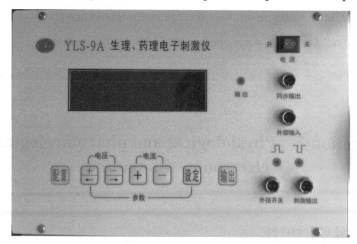

Figure 9-3-1   YLS-9A Physiological and pharmacological electronic stimulator

Instrument features:

(1) Bidirectional pulse: Bidirectional pulse solves the problem of long-term use of a polarized stimulus to generate polarization reactions around the electrode, thereby protecting tissues such as nerves, muscles, and blood vessels in contact with the electrode and avoiding tissue polarization effects.

(2) High voltage: High voltage can be used for strong stimulation of animals, such as convulsions, irritation, stabbing, and stimulation of large animals, such as pigs, dogs, monkeys, rabbits, etc., solving the problem of low stimulation voltage in some biological signal acquisition and processing systems.

(3) Current limit: On the one hand, it protects the stimulus object from high current damage, and on the other hand, it protects the instrument from current damage. When the output current exceeds the current limit value, the instrument automatically reduces the pulse amplitude to ensure that the current does not exceed the set value.

(4) Gradient Boosting: When set to continuous wave variable voltage output mode, the output will automatically boost according to the original set value and incremental interval, as well as incremental automatic boosting output (or decompression output), which is very convenient for pain and anger experiments.

(5) External trigger output: External trigger output is to output one or a set of signals of the same polarity at the output terminal after inputting a pulse signal or a set of pulse signals to the outside. As its output voltage and current are adjustable, it plays a role in signal amplification and waveform shaping.

(6) The portable structure is convenient for movement and stacking.

[Main technical indicators]

Square wave output types: single wave output, single wave intermittent output, continuous wave output, continuous wave intermittent output, continuous wave transformer output, external wave input, transformer current output.

Square wave parameters: Voltage: $1 \sim 200$ V increments of 1 V.

Current:

$0.01 \sim 2.00$ mA, adjustable current limit (configuration 8 is 4.00 mA), adjust step size to 0.01 mA.

Wave width: 50 μs to 4.99999 s.

Gap: 50 μs to 4.99999 s.

Trigger delay: 0 or 20 μs $\sim$ 4.9999 s.

Trigger signal voltage: $\pm 2 \sim 12$ V.

Intermittent: 1 ms $\sim$ 999.999 s.

Pulse front rise time ≤ 1 μs.

Power supply voltage: 220V 50 Hz.

Input power: 10 VA.

[Usage method]

Connect the instrument to the power supply with a power cord, plug in the external switch wire and stimulation output wire, and turn on the power switch.

(1) Parameter settings

The setting method starts by pressing the setting button, and the parameter items on the LCD screen will change from yang text display to yin text display. The items that change to yin text display are adjustable items. Continuously pressing the setting button can cycle through the variable items (note that voltage and current limits can be adjusted at any time, but not pre-set).

(2) Use of configuration keys: The instrument has 8 storage setting modes, and users can set commonly used stimulation parameters in each of the 8 configurations in advance. When using, simply press the configuration key to easily access a certain set of experimental parameters.

(3) Use of external switch: The instrument is equipped with a manual switch, which can control the stimulation output while observing the test animal, making it convenient for experimenters and improving the accuracy of the experiment.

(4) Indicator light display: After pressing the output button or the manual switch, the output indicator light will turn on, and the stimulation output terminal will output a square wave according to the set square wave parameters. At the same time, the square wave phase indicator light will also flash according to the output situation.

(5) Output setting and configuration: Except for adjustable voltage and current, other parameters of the instrument cannot be changed in the output state. The instrument cannot output in the set state, and configuration can only be selected in non-output and non-set states.

[Precautions]

(1) After use, please cut off the power and store in a ventilated and dry place.

(2) If there is high pressure inside, please do not disassemble it by yourself to avoid danger.

[Practice questions]

1. The pulse type used in physiological and pharmacological electronic stimulators is _____.

A. unidirectional pulse

B. bidirectional pulse

C. negative pulse

D. positive pulse

2. The YLS-9A physiological and pharmacological electronic stimulator is capable of outputting square waves that do not include _____.

A. positive pulse

B. positive pulse + gap + negative pulse

C. positive pulse + negative pulse

D. negative pulse + gap

[Thinking questions]

What experimental indicators are mainly tested by physiological and pharmacological electronic stimulators?

（李文涛）

Appendix

Appendix 1　Conversion of drug concentration and dosage in pharmacological experiments

1. Dosage unit

The legal units for drug dosage include weight units and capacity units.

Weight units mainly include grams (g), milligrams (mg), micrograms (μg), nanograms (ng), and picograms (pg).

The conversion relationship is: $1 \text{ g}=10^3 \text{ mg}=10^6 \text{ μg}=10^9 \text{ ng}=10^{12} \text{ pg}$.

Capacity units mainly include milliliters (mL), and sometimes liters (L) and microliters (μL).

The conversion relationship is: $1 \text{ L}=103 \text{ mL}=106 \text{ μL}$.

In addition, international units (IU) and units (U) are also part of the legal units of measurement. For traditional Chinese medicine decoction pieces, the dosage is usually measured in grams (g). In prescriptions, the dosage and quantity of drugs need to be written in Arabic numerals to ensure accuracy and consistency.

2. Volume of drug administration

Before injecting medication, the maximum allowable volume of the animals in a specific injection route should be considered firstly (usually in mL). Only after determining the volume can the appropriate concentration of the solution be determined. Generally, the blood volume of an animal accounts for about 1/3 of its body weight. If the volume of intravenous injection of a drug is too large, it may affect the normal function of the circulatory system. So the volume of intravenous injection should be less than 1/100 of the body weight. The volume of extravenous injection (subcutaneous, muscle, and abdominal cavity) should be less than 1/40 of the body weight. For example, in a 20-gram mouse, the tail vein injection should not exceed 0.2 mL, the injection in areas including muscle, subcutaneous, and abdominal cavity should not exceed 0.5 mL.

3. Drug concentration

Drug concentration refers to the amount of drug contained in a certain amount of liquid or solid preparation. The commonly used methods of expressing liquid preparations are as follows:

1) Percentage concentration

Expressed as the number of units of drug per hundred units of solution, abbreviated as %.

(1) Weight/Volume (W/V) method: expressing the number of grams of drug in 100 mL of solution. For example, 5% glucose solution means that 5 grams of glucose are contained in 100 mL of solution. The drug concentration % without special instructions refers to this method.

(2) Volume/Volume (V/V) method: suitable for the preparation of liquid drugs, expressing the number of mL of drug in 100 mL of solution. For example, 75% ethanol solution means that 75 mL of anhydrous ethanol is contained in 100 mL of solution. Or in other words, 75 mL of anhydrous ethanol plus distilled water to 100 mL can make 75% ethanol solution.

2) Proportional concentration

Used to express the concentration of diluted solutions. For example, 1 : 10000 adrenaline solution means 0.01% adrenaline (1 mL contains 0.1 mg adrenaline).

3) Molar concentration

Mole/liter (M or mol/L) refers to the molar amount of solute contained in 1 L of solution, which is called the molar concentration of the solution. For example, 0.1 mol/L NaCl means that 0.1 grams of moles, that is, 5.844 g NaCl (molecular weight of NaCl is 58.44), is contained in 1 liter of solution.

4) Dose conversion

The dose of drugs used in animal experiments is generally calculated in mg/kg (sometimes also in g/kg). When administering the drug, the dose of the drug needs to be converted from the known drug concentration to the equivalent amount of drug solution that should be injected per kg of body weight (for convenience, rats and guinea pigs can also be calculated per 100 g, and mice and toads can be calculated per 10 g of body weight). Sometimes, it is necessary to calculate the appropriate drug concentration according to the drug dose and the amount of drug solution administered. Sometimes it is also necessary to convert between concentrations (such as percentage concentration and molar concentration) for analysis and calculation.

(1) Convert the drug dose mg/kg and the percentage concentration of the drug solution to the amount of drug solution (mL) that should be injected per kg of body weight, and then calculate how much mL of drug solution should be injected for each animal.

Example: The mouse with 22 g of body weight, should be administrated with hydrochloric acid morphine 10 mg/kg by intraperitoneal injection. The drug concentration is 0.1%. How much mL should be injected?

Calculation method: 0.1% hydrochloric acid morphine solution contains 1 mg of drug per mL, 10 mg/kg is equivalent to 10 mL/kg, animal body weight converted to 0.022 kg, 10 mg/kg × 0.022 kg = 0.22 mL. For calculation convenience, the above 10 mL/kg is firstly converted to 0.1 mL/10 g, the body weight of the white mouse is rewritten as 2.2 × 10 g, 0.1 mL/10 g × 2.2 × 10 g = 0.22 mL.

(2) Calculate the drug concentration that should be prepared by the drug dose mg/kg and the set amount of drug solution mL/kg.

Example: Intravenous injection of hydrochloric acid morphine 10 mg/kg in rabbits, Injection volume: 1ml/kg. hatW is the concentration of the drug solution that should be prepared?

Calculation method: 10 mg/kg is equivalent to 1 mL/kg, 1mL of drug solution should contain 10 mg of hydrochloric acid morphine.

1 : 10 = 100 : X, X = 100 (mg) = 1 g.

So the concentration prepared is 1 g in 100 Ml.

That is the concentration of hydrochloric acid morphine is 1%.

（李成檀）

Appendix 2　Composition and preparation of common physiological solutions

Reagent type and main purpose	Normal saline		Ringer's solution			Locke's solution	Ringer-Locke's solution	Tyrode's solution	Krebs solution	Calcium-free solution
	Cold-blooded animals	Warm-blooded animals	Isolated frog heart	Cold-blooded animals	Warm-blooded animals	Warm-blooded animal heart, etc	Warm-blooded animal myocardium, etc.	Warm-blooded animal small intestine, etc.	Tissue block rinsing during cell culture sampling	Isolated aorta
Reagent										
NaCl	6.5	9.0	6.76	6.5	9.5	9.0	9.0	8.0	6.6	69.544
Composition										
$CaCl_2$			0.117	0.12	0.20	0.24	0.2	0.2	0.28	
KCl			0.09	0.14	0.12	0.42	0.2	0.2	0.35	3.578
$NaHCO_3$			0.225	0.2	0.15	0.1–0.3	0.3	1.0	2.1	
NaH_2PO_4			0.1			0.05				
KH_2PO_4									0.162	1.633
$MgCl_2$								0.1		
$MgSO_4 \cdot 7H_2O$									0.294	3.451
CO_2						Filled with gas for 10 minutes				
Glucose				or 1.0	or 1.0	1–2.5	1	1	2.0	
Na_2EDTA										0.05
O_2						Oxygenated	Oxygenated	Oxygenated	Oxygenated	Oxygenated
ddH_2O	1000	1000	1000	1000	1000	1000	1000	1000	1000	1000

Unit: Grams for solids, milliliters for liquids.

（张朋飞）

Appendix 3　Drug dosage form and prescription

| Drug dosage form

Drug dosage form refers to that any drug must be formulated in a form suitable for medical and preventive use according to pharmacopoeia or prescription before being supplied for clinical use. Commonly used dosage forms are divided into liquid dosage forms, solid dosage forms, semi-solid dosage forms, and aerosols according to their forms.

1. Liquid dosage form

(1) Solution

Generally, it is a clear aqueous solution of chemical drugs for oral or external use.

(2) Injection

The first type is solution injection, also known as ampoule, which is a sterilized solution or suspension of drugs used for injection.

The second type is powder injection, commonly known as powder injection. Some drugs are unstable in solution, so their sterilized dry powder is encapsulated in ampoules and prepared into a solution before use.

The third type is emulsion injection, which is mostly used for intravenous infusion and is usually an insoluble solute in water.

The fourth type is suspension injection, which is usually a drug that is difficult to dissolve in water or requires prolonged action time.

(3) Decoction is the liquid obtained by boiling raw herbs (single or compound) in water. This dosage form is commonly used in Chinese herbal medicine and must be prepared fresh.

(4) Mixtures are water-based liquid preparations made by mixing multiple drugs into a transparent or suspended form, intended for oral administration.

(5) Tinctures generally refer to clear liquid preparations made by ethanol extraction or dissolution of raw medicine.

(6) Liquid extract refers to a concentrated liquid dosage form obtained by removing some solvents from the extract of raw medicine.

(7) Emulsion refers to a liquid emulsion which is a uniform and relatively stable

emulsion made by treating two immiscible liquids with emulsifiers.

(8) Lotion mainly refer to insoluble drug suspensions extracted and prepared by appropriate methods for application or cleaning on the skin or cavity.

(9) Syrup refers to a near saturated concentrated sucrose aqueous solution containing drugs, medicinal extracts, or aromatic substances.

(10) Spiritus refers to concentrated ethanol solutions of volatile drugs.

2. Solid dosage form

(1) Tablet: A small circular tablet made by pressing a drug into an excipient. It can be divided into multi-layer tablets, implantable tablets, enteric coated tablets, topical tablets, etc.

(2) Pill: A spherical or spherical solid preparation made by adding appropriate excipients to a fine powder or extract of a drug.

(3) Capsule: A preparation made by encapsulating a drug in an empty hard or soft capsule.

(4) Powder: A dry powder preparation made by uniformly mixing one or more drugs.

(5) Membrane agent: It is made by dissolving or suspending drugs in a solution of polymers, coating and drying them.

(6) Granules: An orally administered formulation made by drying chemical drugs into granules.

3. Semisolid dosage form

(1) Plaster: an external preparation made by mixing medication and an appropriate matrix, with adhesive properties for application.

(2) Ointment: A semi-solid topical preparation made by adding a suitable matrix to a drug.

(3) Suppository: A soft preparation made by mixing medication with a suitable matrix, specifically designed for administration through different cavities in the human body.

(4) Extract: A powder or paste solid dosage form obtained by concentrating the extract of medicinal herbs.

4. Aerosol

refers to a liquid preparation that a drug is packaged together with a propellant (liquefied gas or compressed gas) in a sealed, pressure resistant container with a valve. It is divided into three types: inhaled aerosols, non inhaled aerosols, and topical aerosols.

‖ Prescription

1. The significance of prescription

A prescription is an important written document issued by a physician based on the patient's condition including the dosage, usage, etc. It is used for pharmacists to prescribe and dispense medication according to the prescription. The significance of prescription is to ensure that patients use drugs correctly and safely, achieving the goal of treating diseases.

2. Basic components of prescription

The complete prescription can be divided into six parts, arranged in the following order:

(1) Prescription Item 1

Including the full name of the hospital, the patient's name, gender, age, outpatient or inpatient number, and the date of prescription.

(2) Prescription Head

Prescription writing starts with Rp (or R), which is the abbreviation of Latin Recipe that means "please take".

(3) Prescription Text

Including the name, dosage form, specifications, and dosage of the drug. If there are several drugs in a prescription, each drug should be written on a separate line, and the quantity of drugs should be expressed in Arabic numerals. The dosage should be written after the drug.

(4) Configuration

For a complete prescription, the physician should also specify the dispensing method after prescribing the medication. Simple prescriptions do not have this option.

(5) Medication method

The usual method of medication is represented as sig. or S (abbreviation for Latin signa). The specific usage can be written in Chinese or represented by Latin abbreviations. The content includes prescription drug dosage, usage, daily frequency, etc.

(6) Physician's signature

The physician completes the prescription, carefully checks it to ensure accuracy, and then signs and hands it over to the patient. Pharmacists must carefully review, evaluate, and verify prescriptions. If errors are found, they have the right to return them to the physician for correction. After confirming that there are no errors, they can proceed with the preparation and dispensing of medication, and finally sign on the prescription form.

3. Precautions for prescription writing

(1) The unit of drug dosage shall be written in accordance with the pharmacopoeia regulations. Solid or semi-solid drugs are measured in grams (g), liquid drugs are measured in milliliters (mL). If mg, kg, or IU is used, it must be specified.

(2) The general medication should be prescribed for 2 ~ 3 days (excluding chronic diseases). And it may be extended appropriately for chronic diseases, elderly diseases, or special circumstances, but the physician should specify.

4. Prescription type

There are mainly two types of prescriptions: complete prescriptions and simplified prescriptions. The commonly used prescription type is simplified prescription (Attached table 3-1).

(1) Complete prescription

Physicians design and prescribe complex prescriptions based on the needs of the patient's condition, including main drugs, adjuncts, shaping drugs, flavoring drugs, etc.

(2) Simplify prescriptions

Write drugs that have been made into various dosage forms. Clearly state the name, dosage form, specifications, dosage, daily dose, administration time, and route of administration of a drug in the prescription text.

Attched table 3-1　Latin abbreviations commonly used in prescriptions and their meanings

Abbreviation	Latin	Meaning	Abbreviation	Latin	Meaning
aa	ana	each	M.f.	misce, fiat	Mixed production
a.c	ante cidul	before dinner	N or N.	numero	number
ad	ad	add	p.o	post oibum	after meal
add	adde addatur	add, should add	p.r.n.	pro re nata	If necessary, use
b.i.d	bis in die	2 times one day	q4h	quaque4h ora	each 4 hours
D.t.d	dentur tales doles	same amount	q.i.d	quter in die	4 times one day
gtt	gutta	drop	q.s.	quantum sufficiat	appropriate amount
h.s.	hora somni	before bedtime	Sig. or S.	signa	marking, usage
i.h.	injectio hypodermica	subcutaneous injection	S.O.S.	si opus sit	if necessary
i.m.	injectio intrausculosa	intramuscular injection	S.S.	semisse	half
i.v.	Injectio intravenosa	intravenous injection	St or stat	statim	immediately
M	misce	mix	t.i.d.	ter in die	3 times a day

Prescription exercise:

(1) Tian, male, 46 years old. Roxithromycin Dispersible tablets,150 mg/tablet, twice daily, 1 tablet each time,dosage for 3 days.

(2) Zhang, female, 32 years old. Kaeszolam tablets (Tab.), 1 mg /tablet, taken orally before bedtime, with a dosage of 1 mg for three days.

(3) Li, male, 50 years old. one dexamethasone injection, specification 1mL: 2mg, subcutaneous injection 1 mg.

(4) Wang, male, 68 years old. Take sulfamethoxazole tablets (0.5 g/tablet) and sodium bicarbonate tablets (0.5 g/tablet) orally at the same time, 1 g each time for each drug, twice a day, double the first dose, three days of dosage.

（李　鑫）

Appendix 4　Experimental report writing

[Requirements for experimental report writing]

An experimental report is a summary written by students after completing an experiment, which truthfully records and organizes the purpose, methods, and results of a certain experiment. The experimental report should fully reflect the scientific, creative, and practical nature of the experimental content. The writing requirements for the experimental report are as follows.

1. Experiment name

The experiment name should be clear and accurately reflect the content of the experiment. If observing the anticonvulsant effect of phenobarbital, it can be written as "anticonvulsant effect of barbiturates".

2. Experimental personnel information

Name, class, student ID, experimental time (×× month ×× day, ×× year).

3. Experimental purpose

Briefly explain the main purpose of conducting the experiment, the problems to be solved in the experiment, and the expected results to be achieved.

4. Experimental materials

List the names (models) of the instruments and equipment used in the experiment, experimental consumables, experimental animals (weight, gender), and experimental drugs (concentration), etc.

5. Experimental methods

Briefly describe the experimental methods, technical routes, administration sequence, observation indicators, and data collection methods used in this experiment.

6. Experimental results

Record the raw data in detail according to the different experimental purposes. Organize and classify the original records for statistical analysis. At the same time, record the experimental time, conditions, environment, or special circumstances that occur.

Note: It is not allowed to change or fabricate the original data, and subjective selection or arbitrary selection is prohibited.

7. Analysis and discussion of experimental results

The data collected in the experiment is first subjected to statistical processing. However, the experiment is analyzed and interpreted based on the theoretical knowledge learned in the field, and the relationship between general and specific patterns observed in the experiment is discussed.

8. Conclusion

Based on the analysis and judgment of the experimental results, draw conclusions. The conclusion is a summary judgment of the experimental results. The conclusion should answer the theme proposed by the experiment, which should be concise, logical, and have theoretical significance.

[Example of experimental report]

Experiment X Experimental report on the dose-response relationship of drugs

Class：_____   Teacher：_____

Date：_____

Group member：Name：_____   Student ID：_____

　　　　　　　　Name：_____   Student ID：_____

　　　　　　　　Name：_____   Student ID：_____

　　　　　　　　Name：_____   Student ID：_____

1. Experimental purpose

Understand the dose-response relationship of drugs and the experimental methods for determining dose-response relationships, as well as the drawing of dose-response curves.

2. Experimental materials

3. Experimental methods

4. Experimental process record

Experimental time point	Operation content	Experimental phenomenon	Remarks

5. Main experimental results recording and analysis

Dose-effect curve: Please draw a schematic diagram of the dose-response relationship that appears in the experiment (note that the specific experimental arrangement shall be subject to the teacher's requirements).

Testing indicators: Record the effect values corresponding to each concentration.

Analysis of experimental phenomena.

6. Conclusion

7. Experimental experience (not mandatory)

Please specify the experience gained in this experiment.

（赵春贞）